SECOND EDITION

PCCN CERTIFICATION REVIEW

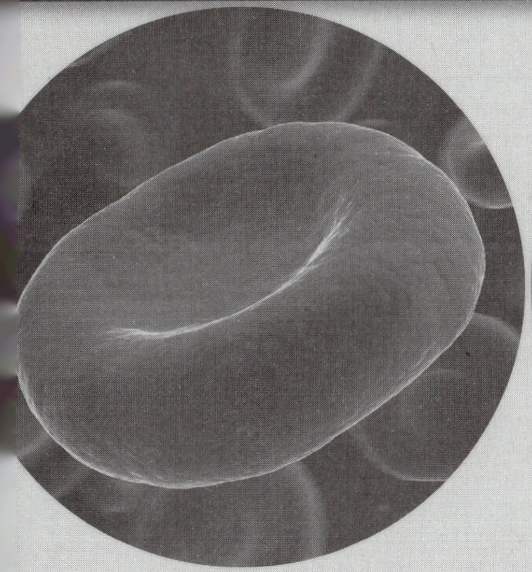

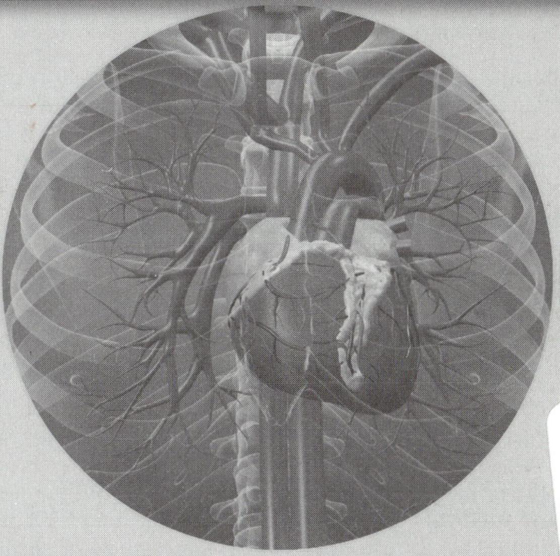

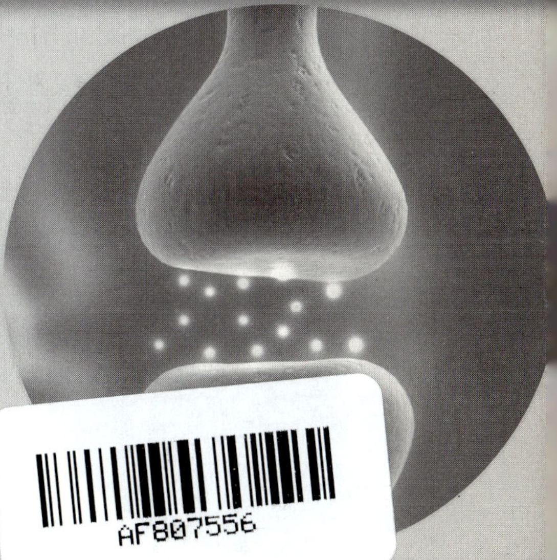

ANN J. BRORSEN, RN, MSN, PHN, CCRN, CEN

KERI R. ROGELET, RN, MSN, MBA/HCM, CCRN

JONES & BARTLETT
LEARNING

World Headquarters
Jones & Bartlett Learning
5 Wall Street
Burlington, MA 01803
978-443-5000
info@jblearning.com
www.jblearning.com

Jones & Bartlett Learning books and products are available through most bookstores and online booksellers. To contact Jones & Bartlett Learning directly, call 800-832-0034, fax 978-443-8000, or visit our website, www.jblearning.com.

Substantial discounts on bulk quantities of Jones & Bartlett Learning publications are available to corporations, professional associations, and other qualified organizations. For details and specific discount information, contact the special sales department at Jones & Bartlett Learning via the above contact information or send an email to specialsales@jblearning.com.

Production Credits
Executive Publisher: Kevin Sullivan
Acquisitions Editor: Amanda Harvey
Editorial Assistant: Rebecca Myrick
Associate Production Editor: Sara Fowles
Marketing Communications Manager: Katie Hennessy
V.P., Manufacturing and Inventory Control: Therese Connell
Composition: Laserwords Private Limited, Chennai, India
Cover Design: Kristin E. Parker
Cover Image: (for all) © Sebastian Kaulitzki/ShutterStock, Inc.
Printing and Binding: Edwards Brothers Malloy
Cover Printing: Edwards Brothers Malloy

To order this product, use ISBN: 978-1-2840-2748-8

Library of Congress Cataloging-in-Publication Data
Brorsen, Ann J.
PCCN certification review / Ann J. Brorsen, Keri R. Rogelet. – 2nd ed.
p. ; cm.
Includes bibliographical references.
ISBN 978-1-4496-9512-5 (pbk.)
I. Rogelet, Keri R. II. Title.
[DNLM: 1. Critical Care–Examination Questions. 2. Nursing Care--Examination Questions. 3. Critical Illness–nursing–Examination Questions. 4. Nursing Assessment–Examination Questions. WY 18.2]
616.028076–dc23

2013001115

6048

Printed in the United States of America
17 16 15 14 10 9 8 7 6 5 4 3 2

Contents

About the Authors

Ann J. Brorsen, RN, MSN, CCRN, CEN

Ann is a nationally known speaker and has presented certification review courses for the PCCN, Adult and Pediatric CCRN, and CEN. Ann has presented programs as diverse as advanced hemodynamics to best practice models for hospital corporations. Ann is a member of Sigma Theta Tau, the American Association of Critical-Care Nurses, the Society of Critical Care Medicine, and the Emergency Nurses Association. Ann also works as a consultant for educational program development and management training for healthcare facilities. Ann continues clinical practice in the ICU, ED, and critical care transport. Ann is also currently the COO and Director of Clinical Applications for Pro Ed in Menifee, California.

Keri R. Rogelet, RN, MSN, MBA/HCM, CCRN

Keri has presented national programs for adult health issues, the Neonatal CCRN, Pediatric CCRN, and Developmental Care. Keri is a regional NRP trainer for the American Academy of Pediatrics and a lead instructor for the S.T.A.B.L.E. program. Keri's professional associations include Sigma Theta Tau, the American Association of Critical-Care Nurses, and the Academy of Neonatal Nursing. In addition, she works as a consultant for pediatric and neonatal product applications. She is currently the CFO and Director of Clinical Development for Pro Ed in Menifee, California.

Contributors

Melissa R. Christiansen, RN, MSN, NP-C, CCRN, CNRN

Melissa has over 23 years' experience as a critical care nurse in neurological, cardiac, and trauma ICUs. She is currently working as a family nurse practitioner in Southern California. Melissa has presented programs on neurologic and neuroscience topics, adult critical care, and emergency nursing certification reviews, as well as courses in post-anesthesia nursing. Melissa is a member of Sigma Theta Tau, the American Association of Critical-Care Nurses, the American Association of Neuroscience Nurses, and the American Academy of Nurse Practitioners.

Jacque E. Jackson, RN, PhD, APRN

Jacque has over 30 years in nursing experience as an educator, manager of cardiovascular and surgical ICUs, CNO, and hospital administrator. He has been a staunch advocate of certification for nurses and utilization of clinical ladders and best practice models for health care.

Reviewers

Mary A. Cowett, RN, RNC-BC
Riverside, California

Vicki Hirshel, RN, BSN, RNC
Riverside, California

Brian N. Ingram, MD
Fairfax, Virginia

Randall C. Jackson, RN, MSN, CCRN
Pittsburgh, Pennsylvania

Acknowledgments

Mary Margaret Forsythe, RN, and Nancy O. Roberts, RN

Mary Margaret and Nancy were two instructors who were ultimate professionals and who believed in their students and the profession of nursing. These women were incredible individuals and will live in the hearts of hundreds of nurses. They passed before their time and are desperately missed.

Karen S. Ehrat, RN, PhD

Karen saw potential in a new grad and made education a joy and a privilege. Her untimely death stole a piece from every soul she touched.

Damien, Minerva, & M'Leah

Angels that taught me every life touches another and remind me why I do what I do.

We are so grateful to all the nurses who provided suggestions for content of this book and to the contributors worked unselfishly and through many a long night. Thank you to the reviewers who gave their time, effort, and suggestions to enhance the content of this manuscript. We would also like to express our gratitude to the editorial staff at Jones & Bartlett Learning.

A.J.B. and K.R.R.

Preface

Congratulations! You are one step closer to achieving certification as a progressive care nurse. Even if you plan to use this book as a study guide for progressive care or acute care nursing, this will be an invaluable resource. A brief introduction to the PCCN credential and test-taking strategies are presented to help you study effectively. This book is updated to reflect the content of the new PCCN Test Plan that takes effect June 26th, 2013. This new Test Plan is somewhat condensed and groups some of the major topics together. We have separated all the major systems into individual chapters to facilitate use of the online program. Please visit http://www.aacn.org to download a copy of the PCCN Test Plan.

There are over 1,000 test questions with rationales in this text that cover a broad range of topics and are representative of the type of questions you will find on the actual examination. The current trend for item writers is to present a question in such a way as to not state any identifiable characteristics, such as a name, age, or gender (if possible). Any name or patient condition presented here is for educational purposes only. Any resemblance to any person, living or dead, is purely coincidental.

With this book purchase you will have access to an online application that allows you to create your own practice tests from the questions written in this book. The questions online are randomly selected and enable you to time yourself and practice as if you were taking the actual examination.

All of us who contributed to the content of this book are dedicated to helping you successfully pass this exam and achieve recognition as a progressive care nurse. Please feel free to contact us if you have any questions or if you would like to schedule a PCCN review course for your facility or group.

Contact Information

Website: http://www.forproed.com
Email: proedcertify@yahoo.com

Section 1

History of the PCCN Credential

Traditionally, nurses have worked in a variety of roles and environments. For most of the 20th century, when nurses graduated from their programs, they had spent many hours in clinical situations and were prepared to practice in any area. Nursing eventually had to adjust from the general practitioner to a nurse who would concentrate practice in one area. Nurses worked in emergency rooms, operating rooms, recovery rooms, obstetrics, and medical–surgical units. Only those nurses who worked in operating rooms or who administered anesthesia were considered specialized. With the advent of emerging technology, the post-World War II population boom, and a trend toward increasingly more acute patients, nursing and hospitals adjusted by placing patients in more sub specialized areas.

One critical issue that arose in the 20th century related to patients with poliomyelitis, who were increasing both in number and special needs. The "iron lung" had been around for years. In the 1930s, the machine cost $1,500, which was also the median cost for a home at that time. Patients who could afford such treatment began to recover, only to develop sequelae that required specialized care. Tilt beds and hot pack treatments were initiated. At one time, even curare was used to combat the severe muscle spasms suffered by polio victims. All of these treatments required time and resources, including larger numbers of nurses.

In 1931, the American Association of Nurse Anesthetist (no "s" on the end) formed. On June 4, 1945, the organization held the first-ever certification examination for a nursing specialty. In 1952, the first accredited program for nurse anesthetists was started.

In 1955, Jonas Salk announced the discovery of a vaccine for polio. The vaccine would help prevent spread of the disease, but thousands of victims still required care. Technology in general was improving and becoming more broadly available. Although the first EKG machines were available in the United States as early as 1909, they were not widely used until the late 1950s.

In the 1960s, many patients required around-the-clock specialized care that required resources and practitioners who were experts or who had a great deal of experience with the particular condition or disease process. Veterans of previous wars and the escalating Vietnam War required increasingly more medical resources. Hospitals began placing cardiac, trauma, burn, and acute medical patients in areas of the hospital designated as providing more "intensive" care. Patient survival rates improved, so the numbers of specialized areas increased.

In 1967, nurses from Nashville Baptist Hospital were frustrated at the lack of educational opportunities for continuing education for intensive care nurses, so they sent inquiries to other nurses to see if interest existed to form an association to provide education to other intensive care nurses. At that time, most of the ICUs served cardiac patients. A year later, more than 400 nurses attended a symposium and affirmed the need for an organization. In 1969, the American Association of Cardiovascular Nurses was formed. In 1971, the name was changed to the American Association of Critical Care Nurses (AACN) in recognition of the broad area covered by critical care.

AACN is now the largest specialty nursing organization in the world. In 1975, the AACN Certification Corporation was established and began offering the CCRN examination. The need for a separate examination for acute care nurses was recognized and the PCCN examination was developed and given in 2004 for the first time at the National Teaching Institute in Orlando, Florida.

We invite you to visit the AACN website at http://www.aacn.org to learn more about the PCCN credential. Thousands of nurses have successfully attained the PCCN credential and we are here to help you become successful. The next section will explain the registration procedure for the examination. You can do it!

REFERENCES

American Association of Critical-Care Nurses [AACN]. (2012). *Homepage*. Retrieved from http://www.aacn.org

American Association of Critical-Care Nurses [AACN]. (2012). *History of AACN*. Retrieved from http://www.aacn.org/WD/publishing/content/pressroom/historyofaacn.content?menu=AboutUs

Smithsonian National Museum of American History. (n.d.). *Polio: How polio changed us*. Retrieved from http://americanhistory.si.edu/polio/howpolio/index.htm

http://www.anesthesia-nursing.com/wina.html

Section 2

Registering for the PCCN Certification Exam

We have included this section to help simplify the registration process for the PCCN exam.

Please note that you do not have to be a member of the American Association of Critical Care Nurses to take this examination. However, at this time there is a discount for members.

First, go to http://www.AACN.org.

Click on "Certification" then select PCCN. The site will guide you to any topic for the PCCN.

Make certain you download the information in the Handbook. Pay close attention to the Test Plan - it is an outline of the test content.

You may register online.

After your application is accepted, you will be given the address of a testing center nearest you, based on your zip code. You do not have to take your exam there. Many nurses have traveled to other states to take the exam. You simply have to take the initiative and set up your appointment at the testing center of your choice.

Make sure to follow all directions from the testing center and arrive early. You can do this!

Section 3

Test-Taking Strategies

When preparing for the PCCN exam, the first thing to do is be absolutely honest with yourself about how you study. If you have good study habits and plenty of time, you are very fortunate. If you are a procrastinator, studying a little bit at a time might help. Nurses have to juggle so many roles that take up their time: parent, child, employee, student, teacher, and so on. One of the biggest struggles is simply finding the time and a place to study. Discovering your learning style will help you find a better way to absorb information. Three types of learners are commonly identified: visual, auditory, and kinesthetic. There is no perfect strategy for learning because every person is unique. Not everyone has a single style of learning; you may use a mix of styles depending on your situation.

Visual learners learn better from reading and writing than from hearing and talking about information. Background noise, such as music or television, is distracting to these types of learners. Finding a quiet space is a problem for some people. You may have to stay awake after family members have gone to bed. Flashcards often work, and some people use colored markers to highlight important information.

Auditory learners learn information effectively by listening and talking. Playing music, listening to audiotapes, or being part of a study group often works.

Kinesthetic learners prefer to learn via a "hands-on" approach. Nurses often learn this way because we have to listen to lectures and then demonstrate skills. This approach focuses on the use of models, manikins, or patients and works well for many healthcare providers. Kinesthetic people are often "antsy" and cannot sit still for long periods of time, so lectures may be difficult for them without frequent breaks. If you are a kinesthetic learner, some of the things that might help while studying include taking frequent breaks, walking around, or riding a stationary cycle.

No matter what your personal learning style, your test-taking skills can be improved. How? Practice! That is why this book was written in a question-and-answer format. Keep practicing the questions until you can answer at least 80% correctly. Research has shown that two-thirds of study time should be spent taking sample tests and only one-third of study time should be spent reviewing content.

Studying, like regular exercise, is good for the brain. As nurses, we must always keep abreast of the professional literature and spend time studying to keep our knowledge and skills up-to-date. In addition, many states require continuing education to renew a professional license. Anything worthwhile takes time, effort, and sacrifice.

There is no way around studying for this certification. There are no shortcuts! If you have been out of school for a while, don't despair! It may be slow going at first, so take things a little at a time. Just like going to the gym, you should make a plan to study in one particular place and at the same time, if possible. This is your space and your time—claim it. Have all your books, tapes, and other study materials handy. If you need snack food, make sure it is not all sugar and include some salty food. Caffeine tends to make people jittery, but if you need it, it may be right for you.

The PCCN Test Plan is a blueprint of the exam's content. The major sections are broken down into subheadings and topics. If you study only a little at a time, you will be fine. One day you may feel like studying right-sided EKGs; the next day you may want to focus on chest tubes. You may download the current content outline at http://www.aacn.org. The current content outline is not included in this book because the exam changes frequently; as such, you should have a copy of the current information.

If you study with a group, you can save a lot of time and effort by breaking up the topics for that study period and having each person present his or her topic(s) and provide handouts and practice questions for the rest of the group. When you can make up a test question about a subject, you really will be prepared. Study for short periods of time, say 30 to 45 minutes, and then take a break. Set small goals, and after you have accomplished each one, reward yourself!

EXAM CONTENT

The PCCN certification exam consists of 125 multiple-choice test questions. Twenty-five of those questions do not count; they are there to be validated. Every question is tried first to see if it is written well and if a certain percentage of people answer it correctly. At this point in the process, those 25 questions can still be "tweaked" for use on future exams, depending on how the test-takers performed on these questions.

Your results are determined by how many answers you get correct and the version of the examination used. Some questions are a bit more difficult than others. If you do not know an answer, take your best guess, because you have at least a chance of guessing correctly. You get points only for questions answered correctly.

STUDY TIPS

A multiple-choice test question consists of three parts: an introductory statement, a stem (question), and options from which you must select the correct answer. The introductory statement provides information about a clinical issue, pathophysiology, or a nursing action or duty.

Stems are worded in different ways. Some stems are in the form of a question; others are in the form of an incomplete statement. Additionally, a stem usually requests one of two types of responses: a positive response or a negative response. The questions you will practice from in this book may have an occasional negative stem to facilitate learning. There are no longer any multiple-multiple-choice questions on the exam!

Key words are important words or phrases that help focus your attention on what the question is asking. Examples of key words include *always, most, first response, earliest, priority, first, on admission, common, best, least, not, immediately*, and *initial*.

You should always be looking for a therapeutic response, as the nurse is always therapeutic. In other words, your initial response as a nurse is always the therapeutic response—you must acknowledge and validate the patient's feelings. Communication skills learned in Nursing 101 are important components of successful test-taking strategies. More than one option may contain a therapeutic response. When in doubt, validate, validate, validate. Always validate feelings before you present information. A medical emergency would, of course, take precedence.

Who is actually the focus of the question? You need to be able to identify this person. Sometimes questions are asked about a friend, a relative, or a significant other instead of a patient. A lot of information in the question may be deliberately distracting. Also, you must, when applicable, validate that person's feelings first.

WHEN IN DOUBT

When answering questions on the examination, remember Maslow's hierarchy of needs and the ABCs (airway, breathing, circulation). When these goals are met, then safety is the priority. After safety, the psychological needs are a priority. Assessment always comes before diagnosis and treatment (intervention). Learning takes place only if the learner is motivated.

Eliminate incorrect options. This gives you a 50% chance of guessing the correct answer. Here are some hints:

- Select the most general, all-encompassing option.
- Eliminate similar options or those that contain words such as "always" or "never."
- If two options say essentially the same thing, then neither is correct. If three of the four options sound similar, choose the one that sounds different.
- Look for the longest option. It is usually the correct answer.
- Watch for grammatical inconsistencies between the stem and options.

IT'S TIME TO TAKE YOUR CERTIFICATION EXAM!

Well, you are finally ready! The night before the exam, get a good night's sleep. Do not cram the night before, although that is easier said than done. Do something relaxing and enjoyable, like going to a movie or out to dinner. Try to avoid caffeine or any other stimulant. Please email or call when you pass the exam so you can be congratulated.

REFERENCES

Kobel Lamonte, M. (2007). Test-taking strategies for CNOR certification. *AORN Journal, 85*(2), 315–332.

Ludwig, C. (2004). Preparing for certification: Test-taking strategies. *Medical-Surgical Nursing, 13*(2), 127–128.

Section 4

Cardiovascular

The cardiovascular section comprises about one-third of each PCCN examination. The review questions presented in this book are representative in style and content similar to those found on the exam. There is basic content that you must know in order to build knowledge and understand concepts. Many questions require a broad knowledge base and employ critical thinking, knowledge integration, professional caring, and ethical practice.

Questions may be presented in different ways to help you retain content. Questions may be short and require simple recall of facts; some questions may be presented in the form of brief scenarios.

Rationale for answers is sometimes one simple sentence, other times the explanation is quite lengthy.

Keep practicing until you can score at least 80%.

SECTION 4: CARDIOVASCULAR QUESTIONS

1. **Determine the pulse pressure for a patient who has a pulse of 78, a BP of 120/85, and a respiratory rate of 16.**
   A. 42
   B. 7
   C. 35
   D. 103

2. **Which of the following percentages would be considered a normal value for an ejection fraction (EF)?**
   A. 25%
   B. 30%
   C. 42%
   D. 60%

3. **Your patient exhibits ST segment depression on his EKG along with moderate, substernal chest pain. These findings indicate a possible**
   A. Anteroseptal MI
   B. Myocardial ischemia
   C. Lateral wall MI
   D. Pericardial tamponade

4. **Which of the following statements is true about events that occur during a normal cardiac cycle?**
   A. Metabolism in the heart is unchanged during diastole
   B. Metabolism in the heart is decreased during diastole
   C. An increase in cardiac output increases diastole
   D. The mitral and aortic valves are open during diastole

5. **What is the mean arterial pressure (MAP) for a patient with a blood pressure of 122/60 and a heart rate of 70?**
   A. 78
   B. 52
   C. 81
   D. 40

6. **Calculate the cardiac output for a patient with a heart rate of 78 and a stroke volume of 60 ml.**
   A. 18%
   B. 4.68 L/min
   C. 1,800 ml/min
   D. 2.34 Liters

7. **Unstable angina usually associated with left anterior descending (LAD) coronary artery lesions is known as**
   A. Prinzmetal's angina
   B. Wellen's syndrome
   C. Crescendo angina
   D. Ludwig's angina

8. **Stroke volume is comprised of which of the following factors?**
   A. Viscosity, blood volume, and impedance
   B. Cardiac output, heart rate, and compliance
   C. Contractility, preload, and afterload
   D. Systemic impedance, heart rate, and compliance

9. **During evaluation of CVP pressure monitoring tracing, the c wave represents**
   A. Mechanical atrial diastole
   B. The decrease in RA volume during relaxation
   C. Emptying of the right atrium into the right ventricle
   D. Increased RA pressure from closure of the tricuspid valve

10. **Exceptional and extreme mental stress, anger and resentment in a post-menopausal woman may cause**
    A. Takosubo cardiomyopathy
    B. Post-partum hemorrhage
    C. Dilated cardiomyopathy
    D. Increased dopamine release

11. **A low CVP reading may represent**
    A. Pulmonary hypertension
    B. Increased contractility
    C. Biventricular failure
    D. Cardiac tamponade

12. **Right ventricular preload in the heart is measured by the**
    A. Left atrial pressure
    B. Pulmonary artery systolic pressure

C. Central venous pressure
D. Pulmonary artery occlusive pressure

13. Your patient was admitted to the progressive care unit (PCU) for chest pain that occurred while he was sleeping and has not resolved. He was diagnosed with Prinzmetal's angina. This form of angina
A. Is caused by a blockage of the circumflex artery
B. Is a benign form of angina
C. Is usually caused by a coronary vasospasm
D. Will always resolve with administration of nitroglycerin

14. You are using the PQRST method of pain assessment for your patient complaining of chest pain. The "S" in this mnemonic stands for
A. Sensitivity
B. Severity
C. Standard
D. Symptoms

15. The normal range for a serum amiodarone is ___ to ____ mcg/ml.
A. 0.5 to 1.5 mcg/ml
B. 1 to 2.5 mcg/ml
C. 1.5 to 3 mcg/ml
D. 2 to 3.5 mcg/ml

16. How does STEMI differ from NSTEMI?
A. Only STEMI involves myocardial cell death
B. NSTEMI has no ST elevation
C. The cardiac enzymes are elevated only in STEMI
D. The cardiac enzymes are elevated only in NSTEMI

17. Which of the following parameters is considered diagnostic of a STEMI on the 12-lead EKG?
A. A STEMI must be diagnosed by the cardiac enzymes results, not an EKG
B. A STEMI has a 1-mm ST elevation with or without a pathologic Q wave
C. A STEMI must have a 5-mm ST elevation of the affected coronary artery
D. A STEMI does not have a pathologic Q wave

18. Calcium channel blockers act primarily on
A. Serotonin uptake
B. Arteriolar tissue
C. Lung receptors only
D. Reduction of cardiac output

19. Decreased preload may result from
A. Hyperthermia
B. Hypothermia
C. Sympathetic stimulation
D. Vasoconstriction

20. **Which of the following conditions would decrease afterload?**
    A. Use of nitrates
    B. Hypothermia
    C. Aortic stenosis
    D. Hypertension

21. **The most sensitive cardiac marker is**
    A. CK-MB
    B. Creatine kinease
    C. Troponin T
    D. Tropinin IIa

22. **If your patient has a CK-MB concentration greater than 5% of the total CK, this finding is indicative of:**
    A. Large muscle damage
    B. Tissue ischemia
    C. Mild muscle injury
    D. Myocardial necrosis

23. **Which of the following substances is released when the myocardium is stretched?**
    A. Brain natriuretic peptide (BNP)
    B. Myoglobin
    C. C-reactive protein
    D. Troponin T

24. **A biomarker that is not cardiac-specific but can be elevated by falls, cardiopulmonary resuscitation, and injections is**
    A. C-reactive protein
    B. Myoglobin
    C. INR
    D. BNP

25. **To monitor the effectiveness of anticoagulant therapy, the international normalized ratio (INR) is frequently used. For a patient with atrial fibrillation, a therapeutic range for INR would be**
    A. 3.5–4.5
    B. 1.5–3.0
    C. 2.0–3.0
    D. 5.0–6.1

26. **A biomarker that indicates an inflammation is present is**
    A. C-reactive protein
    B. CK-MB isoenzyme
    C. White blood count
    D. Troponin 1

27. **When assessing your new patient, you auscultate a blowing, high-pitched murmur at the apex and it appears to radiate to the left axilla. This murmur is probably indicative of**

A. Tricuspid stenosis
B. Mitral insufficiency or regurgitation
C. Aortic stenosis
D. Hypertrophic cardiomyopathy

28. **A cardiac murmur that has maximal intensity at the base of the heart (commonly at the second intercostal space, right sternal border) and radiates to the apex and neck is the murmur of**
A. Mitral stenosis
B. Pulmonary insufficiency or regurgitation
C. Aortic stenosis
D. Tricuspid stenosis

29. **An early diastolic murmur with maximal intensity at the fourth intercostal space, left sternal border, is a murmur of**
A. Mitral stenosis
B. Pulmonary insufficiency or regurgitation
C. Aortic stenosis
D. Tricuspid stenosis

30. **Which of the following statements about angina is true?**
A. If the patient is to undergo a PCTA, it is not necessary to inquire about allergies
B. Troponins and CK-MB isoenzymes are not elevated in patients with stable angina
C. Angina that has not increased in frequency or severity over time is known as variant angina
D. Stable angina is a resting, non-symptomatic angina

31. **The S_2 heart sound is created by**
A. Opening of the aortic and mitral valves
B. Closure of the pulmonic and aortic valves
C. Opening of the pulmonic and mitral valves
D. Closure of the pulmonic and tricuspid valves

32. **Diuretics are used in the treatment of CHF. A diuretic that reduces urinary calcium losses is**
A. Diamox
B. Chlorothiazide
C. Furosemide
D. Spironolactone

33. **The primary use of nesiritide (Natrecor) would be**
A. To depress cGMP production
B. To cause smooth muscle constriction
C. To depress cellular transport
D. To cause vascular smooth muscle vasodilation

34. **What are the most valuable pieces of information evaluated with a 12-lead EKG?**
A. Rate, rhythm, and arrhythmias
B. Rate, rhythm, axis, hypertrophy, and infarction

C. Rate, arrhythmias, and infarction
D. Rhythm, ischemia, and axis

35. **During your assessment of your patient on IV amiodarone, you note weakening bilateral hand grips, increased patient fatigue, and the patient reports muscle aches. After reporting your findings to the physician, which of the follow lab tests should you expect to be ordered?**
A. Urine analysis
B. Hemogram
C. T3 and T4 levels
D. None, these findings are normal and expected

36. **ST elevation in EKG leads V_1-V_3, syncopal episodes and a RBBB may indicate**
A. Takosubo syndrome
B. Hypertrophic cardiomyopathy
C. Brugada syndrome
D. Alcohol induced cardiomyopathy

37. **Pulsus alternans is most often noted with**
A. Mitral stenosis
B. Constrictive pericarditis
C. Left ventricular failure
D. Aortic stenosis

38. **Stimulation of the right vagus nerve in turn stimulates the**
A. Sinoatrial (SA) node
B. Mandibular branch of the trigeminal nerve
C. Acetylcholine reabsorption
D. Chemoreceptors in the carotid arch

39. **Cyanosis of the skin, mucous membranes, and nail beds can occur when deoxygenated hemoglobin is present within the circulation. This cyanosis may be observed when which of the following levels of deoxygenated hemoglobin is reached?**
A. 5 g/100 ml
B. 50 g/500 ml
C. 50 g/250 ml
D. 1.5 g/150 ml

40. **Your patient was diagnosed with left-sided heart failure. On an EKG, left-sided heart failure results in**
A. Tall, peaked P waves
B. Wide, notched P waves
C. Changes in ST segments
D. A prolonged Q wave

41. **Your new patient has been diagnosed with acquired valvular heart disease. The primary cause of acquired valvular heart disease is**
A. Heredity
B. Drug abuse

C. Rheumatic fever

D. Fetal alcohol syndrome

The following three questions are about Levophed. We asked about 300 PCCN review attendees to write down names of medications they think should be included on the PCCN exam because they frequently are used in the progressive care unit. We were very surprised when a large percentage of nurses suggested Levophed. Levophed is usually administered only in ICUs and CCUs. We do not know if the audience was comprised of a lot of nurses who also work in an ICU/CCU setting or if they were just curious. It never hurts to learn something that will help a patient, regardless of whether or not it may be on an exam. So far, no questions about Levophed have been reported on a PCCN exam.

42. Which of the following statements regarding norepinephrine bitrate (Levophed) is correct?

A. The maximum adult dose of Levophed is 40 mcg/min

B. The intravenous duration of action is 10 minutes

C. Dosage >2 mcg/min causes negative inotropic and chronotropic effects

D. Initial dosing of Levophed begins at 0.5 to 1 mcg/min

43. Hyperpyrexia is a potential life-threatening adverse reaction if Levophed is administered concurrently with which of the following classifications of drugs?

A. Alpha blockers

B. Beta-blockers

C. MAO inhibitors

D. Nitrates

44. You are explaining to a new nurse why there is a physician order to keep phenotolamine mesylate (Regitine) at the bedside of a patient receiving Levophed. Which of the following statements is true regarding the use of Regitine?

A. Regitine causes vasodilation in tissues damaged by extravasated IV fluids to correct and prevent necrosis and sloughing

B. Regitine is given only once IV around the extravasation site

C. Regitine is used for vasoconstriction in patients given excessive nitroglycerin

D. Reconstituted Regitine is stable at the bedside for 48 hours

45. A 20 year old football player was admitted to your unit following an episode of chest pain. The EKG monitor now reveals PVCs and runs of tachycardia. Lidocaine is ordered. Which of the following symptoms of lidocaine toxicity requires immediate intervention?

A. A respiratory rate of 7

B. A narrowing QRS

C. A heart rate of 70

D. Hypertonicity

46. Today you are precepting a student nurse. You are preparing to administer Lasix, 40 mg IV. The student asks you how fast the IV dose may be administered. You explain that Lasix must be given slowly because

A. Lasix may cause nausea

B. A rash may develop

C. Hyperkalemia may occur
D. A rapid infusion can lead to hearing loss

47. Your patient with an implanted cardiac defibrillator should have thresholds checked frequently during administration of which of the following medications?
A. Amiodarone
B. Nesiritide
C. Nitrogylcerin
D. Anisindione

48. Symptoms of right-sided heart failure include
A. Orthopnea
B. Elevated left atrial pressure
C. Hepatomegaly
D. Pulmonary edema

49. A 56 year old female was initially admitted to your PCU for severe dyspnea and has been diagnosed with congestive heart failure. After further study it was determined that she has restrictive cardiomyopathy. A common cause of restrictive cardiomyopathy is
A. An unknown viral infection
B. Glycogen storage disease
C. A history of diabetes
D. Unknown

50. You are mentoring a new nurse in the PCU. The patient you will be caring for is receiving lidocaine via a continuous infusion. The nurse must be taught that lidocaine may cause adverse effects such as
A. Hyperexcitability
B. CNS toxicity
C. Ventricular tachycardia
D. Premature atrial complexes

51. If the inferior wall of the heart is infarcted, the leads that will most directly reflect the injury are leads
A. I and aVL
B. II, III, and aVF
C. V_1–V_2
D. V_5–V_6

52. You are teaching your patient about her Coumadin (warfarin) therapy. Part of your teaching must include foods to avoid. Which of the following foods should be avoided?
A. Broccoli, soybean oil, spinach
B. Olive oil, peanut butter, kale
C. Avocado, broccoli, peas
D. Broccoli, green beans, spinach

53. Right-sided congestive heart failure signs and symptoms include
A. Respiratory distress and hepatomegaly
B. Rapid capillary refill and absent jugular venous distension
C. Mitral stenosis and abdominal tenderness
D. Decreased CVP and strong femoral pulses

54. Increased afterload would be present in a patient with which of the following conditions?
A. Polycythemia
B. Aortic insufficiency
C. Hypovolemia
D. Sepsis

55. Your patient was diagnosed with left ventricular failure. Early signs of left ventricular failure are
A. Central cyanosis and dry cough
B. Tachypnea and tachycardia
C. Diffuse chest pain and diaphoresis
D. Pedal edema and ascites

56. While auscultating heart sounds on your new patient, you hear an S_3 heart sound. The third heart sound occurs as a result of
A. Active atrial contraction
B. Aortic stenosis
C. Closure of the aortic and pulmonic valves
D. Increased blood flow across the AV valves

57. An anterior wall infarction may be seen in leads
A. V_4, R
B. V_5–V_6
C. V_7–V_9
D. V_2–V_4

58. Which of the heart valves is most rarely affected by infective endocarditis?
A. Tricuspid
B. Pulmonic
C. Mitral
D. Aortic

59. Which of the following medications should be monitored for cyanide toxicity and avoided in patients with renal problems?
A. Propranolol
B. Sodium nitroprusside
C. Dopamine
D. Verapamil

60. **Your patient had a syncopal episode at work. When he arrived in the PCU, he became apneic and bradycardic. After a dose of atropine and one minute of assisted ventilations, he resumed a normal sinus rhythm and normal respirations. At first, it was thought the patient had the flu. When an IV was started for fluid replacement, excessive bleeding was noted at the IV site. Further examination and tests revealed slight hepatomegaly and hepatitis. Labs showed high numbers of bands and an elevated platelet count. A diagnosis of myocarditis was made. A likely causative agent for this condition is**
    A. Group B Streptococcus
    B. *Escherichia coli*
    C. Coxsackie B1 virus
    D. Halothane toxicity

61. **You are treating an elderly woman with suspected sepsis. Her blood pressure is 94/54, heart rate is 120, respiratory rate is 20, and O_2 saturation is 86% on room air. Before initiating an infusion of dopamine, which of the following actions is a priority for the nurse?**
    A. Obtain consent for a central line
    B. Prepare to infuse dobutamine and dopamine together
    C. Verify the number of isotonic crystalloid boluses already given to the patient
    D. Ensure phentolamine mesylate is at bedside

62. **You are mentoring a new nurse in your progressive care unit who is caring for a patient receiving a dopamine drip. The order is to titrate the dopamine to keep the systolic blood pressure over 80 mmHg. You note that the nurse is titrating the drip every 2 to 3 minutes. You should**
    A. Praise the nurse for her diligence
    B. Verify the order for systolic blood pressure
    C. Suggest that titrations be done only in 15-minute increments
    D. Advise the nurse to wait at least 5 minutes between titrations

63. **Your patient was diagnosed with SVT. He will be discharged on oral amiodarone to control his SVT. Which of the following discharge instructions is true?**
    A. Continue normal outside activities without restrictions
    B. Continue original theophylline regimen
    C. Avoid grapefruit
    D. Expect an increase in urine output

64. **A 45 year old male was transported to the ED then admitted to your unit because of changes in mentation, development of ascites, orthopnea, paroxysmal nocturnal dyspnea, and excessive fatigue. On physical examination, you note S_3 and S_4 gallops, basilar crackles, and the EKG shows sinus tachycardia. These symptoms are usually indicative of which of the following types of cardiomyopathy?**
    A. Restrictive cardiomyopathy
    B. Dilated cardiomyopathy
    C. Alcohol-induced cardiomyopathy
    D. Hypertrophic cardiomyopathy

65. Your patient requires an infusion of dobutamine. Dobutamine improves cardiac output primarily by

A. Increasing afterload
B. Increasing heart rate
C. Decreasing preload
D. Improving contractility

66. Atropine was given to your patient during an episode of bradycardia that resulted in a heart rate decreasing to the 20s. The patient had just been deeply suctioned. The low heart rate was unresponsive to oxygen support, so assisted ventilation via a bag-valve mask was provided. The heart rate improved to prebradycardic levels. Which of the following potential complications of atropine administration may now occur?

A. Diuresis
B. Hypertension
C. Rebound bradycardia
D. Headache

67. Your patient with recurrent VT was started on intravenous amiodarone today. Which of the following signs should the PCU nurse monitor closely during administration of the initial loading dose?

A. Urine output and parathyroid levels
B. Urine output and liver function tests
C. Thyroid levels and hypertonicity
D. Observe for greenish discoloration of the skin and monitor thyroid levels

68. In addition to heart rate and urine output, which of the following laboratory values should be monitored closely for a patient taking diazoxide and furosemide for hypertension?

A. Glucose levels
B. Bilirubin levels
C. Calcium levels
D. INR levels

69. A complication of high-contrast mediums used for cardiac catheterizations is

A. Hypoglycemia
B. Hypernatremia
C. Polycythemia
D. Seizures

70. Which of the following statements is true about pericardial effusions?

A. Diastolic filling is increased
B. On CXR, a "water bottle" silhouette is noted
C. The voltage of the QRS complex is increased
D. This is a painless, hard-to-diagnose condition

71. Your patient is 48 years old and is being discharged to the care of his primary healthcare provider following treatment for a small pulmonary embolus. He will be continuing anticoagulant therapy. You are reinforcing previous teaching about his medication. Your patient takes numerous herbal remedies daily. Which ones should he avoid while he is taking an anticoagulant?

A. Dong quai, gingko biloba, saw palmetto
B. Aloe extract, bilberry, broccoli
C. Calendula, clove, allspice
D. Fenugreek, licorice, leeks

72. Cardiac glycosides are often used in the treatment of heart failure. A major effect of this classification of medications is

A. Increased conductivity
B. Positive chronotropism
C. Its usefulness as a ventricular antiarrhythmic
D. Inotropism

73. Which drug listed below contains a high concentration of iodine?

A. Lidocaine
B. Amiodarone
C. Aminophylline
D. Digoxin

74. A pansystolic murmur is audible with

A. Pulmonic insufficiency
B. Tricuspid insufficiency
C. Atrial stenosis
D. Mitral stenosis

75. A reflex tachycardia caused by stretch of right atrial receptors is known as the

A. Herring–Sines law
B. Bainbridge reflex
C. Starling's law
D. Renin–angiotensin system

76. Your 27 year old patient has been consuming large quantities of power drinks and has been having intermittent episodes of SVT. Today she was admitted to your unit because she had a syncopal episode at dance class and requires therapy for the SVT. Which of the following medications is specific to the treatment of sustained supraventricular tachycardia?

A. Atropine
B. Theophylline
C. Amiodarone
D. Adenosine

77. The most commonly used type of ventricular assist device is the

A. RVAD
B. VAD
C. BIVAD
D. LVAD

78. Indications for use of a ventricular assist device are

A. Extensive organ damage
B. As destination therapy
C. Prolonged cardiac arrest
D. Dysrhythmias

79. Which of the following statements is true regarding the fourth heart sound (S_4)?

A. S_4 occurs just after the first heart sound
B. The fourth heart sound occurs with ventricular contraction
C. The fourth heart sound is benign
D. The fourth heart sound is always pathologic after 24 hours of life

80. Your patient has Wolff-Parkinson-White syndrome. She has experienced increasing bouts of tachycardia over the past few weeks. Her cardiologist has decided to use overdrive pacing. How do you explain this type of pacemaker to a new orientee you are precepting in the PCU?

A. The pacemaker or AICD is set on demand mode and is asynchronous
B. The pacemaker is at a set constant rate of 80 bpm and is synchronous
C. The pacemaker or AICD is set on demand mode and is synchronous
D. The pacemaker or AICD is set on inhibit mode and is synchronous

81. Your patient has had an AICD for 8 months. He has come to the hospital after a syncopal episode during work today. You note his pulse is very irregular and he is complaining of getting "zapped" often. The patient says he is exhausted from the repeated shocks and asks for pain medication. His EKG shows sinus bradycardia with numerous pacemaker spikes. As a progressive care nurse, you suspect

A. The AICD has a faulty lead
B. The patient has been in the proximity of a large magnetic field
C. The battery in the AICD is losing power
D. The patient has a generator failure of his AICD

82. Your patient had a DDD pacemaker inserted 3 years ago. His college schoolwork has been declining, and he has not been participating in activities with his friends. He now has Pacemaker syndrome. What symptoms do you expect to see with this condition?

A. Fatigue, agitation, forgetfulness
B. Fatigue, dizziness, confusion
C. Fatigue, agitation, dyspnea
D. Fatigue, dizziness, syncope

83. The most common infection in patients with a ventricular assist device is

A. Septicemia
B. Pericarditis
C. Pneumonia
D. Pericardial effusion

84. Quincke's sign is usually observed in patients who have a diagnosis of

A. Mitral stenosis
B. Endocarditis

C. Aortic insufficiency
D. Pericarditis

85. Which of the following hemodynamic changes will occur in a patient with a cardiac tamponade?
A. Cardiac output increases
B. Stroke volume increases
C. Stroke volume decreases
D. Heart sounds are easily auscultated

86. Beck's triad is a combination of symptoms useful in diagnosing a cardiac tamponade. These symptoms include
A. Increased pulse pressure, increased JVD, and tachycardia
B. A pericardial friction rub, hypertension, and RV failure
C. LV failure, tachycardia, and hypertension
D. Distended neck veins, muffled heart sounds, and hypotension

87. If a dopamine infusion infiltrates, the suggested treatment is to inject which of the following medications into the affected area?
A. Epinephrine
B. Phentolamine
C. Lidocaine
D. Atropine

88. Your patient has developed diffuse chest pain and tachycardia. Upon auscultation you hear muffled heart sounds and note an increased JVD. You suspect the patient has developed a cardiac tamponade. If your patient does have a cardiac tamponade, which of the following findings would you expect on a chest X-ray?
A. A dilated superior vena cava
B. A pneumothorax
C. Narrowed mediastinum
D. Delineation of the pericardium and epicardium

89. Today your patient was diagnosed with left ventricular failure. Early signs of left ventricular failure include
A. Hypoxemia and peripheral cyanosis
B. Tachypnea and tachycardia
C. Dyspnea and profuse sweating
D. Central cyanosis and paradoxical respirations

90. A patient was admitted to the PCU with aortic insufficiency. During his initial assessment, you note the popliteal BP is higher than the brachial BP by at least 40 mmHg. This phenomenon is known as
A. DeRoge's sign
B. Hill's sign
C. Holmes' sign
D. Rochelle's sign

91. A fellow nurse and her family just returned from a vacation in Europe. She has been complaining to her husband about leg cramping for the past 3 days. The hospital's nurse practitioner sent her to the ED for further evaluation and subsequent admission to the PCU. During your initial assessment you found the patient sitting on the side of the bed, leaning forward. She states the position relieved her newly developed chest pain. She also states that the pain is worse on inspiration. You notify the PCU hospitalist, and he orders a CXR and lab work. The sed. rate and WBCs are elevated. This patient most likely is suffering from

A. A thoracic aneurysm
B. Pericarditis
C. Pulmonary hypertension
D. A pulmonary embolus

92. Your patient is in fulminant CHF. What is the purpose of administering vasoactive and inotropic medications to this patient?

A. Decrease preload, decrease afterload, increase contractility
B. Increase preload, increase afterload, decrease contractility
C. Increase myocardial oxygen demand, decrease contractility, increase afterload
D. Decrease myocardial oxygen demand, decrease contractility, increase preload

93. Your patient was found in his room in full arrest. After starting CPR and placing the patient on a monitor, you discover the patient is in ventricular fibrillation. Your next priority is to

A. Cardiovert the patient with 200 Joules
B. Administer 1 mg of 1:10,000 epinephrine IV
C. Administer 300 mg of amiodarone IV
D. Defibrillate the patient with 200 Joules with a biphasic defibrillator

94. Which of the following drugs is classified as both a negative chronotrope and a positive inotrope?

A. Amiodarone
B. Digoxin
C. Pronestyl
D. Epinephrine

95. Your patient just had a temporary atrial pacemaker placed. On the EKG you note pacemaker spikes that are not followed by P waves. Which of the following nursing actions should be performed at this time?

A. Turn off the pacemaker
B. Make certain the pacemaker is in the demand mode
C. Increase the milliamperes
D. Do nothing—the pattern is normal

96. Which of the following statements is true regarding a type I aortic aneurysm?

A. Type I aneurysms are the rarest form of aneurysm
B. Type I aneurysm tears begin in the ascending aorta

C. Type I aneurysm tears are in the intimal lining
D. Type I tears are in the descending aorta

97. **Type III aneurysms**
A. Begin in the thoracic arch
B. Are the rarest form of aneurysm
C. Involve intimal tears
D. Occur in the descending aorta

98. **A risk factor for an aortic aneurysm would not include**
A. Connective tissue disorders
B. Medial necrosis of the aorta
C. Hypotension
D. Coarctation of the aorta

99. **Your patient was admitted to the PCU for an intractable cough about an hour ago. He is now complaining of diffuse abdominal pain. On assessment you notice a pulsatile mass in his abdomen. The next action you should take is to**
A. Palpate the mass to determine its size
B. Immediately report this finding to the physician
C. Auscultate the mass
D. Prepare the patient for a biopsy of the mass

100. **Your patient has pericarditis and the physician has prescribed colchicine. Your patient teaching should include dietary restrictions. Which food should the patient avoid if taking colchicine?**
A. Diet Coke
B. Pears
C. Grapefruit
D. Bananas

101. **If a patient becomes tachycardic, what happens to the QT and RR intervals?**
A. No change occurs
B. The QT interval lengthens and the RR interval remains constant
C. The QT interval shortens and the RR interval lengthens
D. The QT and the RR intervals shorten

102. **Your 54 year old patient with asthma has been started on Plavix post-newly-diagnosed non-Q-wave MI. Which adverse drug reaction would you advise this patient to report immediately to the physician?**
A. Bronchospasms
B. Pneumonia
C. Apnea
D. Hemoptysis

103. **When should you suspect a patient has suffered a right ventricular MI?**
A. When the patient has right arm pain or paresthesias with substernal chest pain
B. When the patient has an inferior wall MI with suspected posterior involvement
C. When angina is pain unrelieved with sublingual NTG
D. With EKG changes in leads V_5 and V_6

104. Your patient has been on dofetilide for a week while being treated for unstable atrial fibrillation. Which of the following electrolyte levels should be monitored closely?

A. Potassium and sodium
B. Sodium and magnesium
C. Potassium and magnesium
D. Magnesium and chloride

105. Your 60 year old patient is being monitored post-streptokinase administration for a thrombolytic stroke 2 days ago and current anticoagulation therapy. You are called to the room by his family after he complained of a severe headache due to "someone is trying to drill into my head." You would suspect these symptoms are an adverse effect to which drug?

A. Aspirin
B. Angiomax
C. Plavix
D. Lovenox

106. Your patient suffered a myocardial infarction with resultant cardiopulmonary resuscitation 3 days ago. Which of the following medications would most likely be contraindicated at this time?

A. Lidocaine
B. Amiodarone
C. Potassium chloride
D. Dofetilide

107. On an EKG, upright QRS in leads V_1 and V_2 indicate which of the following types of bundle branch block?

A. Right
B. Left
C. Dual bundle branch block
D. Only leads aVF and III diagnose bundle branch blocks

108. Your patient had an MI with second-degree heart block. She just had a VVI pacemaker inserted. What does the first V indicate?

A. Paced, ventricular
B. Paced, inhibited
C. Ventricular inhibited
D. Ventricular

109. What does the second V in a VVI pacemaker indicate?

A. Ventricular paced
B. Ventricular inhibited
C. Ventricular sensed
D. Ventricular programmed

110. Quinidine and hypomagnesemia can both lead to which of the following conditions?

A. Monomorphic ventricular tachycardia
B. Torsade de pointes

C. Ventricular fibrillation
D. Atrial tachycardia

111. A patient was started on esmolol for severe hypertension refractive to other drug regimens. Esmolol is incompatible with which of the following medications?
A. Cimetidine
B. Furosemide
C. Penicillin G potassium
D. Midazolam

112. Dilated cardiomyopathy is characterized by dilation of the ventricles and impaired systolic function. Common causes are valvular heart disease and ischemic heart disease. Other causes are idiopathic. The most common cause of idiopathic dilated cardiomyopathy is
A. Autoimmune
B. Alcohol
C. Genetic
D. Familial

113. The physician ordered Ofirmev to help with pain control on your post-CABG patient. Which statement is true concerning the use of this medication?
A. Ofirmev can be given IVP
B. Ofirmev should be diluted prior to administration
C. Ofirmev dosing for a patient weighing <50 kg should be calculated at 10 mg/kg
D. The maximum daily dose of Ofirmev is 4,000 mg for a patient weighing >50 kg

114. Which of the following is considered an end effect of CHF?
A. Atrial fibrillation
B. Increased renal perfusion
C. Pulmonary venous shrinkage
D. Systemic venous engorgement

115. The type of cardiomyopathy that is characterized by replacement of normal cells by fatty tissue is known as
A. Restrictive cardiomyopathy
B. Hypertrophic cardiomyopathy
C. Arrhythmogenic cardiomyopathy
D. Dilated cardiomyopathy

116. Your patient has been experimenting with multiple drugs. She was admitted to your unit after a cocaine overdose. The patient has had an anterolateral myocardial infarction. Where do you expect to see changes on the 12-lead EKG?
A. Leads V_1, V_2, I, and AVL
B. Leads V_2, V_3, V_4, I, and AVL
C. Leads V_2, V_3, V_4, II, III, and AVF
D. Leads V_1, V_2, II, III, and AVF

117. A patient is receiving propranolol IV for SVT and hypertension. Which of the following are life-threatening side effects of propranolol administration?
A. Laryngospasm and bronchospasm
B. Complete heart block and dizziness

C. Respiratory depression and cardiovascular collapse
D. Polymorphic VT and dyspnea

118. Regurgitation systolic murmurs are associated with
A. Aortic stenosis
B. Pulmonic valve disease
C. Ventral septal defect
D. Atrial septal defects

119. A 65 year old female was admitted to the PCU for treatment of intermittent chest pain and severe hypertension. A nitroglycerin drip was ordered. Which of the following is true regarding nitroglycerin administration?
A. Use only plastic IV tubing
B. Nitroglycerine may be piggy-backed to Isolyte P
C. Nitroglycerine should be filtered prior to delivery
D. Have normal saline or other volume expander available at bedside

120. What do abnormal Q waves signify on a 12-lead EKG?
A. Partial thickness death of myocardium
B. Complete thickness infarction of myocardium
C. They are of no significance
D. Repolarization of the myocardium

121. The most common new onset dysrhythmia seen in a patient with a diagnosis of pulmonary edema is
A. Paroxysmal atrial tachycardia
B. Supraventricular tachycardia
C. Sinus rhythm with an RBBB
D. Atrial fibrillation

122. What are some common reasons for pacemaker insertion?
A. Tachycardia, Wenckebach, and bradycardia
B. Symptomatic bradycardia, overdrive pacing, and acute MI with sinus dysfunction
C. Complete heart block, Wenckebach, and tachycardia
D. Bundle branch block, Wenckebach, and tachycardia

123. Right ventricular afterload may be reduced by
A. A hypoxic state
B. Hypoventilation
C. Inhaled nitric oxide
D. Administration of epinephrine

124. Mr. C. was admitted to the PCU with cough, fever, chills, anorexia, malaise, and headache. He currently has a pericardial friction rub and has a history of rheumatic fever. While examining Mr. C., you note fine, dark lines in his nail beds and some flat lesions on his palms. These flat lesions are known as
A. Janeway lesions
B. Osler's nodes
C. Roth spots
D. Pella's sign

125. A definitive diagnosis of myocarditis can be made via

A. Transmural catheterization
B. Transesophageal ultrasound
C. Transcutaneous ultrasound
D. Endomyocardial biopsy

126. Adverse effects of procainamide include

A. Depressing the excitability of cardiac muscle
B. Junctional tachycardia
C. Slowing conduction in the atria
D. Severe hypotension

127. A patient received 4 mg of morphine IV and now is unresponsive; his respiratory rate and depth are diminished. The antagonist for morphine is

A. Naloxone
B. Atropine
C. Regitine
D. Epinephrine

128. Your patient has changes in mentation, development of ascites, orthopnea, paroxysmal nocturnal dyspnea, and excessive fatigue. On physical examination, you note S_3 and S_4 gallops, basilar crackles, and the EKG shows sinus tachycardia. These symptoms are usually indicative of which of the following types of cardiomyopathy?

A. Restrictive cardiomyopathy
B. Dilated cardiomyopathy
C. Alcohol-induced cardiomyopathy
D. Hypertrophic cardiomyopathy

129. The type of echocardiography used to evaluate the motion of the cardiac valves and detect pericardial fluid is known as ____________ echocardiography

A. M-mode
B. Two-dimensional
C. Contrast
D. Continuous-wave Doppler

130. The type of echocardiography that shows the quantity of flow across an obstruction is called

A. Two-dimensional echocardiography
B. Continuous-wave Doppler echocardiography
C. M-mode echocardiography
D. Contrast echocardiography

131. Dobutamine is used to improve cardiac output primarily by

A. Causing profound peripheral vasodilation
B. Acting on alpha-adrenergic receptors in the heart
C. Acting on beta1 adrenergic receptors in the heart
D. Acting on both alpha-and beta-adrenergic receptors in the cardiovascular tissue

132. Alpha-adrenergic effects of norepinephrine include

A. Increased force of myocardial contraction
B. Peripheral arteriolar vasoconstriction
C. Increased AV conduction time
D. Central venous vasodilation

133. Your patient is on lisinopril (Zestril) for hypertension after suffering a septal MI. A vial of epinephrine 1:1,000 is kept at the bedside should the patient exhibit which of the following symptoms?

A. Angioedema
B. Pyelonephritis
C. Cholestatic jaundice
D. SIADH

134. Nifedipine is classified as a

A. Calcium channel blocker
B. Beta-blocker
C. MAO inhibitor
D. Catecholamine

135. You are preparing to give adenosine to a patient in SVT. Why is it important that adenosine be given rapidly?

A. If given slowly, the adenosine will probably fail to convert the SVT
B. Adenosine is incompatible with adrenalin
C. If given slowly, adenosine may cause systemic vasodilation and reflex tachycardia
D. If given slowly, adenosine may cause blurred vision

136. A heart murmur associated with acute valvular regurgitation is called

A. S_3
B. S_2
C. S_1
D. S_4

137. Your patient was diagnosed with refractive SVT that did not respond to either adenosine or cardioversion. She is being monitored before being transported for ablation therapy. Tachyarrhythmias that are refractive to conventional therapies may have to be treated with radio-frequency ablation. This treatment is usually successful on reentry tachyarrhythmias. The radio frequency destroys myocardial tissue via

A. Radiation
B. Heat
C. Cold
D. An overriding signal to ablate the pacemaker

138. A high CVP reading may be caused by

A. Nitroglycerin administration
B. Increased contractility
C. Hypovolemia
D. Cardiac tamponade

139. **New-onset atrial fibrillation frequently develops as sequelae to**
   A. Pulmonary edema
   B. Left heart failure
   C. Use of PPIs
   D. Tricuspid regurgitation

140. **Intravenous hydralazine is incompatible with**
   A. Furosemide
   B. Hydrocortisone
   C. Potassium chloride
   D. Heparin

141. **Nesiritide is an appropriate drug to help treat which of the following heart conditions?**
   A. Constrictive pericarditis
   B. Acute decompensated congestive heart failure
   C. Chronic obstructive cardiomyopathy
   D. Pericardial tamponade

142. **Dofetilide (Tikosyn) should not be administered to any patient with the following cardiac abnormality**
   A. Atrial flutter
   B. Prolonged QT interval
   C. Ventricular tachycardia
   D. NSR postconverted atrial fibrillation

143. **Which of the following medications is used to specifically treat atrial fibrillation?**
   A. Dofetilide
   B. Mexiletine
   C. Sotalol
   D. Flecainide

The following questions are representative of the current Guidelines for Cardiopulmonary Resuscitation from the American Heart Association. Whenever the PCCN exam is administered, there is an expectation that the individual is knowledgeable about these guidelines and current content.

144. **Under the new 2010 American Heart Association guidelines for chest compressions, the rescuer should compress the sternum of an adult to a depth of**
   A. 1 inch
   B. 1½ inches
   C. 2 inches
   D. 3 inches

145. **The BLS sequence for adults receiving CPR is**
   A. ABC
   B. CAB
   C. AOB
   D. BAC

146. Which of the following statements is true regarding routine application of cricoid pressure during cardiac arrest?

A. Cricoid pressure is not recommended as a routine action

B. Cricoid pressure should be applied whenever possible during cardiac arrest

C. Cricoid pressure must be used when there are two or more rescuers

D. Cricoid pressure must be applied only by a paramedic, MICN, or a physician

147. The most reliable method of confirming and monitoring correct placement of an ETT is by use of

A. Auscultation

B. Visualization of the cords

C. Use of an end tidal CO_2 monitor

D. Continuous wave capnography

148. The single most-important component of a successful outcome for a patient requiring advanced cardiac life support is

A. Early defibrillation

B. Use of epinephrine in place of vasopressin

C. Therapeutic hypothermia

D. High-quality CPR

149. According to the 2010 American Heart Association Guidelines for CPR and Emergency Cardiovascular Care, which of the following medications is no longer recommended for routine use in the management of PEA or asystole?

A. Epinephrine

B. Adenosine

C. Atropine

D. Vasopressin

150. Withdrawal of life support is a difficult decision. If an adult post–cardiac arrest patient is treated with therapeutic hypothermia, the patient should be evaluated via neurologic signs, biomarkers, electrophysiologic studies, and imaging where available at ________ after cardiac arrest.

A. 24 hours

B. 48 hours

C. 72 hours

D. 96 hours

151. Which of the following statements about drowning victims is true?

A. There is no evidence that water acts as an obstructive foreign body

B. CPR should be performed while the patient is in the water

C. Immediate maneuvers to relieve foreign body airway obstruction should precede BLS

D. Spinal cord injuries are common among drowning victims

152. What is the purpose of a right side 12-lead EKG?

A. It allows a view of the pulmonary blood flow

B. It looks at the inferior wall of the heart

C. It looks at the right ventricle and the posterior of the heart

D. It assesses for left ventricle aneurysm

153. Your patient lives on a nearby Indian reservation. He is retired and on a fixed income without insurance. He is being discharged today after an overnight observational stay for chest pain. In planning his discharge care, which of the following should be considered first to increase compliance with his plan of care once he is home?

A. Arrange for home nursing visits every day for 1 week

B. Ask the physician to consider an over-the-counter antiplatelet medication

C. Schedule his follow-up appointment with the cardiologist in 3 months

D. Suggest a gym membership to begin exercising

154. Mr. G. was diagnosed with unstable angina. He is scheduled for an exercise stress test. He tells you that he has a "bad hip" and an old knee injury that make it difficult for him to walk or stand for more than 20 minutes. You tell him:

A. "You only need to walk for 10 minutes"

B. "You can ride a bike for 20 minutes instead"

C. "I will call the physician and ask for the weight-lift test"

D. "I will call the physician and ask for a stress echocardiography test"

155. Approximately what percentage of coronary artery blockage is needed to cause angina?

A. 45%

B. 60%

C. 75%

D. 90%

156. Which of the following leads is best for monitoring for a RBBB?

A. Lead II

B. Lead I

C. Lead V_1

D. Lead V_6

157. With regard to stable angina, which of the following statements is true?

A. A positive treadmill test will indicate CAD

B. A thallium test will not diagnose LV dysfunction

C. The treadmill test will miss as many as 20% of cases of single-vessel disease

D. CK-MB isoenzymes and troponins will not increase

158. Ms. M. underwent CABG surgery 4 days ago and was transferred to your care yesterday. Today she complains of dull aching around the sternum. You note increased tenderness to touch along the sternal edge and contracted intercostal muscles. You should

A. Contact the physician for an order for a 12-lead EKG, cardiac enzymes, and morphine

B. Culture-swab the wound for bacterial infection

C. Do nothing; her pain is normal

D. Administer morphine and diazepam as ordered

159. The drug of choice to treat AV nodal and atrioventricular reentrant arrhythmias is

A. Amiodarone

B. Clonidine

C. Quinidine
D. Adenosine

160. Your patient was admitted to your unit for observation after falling 10 feet into a ravine. She was diagnosed with systemic lupus erythematosus (SLE) 2 years ago. She suffered a concussion, three fractured ribs, a fractured radius, and a sprained ankle. She is on a Holter monitor and is receiving IV fluids and antibiotics. Which of the following conditions would be exacerbated by the SLE?
A. Hypotension
B. Constipation
C. Pericarditis
D. Polycythemia

161. If the international normalized ratio (INR) is greater than 5.0, the patient is at significant risk of bleeding. A drug that can cause a significant rise in the INR is
A. Ethacrinic acid
B. Penicillin
C. Amiodarone
D. A statin

162. A drug that will significantly decrease the INR would be
A. Naficillin
B. Vitamin K
C. High-dose vitamin C
D. Cyclosporine

163. Your patient is a 54 year old dockworker who was admitted with a non-STEMI inferior wall MI. He is complaining of dyspnea, weakness, bilateral crackles, and demonstrates orthopnea. He has developed an S_3 heart sound. You suspect he has also developed
A. A pulmonary embolus
B. Pulmonary hypertension
C. A fat embolism
D. Cardiogenic shock

164. Your patient suddenly complains of chest pain. You auscultate a new holosystolic murmur at the lower left sternal border. Your patient has probably experienced a
A. Dissecting thoracic aneurysm
B. Pulmonary embolus
C. Ventricular septal rupture
D. Lateral wall MI

165. Your patient has been diagnosed with pericarditis secondary to blunt chest trauma and cardiac contusion after a motor vehicle accident. She asks you how long the pericarditis may last. Your answer will be formulated based on the fact that
A. Acute pericarditis will self-resolve in 1 week
B. Acute pericarditis should self-resolve in 2–6 weeks
C. Acute pericarditis will always result in chronic pericarditis
D. Chronic pericarditis is reoccurring and not associated with any other cardiac symptoms

166. A patient is at high risk for ventricular septal defect or rupture or even a ventricular aneurysm if an infarct occurs in the

A. Left anterior descending artery
B. Left main coronary artery
C. Left circumflex artery
D. Right coronary artery

167. Auto-regulatory control of cardiac vessels becomes impaired if the coronary perfusion pressure drops below

A. 35 mmHg
B. 40 mmHg
C. 50 mmHg
D. 60 mmHg

168. If blood pressure is lower by at least 10–11 mmHg on inspiration than on expiration, this is known as

A. Pulsus alternans
B. Pulse pressure
C. Pulsus paradoxus
D. Pulsus parvus

169. You are providing discharge instructions to your patient with angina. The doctor has ordered nitroglycerine translingual spray, use 2 sprays every 5 minutes as needed for chest pain and use 1 spray prior to strenuous activity. Which of the following statements is true about the use of nitroglycerine translingual spray?

A. The nitroglycerine spray must be administered only under the tongue to be effective
B. Each nitroglycerine spray administers 0.2 mg
C. Effects may last up to 2 hours
D. Prophylactic administration should be taken 5 to 10 minutes before activity

170. Your patient will be discharged to home on transdermal ointment nitroglycerin to control angina symptoms. During your care, the patient informs you that he is looking forward to sitting in his hot tub after he is discharged. What is the best action you should take as a result of the patient's statement about the hot tub?

A. Tell him that due to his condition he should never use his hot tub again
B. Notify the physician and request a change from transdermal to an extended release tablet or capsule
C. Advise the patient to increase the amount of transdermal ointment to compensate for medication lost while in the water
D. Do nothing

171. Your patient, Mr. R., suffered an MI but is now in stable condition in your progressive care unit. Nine family members arrive at the PCU, demanding to see the patient. Your best response would be to

A. Notify social services
B. Identify a responsible family spokesperson and contact him or her
C. Refuse to admit more than one person
D. Call security to remove the visitors

172. Continuing with the scenario in Question 171, after you have identified Mr. R.'s significant other, his estranged wife arrives at the PCU. Mr. R. tells you he does not want contact with his estranged wife. He even writes a note to that effect to be placed on his chart. He also states he wants no information given to the estranged wife. She became belligerent when told of Mr. R.'s wishes and threatened the staff with a lawsuit. The most appropriate nursing action would be to

A. Request an ethics/multidisciplinary care conference to discuss communication and dissemination of the patient's medical status and to review the visitation policy
B. Immediately call the hospital attorney to speak with the wife
C. Give the wife any information she wants, but do not inform the patient that you have done so
D. Request that the patient's physician write a non-visitation order for the wife

173. The major advantage of using an internal mammary artery for cardiac bypass would be

A. Greater ease of harvesting
B. Better postsurgical patency
C. A lowered infection rate
D. A lower rate of reperfusion rhythms

174. Your patient just underwent a percutaneous intervention for stent placement, after which he was returned to your telemetry unit. You note a rash over the patient's trunk and arms. This is probably due to

A. An allergic reaction to contrast dye
B. Petechiae from a fat emboli
C. A reaction to the indwelling stent
D. The underlying endocarditis

175. A sign of necrosis seen on an EKG would include

A. Acute ST elevation
B. A right BBB
C. A left BBB
D. A Q wave in Lead III

176. The most common major impediment to family education regarding placement of a ventricular assist device is

A. Language
B. Technology
C. Time
D. Physician availability

177. The physician has just informed your patient that she needs an LVAD. The patient is crying and says, "I just know I am going to die. What's the point? It must be my time." The patient is obviously quite stressed. The priority for the nurse at this time is to

A. Tell the patient she will not die
B. Explore possible suicidal ideation
C. Immediately place the patient in a single room
D. Notify the hospital's spiritual advisor

178. Your patient has just transferred from the ICU to your unit. The patient had an abdominal aortic aneurysm repair 2 days ago. He is somewhat restless, and his vital signs are stable. He keeps pointing at the lumbar area of his back and saying that he has discomfort in that area. This may indicate

A. A blister from the surgical ground pad
B. Need for repositioning
C. Irritation from the dressing
D. Retroperitoneal bleeding

179. The definitive invasive diagnostic procedure to diagnose an aortic dissection is a(n)

A. Left lateral recumbent CX
B. Computerized tomography (CT) scan
C. Transesophageal ultrasound
D. Aortogram

180. You are discussing EKG interpretation with your nursing student. She asks you why there is such a difference in the size of the P and QRS waves. You tell her:

A. "The P wave represents repolarization of the atrium and the QRS the depolarization of the ventricles; the size difference is related to lead placement."
B. "The P wave represents repolarization of the atrium and the QRS the repolarization of the ventricles; the size difference is related to the muscle mass involved in the polarization."
C. "The P wave represents depolarization of the atrium and the QRS the depolarization of the ventricles; the size difference is related to the muscle mass involved in the polarization."
D. "The P wave represents depolarization of the atrium and the QRS the repolarization of the ventricles; the size difference is related to the lead placement."

181. Your patient with obstructive jaundice has no prior history of cardiac arrhythmias. He asks why he is on a cardiac monitor. Your best response is

A. "You may develop a slower heart rate. This monitor will alert staff to any dangerous drop in your heart rate."
B. "You may develop sinus tachycardia, and the monitor will alert staff to any increase in your heart rate."
C. "You will develop atrial flutter, and the monitor will alert staff to changes in your heart rate."
D. "You may develop ventricular tachycardia and the monitor will alert you to changes in your heart rate."

182. Your patient was admitted for pneumonia. He is 2 years post heart transplant. When you place the EKG monitoring leads, you note sinus tachycardia with PVCs and a 2-mm ST elevation. The patient denies pain. This finding is

A. Impossible
B. Normal
C. Indicative of an RBBB
D. Indicative of an inferior MI

183. A patient who is status post heart transplant may have significant bradycardia. The drug of choice in such cases is

A. Atropine
B. Isuproterenol
C. Apresoline
D. Adenosine

184. Your patient is 36 hours status post right femoral bypass graft. The patient complains of pain with even slight movement of the limb. You suspect

A. An arterial obstruction
B. A DVT
C. A venous obstruction
D. A leg cramp from prolonged bed rest

185. Your patient received streptokinase about 30 minutes ago for a lateral wall STEMI. You would expect which of the following events to occur?

A. Lowered CPK isoenzymes
B. Reperfusion rhythms
C. Transient increased chest pain
D. Mild CHF

186. A quadriplegic patient has undergone a CABG and has had no complications. You are about to teach his wife how to change the chest dressings and the graft site dressings on the legs. Principles of teaching include

A. Teaching all the information at once
B. Teaching the information as fast as possible
C. Explaining the rationale for the procedure, and then demonstrating it
D. Speaking slowly so that the patient can hear

187. Your patient had a cardiac arrest. You are doing CPR near his implanted ICD generator. If the ICD defibrillates, you would feel

A. A powerful shock
B. Nothing
C. Mild tingling
D. A mild shock

188. When you receive report on your patient, you are told his ICD was reset. You notice a large magnet on the table outside the room. What is the purpose of this magnet?

A. It inhibits all output from the ICD
B. It inhibits the shocking portion only of the ICD
C. It inhibits the pacemaker function of the ICD
D. It allows timing of the ICD to be set

189. Tachyarrhythmias that are refractive to conventional therapies may have to be treated with radio-frequency ablation. This treatment is usually successful on reentry tachyarrhythmias. The radio-frequency destroys myocardial tissue via

A. Radiation
B. Heat

C. Cold

D. An overriding signal to ablate the pacemaker

190. Your patient has atrial fibrillation and needs to be cardioverted. The patient was medicated for pain and anxiety with morphine and Versed. Which additional medication will help the process of cardioversion from atrial fibrillation to a normal sinus rhythm?

A. Digitalis

B. Amiodarone

C. Pronestyl

D. Ibutilide

191. During insertion of a CVP catheter, your patient has a short run of V-tach and shows unifocal PVCs. Your immediate response should be to

A. Administer lidocaine 1 mg/kg

B. Hang an amiodarone drip

C. Notify the physician who is inserting the catheter

D. Immediately have the physician completely withdraw the catheter

192. During shift report, you are told that your patient has a 90% occlusion to the circumflex coronary artery. Which type of myocardial infarction is this patient at greatest risk of developing?

A. Lateral wall infarction

B. Anterior wall infarction

C. Posterior wall infarction

D. Septal wall infarction

193. Your patient suffered a myocardial infarction as a result of 100% occlusion of the left anterior descending and circumflex artery. Although cardiac catheterization returned some blood flow to the left side of her heart, you note a new murmur at the fifth intercostal space, midclavicular line. You suspect

A. Tricuspid valve stenosis

B. Mitral valve regurgitation

C. Pulmonic stenosis

D. Aortic regurgitation

194. Which of the following nursing actions would be important in the care of a patient with occlusive disease of the terminal aorta and a nonhealing wound on the left foot?

A. Elevate the legs

B. Place the patient in high Fowler's position

C. Maintain normothermia

D. Fluid restriction

195. A 30 year old male who lost control of his motorcycle while riding in the rain was admitted to your unit. At the time of the accident, he was wearing a helmet and protective gear. He suffered a fractured left femur, a fractured rib, a cervical sprain, and road rash on his face and neck. He is admitted with a blood pressure of 84/44, HR 100, RR 26 and shallow, T 98.4° F. His 12-lead EKG shows ST elevation in the anterior leads. His CXR shows a normal cardiac silhouette and no infiltrates.

His Hgb is 9.0, and his Hct is 32. MB is 18%. The patient is restless and complains of pain in the chest and left leg. Which condition would you anticipate?

A. Systolic dysfunction
B. Hypovolemic shock
C. Pulmonary hypertension
D. Pulmonary edema

196. **Four days ago, Mrs. G., who is 70 years old, was admitted to your unit status post laparotomy for an unknown abdominal mass. During the surgery, she had minimal blood loss and an uneventful course. The patient's history includes smoking since she was 15 (unknown number of packs per day), Type II diabetes, a permanent pacemaker, an anterior MI, and a right-sided stroke 20 years ago with no deficits.**

Three days ago, Mrs. G. had a hypotensive episode; her BP dropped to 82/48, and her heart rate was 70. The hospitalist ordered dobutamine and the blood pressure increased until the MAP was 72.

Today, Mrs. G. remains on the dobutamine at 2 mcg/kg/min. Her BP is 108/60, MAP 76, heart rate 70. Attempts at weaning dobutamine have failed—her blood pressure drops precipitously if the dobutamine dosage is lowered.

What do you think is the cause of Mrs. G.'s initial hypotensive episode?

A. Hypovolemic shock
B. Previous MI
C. Rapid rewarming postoperatively
D. Cell mediated response

197. **Which physical finding is significant for carotid stenosis?**

A. Heberden's nodules
B. Systolic murmur Grade IV/VI
C. Carotid bruit
D. Broussard's nodules

198. **Which 12 lead EKG changes would you expect to see in a patient with COPD?**

A. Low-voltage P waves, tachycardia
B. Tall P waves, left ventricular hypertrophy
C. Tall, peaked P waves, right ventricular hypertrophy, low-voltage QRS
D. Low-voltage QRS, left atrial hypertrophy

199. **While caring for your patient on nesiritide, you note a decrease in urine output. Which of the following lab results should you immediately report to the physician?**

A. BUN/Creatinine ratio >20
B. Serum bicarbonate 25 mEq/L
C. Urine osmolality of 1,000 mOsm/L
D. Urine specific gravity of 1.005

200. **Integrilin (eptifbatide) is indicated for which of the following conditions?**

A. DVT
B. Pulmonary embolism
C. Acute coronary syndrome (ACS)
D. Occlusive cerebrovascular accident

201. **You overhear your patient discussing his aortic stenosis with his family. He states, "It can't be that bad, because the murmur isn't that loud." Your best response is**
A. Do not say anything, it would be considered eavesdropping
B. Interrupt and say that nothing has been confirmed yet
C. Give the patient an iPad and tell him to search the Internet
D. Use the opportunity to teach the patient by asking if you can clarify his understanding of his disease process

202. **Mr. B. was admitted to your unit to rule out myocardial infarction 2 days ago. He has a history of GERD and stomach ulcers. He is due to be discharged today on digoxin and oral antacids. You review his A.M. labs prior to beginning your physical assessment. Lab results are as follows**

WBC 11,000/mm^3	RBC 5.2 mil/mm^3	PLT 350,000/mm^3
Hgb 13 g/dL	Hct 48 mL/dL	
Potassium 4.5 mEq/L	Total calcium 13.5 mg/dL	Magnesium 1.87 mg/dL
Sodium 140 mEq/L	Chloride 104 mEq/L	

You would probably expect to see which of the following signs and symptoms during your assessment of Mr. B.?
A. Hypotension, prolonged QT interval, junctional tachycardia
B. Bradycardia, confusion, hypertension, decreased grasp strength
C. Muscle spasms, hypertonicity, ventricular tachycardia
D. Second-degree Type 2 heart block, shortened QT interval, hypotension

203. **You are caring for a 7-day postoperative CABG patient. He remains severely hypocalcemic despite calcium supplementation. Which of the following complications is this patient at greatest risk for developing?**
A. Bleeding
B. Muscle tetany
C. Flattened T waves
D. Deep vein thrombosis

204. **Peripartum cardiomyopathy is a form of**
A. Restrictive cardiomyopathy
B. Hypertropic cardiomyopathy
C. Viral cardiomyopathy
D. Dilated cardiomyopathy

205. **Your patient was admitted for ascites, orthopnea, paroxysmal nocturnal dyspnea, and excessive fatigue. On physical examination, you note S_3 and S_4 gallops, basilar crackles, and the EKG shows sinus tachycardia. These symptoms are usually indicative of which type of cardiomyopathy?**
A. Dilated
B. Restrictive
C. Alcohol-induced
D. Hypertrophic

206. Your patient has a newly placed stent. You overhear the cardiologist state that ticagrelor (Brilinta) is going to be started. What order do you expect to see when you check the chart?

A. Begin Brilinta 180 mg PO once per day immediately
B. Begin Brilinta 90 mg IV once per day in 3 days
C. Give Brilinta 180 mg PO now, then begin 90 mg PO BID in 5 days
D. Begin Brilinta 90 mg PO BID in 10 days

207. Your patient is on ticagrelor (Brilinta). What other drug should always be taken concurrently with ticagrelor (Brilinta)?

A. Aspirin
B. Nitroglycerin
C. Digoxin
D. Plavix

208. You are preparing to give Mrs. D. her 0900 dose of Coumadin as part of her atrial fibrillation management. You are reviewing her A.M. labs prior to administration of the medication. Which lab result would cause alarm?

A. PTT 72 seconds
B. PLT 180,000/mm^3
C. APTT 38 seconds
D. PT 28 seconds

209. Yesterday, your patient was shoveling snow when he became short of breath and felt diffuse chest discomfort. When he went inside for lunch, the pain disappeared. He later resumed shoveling snow and felt more fatigued than ever. Today, he was admitted to your unit with orthopnea and profound dyspnea. He is constantly saying, "I'm 58 years old and have been outside all my life. I'm not sick enough to be in here." His girlfriend reports that over the past 3 weeks, the patient has been more tired than usual, even when performing small tasks around the house.

His assessment findings are as follows:
EKG: Borderline ST at 100 with rare PACs
Manual cuff BP 142/74
Skin warm, pale
Capillary refill 4 seconds, 2+ pitting edema (pretibial)
RR 20, breath sounds: crackles in posterior lobes
O_2 2 L/min via NC
ABGs were drawn, but results are unavailable
Mentation: Alert, oriented 3 4

This patient has probably developed
A. Mild pericarditis
B. Pulmonary edema (noncardiac)
C. Chylothorax
D. Left ventricular failure

210. **Mrs. N. is 64 years old and has a history of COPD. Today, she was admitted with an inferior wall MI. About 30 minutes ago, she complained of increasing shortness of breath. When she changed her position, the dyspnea abated. She is again complaining of dyspnea, and you perform a 12-lead EKG because your unit monitor allows monitoring of only leads II and MCL1. The EKG shows lead V_1–V_4 ST-segment depression. Other physical and laboratory findings are as follows:**

EKG: Sinus arrhythmia at 93
Manual cuff BP 102/60
Skin pale, cool, clammy; sacral edema, pedal and pretibial edema
RR 22, breath sounds: bilateral crackles
O_2 2 L/min via NC
ABGs: pH 7.38, pCO_2 48, PaO_2 66, HCO_3 34
Mentation: Alert, oriented 3 4

What is the interpretation of the ABGs?

A. Uncompensated metabolic acidosis
B. Compensated respiratory acidosis
C. Uncompensated metabolic alkalosis
D. Compensated respiratory alkalosis

211. **Continuing with the scenario from Question 210, Mrs. N. is probably developing**

A. Pulmonary effusion
B. Left ventricular failure
C. Pericarditis
D. Congestive heart failure

212. **Your patient is a 45 year old ironworker. He was admitted for cardiomyopathy. His initial ejection fraction was 21%, and he has been confused most of the time since his admission yesterday. On admission, his EKG showed ST depression in leads V_1–V_4. He has been more dyspneic and is getting restless. Current vital signs and parameters are as follows:**

EKG: ST at 116
Manual cuff BP 102/70
Skin pale, cool
Temp 99° F
Bilateral pretibial and pedal edema
Sacral edema also present
RR 30, breath sounds clear, slightly diminished RLL
O_2 4 L/min via mask
Mentation: Oriented to self, confused at times

From which condition does this patient appear to be suffering at this time?

A. An anterior MI
B. Inferior wall MI
C. Biventricular failure
D. Right ventricular failure

213. The type of myocardial infarction that involves the entire thickness of myocardium in a region is called

A. Subendocardial
B. Anteroseptal
C. Transmural
D. Inferior wall

214. Your patient with an implanted cardiac defibrillator should have thresholds checked frequently during administration of which of the following drugs?

A. Amiodarone
B. Nesiritide
C. Nitroglycerin
D. Anisindione

215. Increased preload may be caused by

A. Hemorrhage
B. Hyperthermia
C. Renal problems
D. Vomiting

SECTION 4: CARDIOVASCULAR ANSWERS

1. **Correct answer: C**
   A pulse pressure is the difference between the systolic blood pressure and the diastolic blood pressure—in this case, 35. This measurement is significant because if the patient has a narrow pulse pressure, it would indicate systemic compensatory vasoconstriction due to a decrease in arterial pressure (the stroke volume falls and the systolic pressure decreases). Another way to look at this phenomenon is to think of the high systemic vascular resistance causing an increase in diastolic pressure.

2. **Correct answer: D**
   The ejection fraction should be over 50%. This is the amount of blood ejected from the left ventricle compared to the total amount available. This amount is expressed as a percentage. For example, if the ventricle contains 90 ml of blood and 50 ml are ejected, the amount would be represented as a percentage, in this case 55%. An ejection fraction of 35% or less indicates a problem with contractility, outflow, or filling.

3. **Correct answer: B**
   ST segment depression usually indicates myocardial ischemia. This patient also exhibited substernal chest pain, another finding seen with ischemia.

4. **Correct answer: B**
   Metabolism of the heart is decreased during diastole, which comprises about one-half of the cardiac cycle at birth. Shortly after birth the diastolic phase lengthens to comprise two-thirds of the cardiac cycle. An increase in cardiac output decreases diastole because more time is necessary to eject contents.

5. **Correct answer: C**
   The MAP is a mean pressure that takes into account that the diastolic phase of the cardiac cycle comprises two-thirds of the cycle. The calculation for the MAP is MAP = 2(DBP) + (SBP) / 3; in this case, 81. If you took the average of the two pressures, it would not account for the importance of the diastolic phase. The heart rate is not entered into this calculation. Patients should maintain a MAP of at least 60 to ensure perfusion to the brain and kidneys.
   When the heart rate is over 100, the diastolic phase may be less than one half the cardiac cycle. Electronic machines are calibrated to take variables into consideration and the digitally displayed MAP readings are highly accurate.

6. **Correct answer: B**
   Normal cardiac output should be 4 to 8 L/min. The formula for calculating this value is: CO = HR × SV. In this case, 78 (HR) × 60 (SV) = 4,680 ml/min. Converted to liters, this value would equal 4.68 L/min.

7. **Correct answer: B**
   Unstable angina usually associated with left anterior descending (LAD) coronary artery lesions is known as Wellen's syndrome. Characteristic changes include inverted symmetric T waves and/or biphasic waves with little or no ST elevation and the absence

of Q waves. However, the most dangerous aspect of this syndrome is that the EKG changes appear only when the patient is pain free. Sometimes, staff may believe the resolution of pain means the patient can be scheduled for a stress test. The stress test may initiate an impending MI, so it must not be performed. When a patient has Wellen's syndrome, an MI may occur in as little as a few minutes to a few days.

8. **Correct answer: C**
   Stroke volume is comprised of contractility, preload, and afterload. Viscosity, blood volume, and impedance represent the components of afterload. Myocardium is sensitive to changes, especially increased afterload. With only minute changes in afterload, the stroke volume can fall significantly.

9. **Correct answer: D**
   During CVP pressure monitoring, the c wave represents the increase in RA pressure from closure of the tricuspid valve.

10. **Correct answer: A**
    Exceptional and extreme mental stress, anger and resentment in a post-menopausal woman may cause Takosubo cardiomyopathy ("broken heart" syndrome). Excessive catecholamine release may stun or completely exhaust the mid-section and tip the heart. Troponin and creatinine kinase levels are only very slightly elevated. EKG changes may show initial ST elevation and short QT. For a few days the QT may be prolonged with large, deep negative T waves. Recovery may take weeks and show a flipped T wave and normal QT. Treatment is via supportive care relief of stress.

11. **Correct answer: B**
    A low CVP reading may represent increased contractility. The heart is able to eject its contents more easily, reducing the pressure in the right atrium.

12. **Correct answer: C**
    Right ventricular preload in the heart is measured by the central venous pressure (CVP). The normal range for a CVP is 2–8 mmHg. The CVP is also known as the right atrial pressure (RAP).

13. **Correct answer: C**
    Prinzmetal's angina is also known as variant angina and is usually caused by a coronary vasospasm. It may occur at rest, long after exercise, or during sleep.

14. **Correct Answer: B**
    The S in the PQRST pain assessment algorithm stands for Severity.
    The PQRST pain assessment method is used to collect assessment data regarding chest pain in a logical manner that ensures complete assessment data is gathered.

    - The P in the acronym stands for "provokes." Does any activity specifically provoke the pain?
    - Q represents the "quality of the pain." Typical adjectives used include sharp, stabbing, squeezing, pressure, tightness, dull, indigestion-like, and pulsating.
    - R is "radiation," meaning that pain starts at one location and ends at another location. For example, pain may radiate from the chest to the jaw, a specific arm, the back, and/or abdomen.

- S stands for "severity of the pain." Some patients may have altered pain sensation from other disease processes such as diabetes, neuropathies, and multiple scleroses and may not present with typical symptoms for a myocardial infarction.
- T stands for "time." The duration of the pain is important when considering antithrombolytics as treatment, because this is highly time sensitive and will impact success of the treatment.

15. **Correct answer: B**
    The normal range for a serum amiodarone level is 1 to 2.5 mcg/ml.

16. **Correct answer: B**
    STEMI and NSTEMI are both myocardial infarctions. The essential fact is that the NSTEMI does not have ST elevation on the EKG tracing and is identified by the cardiac enzymes. The STEMI diagnosis is based on symptoms, clinical examination, and the EKG tracing. Treatment is not delayed for the patient presenting with STEMI.

17. **Correct answer: B**
    A 1-mm ST elevation, with or without a pathologic Q wave, is diagnostic for STEMI. A large R wave in lead V_1 or V_2 may indicate a posterior wall MI. An NSTEMI has no ST elevation and must have cardiac enzymes for diagnosis.

18. **Correct answer: B**
    Calcium channel blockers act primarily on arteriolar tissue. Large lumen vessels in the arterial system are affected. The advantage of this action is that both systolic and diastolic pressures are reduced and the patient will not have a drop in blood pressure. The blood pressure may be lowered slightly and cause a reflex baroreceptor response to speed up the heart rate to maintain cardiac output.

19. **Correct answer: A**
    Decreased preload may result from hyperthermia (vasodilation), diuresis, hemorrhage, surgery, vomiting, and diarrhea. Any condition(s) that may result in a loss of fluid within the intravascular space will decrease preload.

20. **Correct answer: A**
    The vasodilatory action of nitrates will decrease afterload.

21. **Correct answer: C**
    The most sensitive cardiac markers are Troponin T and troponin I. These biomarkers show injury to myocytes, not just cell death. Troponin T can be elevated with skeletal muscle injury. Troponin I is diagnostic of an MI and can be falsely elevated in renal insufficiency.

22. **Correct answer: D**
    If your patient has a CK-MB concentration greater than 5% of the total CK, this finding is indicative of myocardial necrosis.

23. **Correct answer: A**
    Brain natriuretic peptide (BNP) is released when the myocardium is stretched. BNP is a substance secreted from the ventricles in response to changes in pressure that occur when heart failure develops and worsens. False high levels tend to be found in females, the elderly, patients with hypertension, and patients who take nesiritide. False low levels can occur in obese patients because the BNP collects in adipose tissue and clears slowly.

BNP levels below 100 pg/mL indicate no heart failure
BNP levels of 100–300 pg/mL suggest heart failure
BNP levels above 300 pg/mL indicate mild heart failure
BNP levels above 600 pg/mL indicate moderate heart failure
BNP levels above 900 pg/mL indicate severe heart failure

Please note that the BNP levels are measured in picograms (pg), not milligrams (mg). A picogram is one billionth of a milligram or one trillionth of a gram.

24. **Correct answer: B**
A biomarker that is not cardiac specific but can be elevated by falls, cardiopulmonary resuscitation, and injections is myoglobin. Serum myoglobin is a test that measures the amount of myoglobin in the blood. Myoglobin is a protein in heart and skeletal muscles. Muscles use up available oxygen. Myoglobin has oxygen attached to it, so additional O_2 is available to muscles. If the muscle is damaged, myoglobin is released and excreted by the kidneys. In large amounts, kidney damage may occur. If the patient has suffered an infarct, myoglobin levels peak about 8 hours after infarct, rapidly returning to normal in about 18–24 hours.

25. **Correct answer: C**
For a patient with atrial fibrillation, a therapeutic range for INR would be 2.0–3.0. For prosthetic valves, the therapeutic range would be 2.5–3.5.

26. **Correct answer: A**
A biomarker that indicates an inflammation is present is C-reactive protein. C-reactive protein is produced by the liver. Blood is mixed with an antiserum which attaches to a specific protein. Levels of CRP may not be increased in people with rheumatoid arthritis and lupus. Some additional causes of elevated C-reactive protein levels are: cancer, connective tissue disease, inflammatory bowel disease, rheumatic fever, tuberculosis, the last half of pregnancy or with the use of oral contraceptives, and possible uremia.

27. **Correct answer: B**
If you auscultate a blowing, high-pitched murmur at the apex and it appears to radiate to the left axilla, this murmur is probably indicative of mitral insufficiency or regurgitation.

28. **Correct answer: C**
A cardiac murmur that has maximal intensity at the base of the heart (commonly at the second intercostal space, right sternal border) and radiates to the apex and neck is the murmur of aortic stenosis.

29. **Correct answer: D**
An early diastolic murmur with maximal intensity at the fourth intercostal space, left sternal border, is a murmur of tricuspid stenosis.

30. **Correct answer: B**
The following statement is true about angina: Troponins and CK-MB isoenzymes are not elevated in patients with stable angina. These biomarkers are also not elevated in unstable angina.

31. **Correct answer: B**
The S_2 heart sound is created by closure of the pulmonic and aortic valves. S_2 is best heard in the upper left sternal border or pulmonic area.

32. **Correct answer: B**
Chlorothiazide reduces urinary calcium losses and does not result in profound potassium losses.

33. **Correct answer: D**
The primary use of nesiritide (Natrecor) would be to cause vascular smooth muscle vasodilation. It is a b-type natriuretic peptide that stimulates cGMP production. Like ATP, cGMP is used to increase more specialized cellular energy conversion, resulting in smooth muscle relaxation.

34. **Correct answer: B**
Rate, rhythm, axis, hypertrophy, and infarction are the most valuable areas examined in a 12-lead EKG.

35. **Correct answer: C**
Muscle aches, muscle weakness, and fatigue are findings associated with drug-induced hyperthyroidism associated with amiodarone administration. T3 and T4 levels should be checked. Additional labs expected to be ordered would include serum amiodarone levels, CBC, LFT, and coagulation studies. Amiodarone toxicity may lead to agranulocytosis, anemia, neutropenia, pancytopenia, and liver injury resulting in increased bleeding disorders

36. **Correct answer: C**
ST elevation in EKG leads V_1-V_3, syncopal episodes and a RBBB may indicate Brugada syndrome. This is a genetic disease found equally in boys and girls, but more prevalent in young men. The heart is structurally normal, as can be the EKG when tested. Patients may develop polymorphic ventricular tachycardia (without a prolonged QT) or other ventricular arrhythmias. Patients have syncopal episodes if the episode is brief or cardiac arrest if the episode is sustained. Fever and some medications may increase the incidence. Specific drugs used to initiate symptoms and diagnose Brugada are flecainide, ajmaline, and procainamide. The only treatment is use of an AICD.

37. **Correct answer: C**
Pulsus alternans occurs in left ventricular failure when a weakened myocardium cannot maintain an even pressure with each contraction. The pulses alternate between strong and weak. This condition is also seen in CHF.

38. **Correct answer: A**
When the parasympathetic and sympathetic nervous systems stimulate the right vagus nerve, the SA node is affected and slows the heart rate. Acetylcholine is a neurotransmitter.

39. **Correct answer: A**
Cyanosis may be observed when at least 5 g/100 ml of deoxygenated hemoglobin is present in circulation.

40. **Correct answer: B**
On an EKG, left-sided heart failure results in wide, notched P waves. A tall, peaked P wave is indicative of right-sided heart failure. Changes in ST segments (or T waves) usually indicate myocardial ischemia.

41. **Correct answer: C**
Rheumatic fever remains the most common cause of acquired valvular disease. The valves are a perfect place for bacteria to colonize, and the blood is a perfect medium for bacterial growth. The causative organism is beta-hemolytic streptococcus.

42. **Correct answer: D**
Initial dosing of Levophed begins at 0.5 to 1 mcg/min. Levophed has a rapid onset with a duration of 1–2 min. At doses <2 mcg/min, Levophed causes positive inotropic and chronotropic effects. Once dosing is >4 mcg/min, arterial and venous vessels constrict, leading to increased blood pressure. Although usual maintenance dosing is 2 to 12 mcg/min, dosing may be titrated up to a maximum of 30 mcg/min to maintain blood pressure.

43. **Correct answer: C**
Hyperpyrexia is a potential life-threatening adverse reaction if Levophed is administered with medications classified as MAO inhibitors. Concurrent alpha blocker administration leads to decreased vasopressor effects. Beta-blocker administration may lead to decreased effects of both drugs. Levophed administration with nitrates will also lead to decreased effects of both drugs.

44. **Correct answer: A**
Regitine is kept at the bedside of patients on IV norepinephrine and dopamine in case IV extravasation occurs. The Regitine causes vasodilation in tissues to correct and prevent necrosis and sloughing. The solution should be used immediately. Never store the unused portion. In case of extravasation, multiple injections should be given around the IV site and other vascular access obtained. Some facilities do not allow nurses to administer Regitine, so please check policies and procedures for your specific facility.

45. **Correct answer: A**
Lidocaine infusion may cause respiratory arrest. A respiratory rate of 7 indicates impending failure and immediate action is required to provide respiratory support via a resuscitation bag, and staff should prepare for intubation. The infusion should be stopped if respiratory failure occurs, if a widening QRS is noted, or the heart rate drops below 60. The infusion must also be stopped if the patient becomes hypotensive, has difficulty speaking, or experiences numbness and tingling.

46. **Correct answer: D**
Rapid infusion of Lasix can cause ototoxicity and result in tinnitus and hearing loss.

47. **Correct answer: A**
Amiodarone may affect the pacing threshold of implanted cardiac defibrillators, thus the pacing settings should be verified prior and during amiodarone administration. Anisindione is an anticoagulant and administration is contraindicated for a patient with an invasive device such as an implanted cardiac defibrillator.

48. **Correct answer: C**
Symptoms of right-sided heart failure include hepatomegaly. When the right side of the heart fails it is often due to left-sided failure. The right ventricle cannot adequately pump blood out, so filling pressures rise and the blood backs up, resulting in the hepatomegaly. Thus, the CVP and RV pressures are elevated. Additional symptoms can include splenomegaly, ascites, abdominal pain, S_3, S_4, and weight gain.

49. **Correct answer: B**
A common cause of restrictive cardiomyopathy is glycogen storage disease. Amyloidosis is an additional cause of restrictive cardiomyopathy. The myocardium (especially the left ventricle) becomes rigid from fibrosis. This results in inadequate left ventricular filling and increased atrial dilatation. Left ventricular diastolic dysfunction occurs.

Systolic function remains normal in this type of cardiomyopathy. Fluid backs up into the lungs and the patient looks like they have congestive heart failure. There is no cure, and symptoms are treated as they occur.

50. **Correct answer: B**
Signs of CNS toxicity from lidocaine may include agitation, vomiting, drowsiness, and muscle twitching. Later signs may include loss of consciousness, seizures, respiratory depression, and apnea. Cardiac toxicity may develop and cause hypotension, bradycardia, heart block, and may lead to cardiovascular collapse.

51. **Correct answer: B**
Leads II, III, and aVF show damage to the inferior wall of the heart. Leads I and aVL show damage to the higher areas of the lateral wall. V_1 and V_2 show septal wall damage. V_5 and V_6 show damage to the apical area.

52. **Correct answer: A**
Many foods should be avoided when taking warfarin. Those highest in vitamin K (the antagonist to warfarin) are broccoli, Brussels sprouts, cabbage, spinach, turnip greens, endive, scallions, and parsley. Additional foods to be avoided are red leaf lettuce, watercress, oils such as soybean and canola, and salads in general. All these foods decrease the effectiveness of warfarin.

53. **Correct answer: A**
This question is a slightly different way of asking about the symptoms of right heart failure. It is imperative that students are very familiar with symptoms of both right and left heart failure. Right-sided heart failure signs and symptoms include respiratory distress and hepatomegaly. The respiratory distress is the result of blood's failure to flow to the lungs, causing hypoxemia. As blood backs up into the hepatic system, hepatomegaly and splenomegaly may result.

54. **Correct answer: A**
Polycythemia increases afterload due to the excess circulation of red blood cells. Hypovolemia and sepsis decrease afterload, as does aortic insufficiency. Aortic stenosis increases afterload, as do peripheral vasoconstriction and hypertension.

55. **Correct answer: B**
Early signs of left ventricular failure are tachypnea and tachycardia. Severe left ventricular failure also causes dyspnea.

56. **Correct answer: D**
The third heart sound, S_3, occurs when increased blood flow travels across the AV valves secondary to rapid passive ventricular filling from the atria. This is easy to remember if you associate the S_3 sound with fluid. It is prominent in CHF, mitral valve insufficiency, anemia, and left-to-right shunts like ASD and VSD

57. **Correct answer: D**
Leads V_2–V_4 indicate damage to the anterior wall of the heart. Leads V_4 and R indicate right ventricular damage. V_5 and V_6 indicate apical injury. Leads V_7–V_9 are specific to the posterior wall.

58. **Correct answer: B**
The pulmonic valve is rarely affected by infective endocarditis. The mitral valve is the most common site affected by infective endocarditis. The aortic valve is the next most

common valve affected. The tricuspid valve is often involved secondarily as a result of IV drug abuse.

59. **Correct answer: B**
Patients receiving sodium nitroprusside should be monitored for cyanide toxicity, and use of sodium nitroprusside should be avoided in patients with renal problems. Cyanide toxicity may result in tachycardia and severe hypotension. Monitor venous O_2 concentration and acid–base balance. If nitroprusside extravasates from an IV, it will cause tissue sloughing and necrosis. The RBC cyanide level should be less than 50 mcg/ml.

60. **Correct answer: C**
Myocarditis is clinically defined as inflammation of the myocardium. Coxsackie B1 virus has been more prevalent as a frequent cause of myocarditis. Numerous infections, systemic diseases, drugs, and toxins are associated with the development of myocarditis. Viruses, bacteria, protozoa, and even worms have been implicated as infectious agents. The absolute band count is not sensitive enough to predict sepsis, but a ratio of immature-to-total polymorphonuclear leukocytes <0.2 has a very high negative predictive value.

61. **Correct answer: C**
When starting dopamine, it is important to ensure that hypovolemia has been treated appropriately. In septic shock, the patient may receive as many as 3 to 10 fluid boluses until pulmonary edema is noted or the boluses fail to impact blood pressure. Central venous access is the preferred route. If central access is unavailable, peripheral access is acceptable. However, the site must be monitored closely for infiltration and additional IV access points must be available. Phentolamine mesylate should be available in case infiltration does occur, but it is not the first action to be performed.

62. **Correct answer: D**
First, it is unlikely that a nurse in a progressive care unit would be aggressively titrating a dopamine drip. However, a few PCUs are titrating to this level. We just wanted you to know more about dopamine and rates of titration so in case a question would appear on the test, you would answer it correctly. Dopamine should not be titrated any faster than every 5 minutes because onset of action is 5 minutes and duration is 10 minutes. Titrating more frequently than every 5 minutes may result in greater hemodynamic instability and more difficulty in determining the effective dosage.

63. **Correct answer: C**
Discharge instructions for a patient prescribed amiodarone include avoiding grapefruit and grapefruit juice because they increase blood amiodarone levels. Outside activities should include restricting contact sports and require use of sunscreen and clothing to protect the skin from exposure to sunlight. Amiodarone may impair liver function and lead to thrombocytopenia. Sunlight exposure may lead to a bluish-gray cast to the skin. If the patient normally uses theophylline to treat asthma, the dosage may need to be decreased as amiodarone increases serum theophylline levels. However, in this case, nothing was mentioned about this patient having asthma. Dark urine, respiratory distress, and/or edema should be reported immediately to the physician, as these are signs of renal and pulmonary impairment.

64. **Correct answer: B**
This patient has dilated cardiomyopathy that is causing systolic dysfunction. Patients with this type of cardiomyopathy will have S_3 and S_4 gallops, and the EKG may show

atrial fibrillation, ventricular dysrhythmias, or a sinus tachycardia most of the time. The patient may have a systolic murmur of the AV valves. The patient will probably also have peripheral edema or ascites, hepatomegaly, and pale, cool extremities. It is possible to have changes in mentation. Hypertrophic and restrictive cardiomyopathies are diastolic dysfunctions.

65. **Correct answer: D**
Dobutamine improves cardiac output primarily by increasing cardiac contractility. Unlike dopamine, dobutamine does not increase heart rate and can be used in tachycardic patients.

66. **Correct answer: D**
Atropine administration may result in headaches, dizziness, and coma. You should also observe for urinary retention and hypotension and tachycardia due to blocking of parasympathetic receptor sites.

67. **Correct answer: B**
The PCU nurse should monitor closely the urine output and liver function tests of a patient receiving a loading dose of amiodarone. The high concentration of amiodarone may cause renal necrosis and impaired output leading to vascular congestion and respiratory distress. Amiodarone has been linked to hepatocellular damage and impaired liver function. Other side effects include anemia, neutropenia, pancytopenia, and thrombocytopenia. Thyroid levels should also be monitored because amiodarone may cause hypo-or hyperthyroidism. Amiodarone has been linked to bluish-gray pigmentation in long-term patients exposed to sunlight.

68. **Correct answer: A**
Patients taking both diazoxide and furosemide should have their glucose levels monitored closely for possible hyperglycemia. Diazoxide inhibits pancreatic release of insulin and stimulates the liver to release glucose.

69. **Correct answer: B**
The high-contrast mediums used in cardiac catheterizations may cause or contribute to hypernatremia due to their high sodium content.

70. **Correct answer: B**
The classic description of an X-ray showing a pericardial effusion is the "water bottle" silhouette. In patients with a pericardial effusion, QRS amplitude is decreased. Diastolic filling is decreased as well.

71. **Correct answer: A**
Dong quai, gingko biloba, and ginseng can increase bleeding times and should be avoided while taking anticoagulants. Saw palmetto decreases the effectiveness of Plavix.

72. **Correct answer: D**
Cardiac glycosides possess positive inotropic activity, which is mediated by inhibition of sodium-potassium adenosine triphosphatase. Also, cardiac glycosides reduce conductivity in the heart, particularly through the atrioventricular node, and therefore have a negative chronotropic effect. The cardiac glycosides have very similar pharmacologic effects but differ considerably in their speed of onset and duration of action. They are used to slow the heart rate in supraventricular arrhythmias, especially atrial fibrillation, and also are used in patients with chronic heart failure.

73. **Correct answer: B**
The high iodine content of amiodarone can actually exert an effect on the thyroid and produce an antiarrhythmic action. It is always a good idea to ask if the patient has an allergy or sensitivity to iodine prior to administering this medication.

74. **Correct answer: B**
By definition, pansystolic means the murmur is heard throughout systole. The only systolic murmur listed is tricuspid insufficiency. All the others are diastolic murmurs.

75. **Correct answer: B**
A reflex tachycardia caused by stretch of right atrial receptors is known as the Bainbridge reflex. It is believed that the Bainbridge reflex exists to speed up the heart rate if the right side becomes overloaded and helps equalize pressures in both sides.

76. **Correct answer: D**
Adenosine is used for the suppression/elimination of sustained supraventricular tachycardia. It can also be used in diagnostic studies to establish the cause of the SVT. Adverse effects may include transient arrhythmias, flushing, dyspnea, and, rarely, apnea. It is important to note that in approximately 30% of patients, SVT recurs. Caffeine and theophylline act by competitive antagonism to diminish the effect of adenosine.

77. **Correct answer: D**
The left ventricular assist device (LVAD) is the most commonly used because left heart failure is more common and usually precedes right ventricular failure.

78. **Correct answer: B**
Ventricular assist devices (VAD) are used as destination therapy as well as a bridge to transplant. Prolonged cardiac arrest, especially with neurologic damage, is a contraindication to use of a VAD. Extensive organ damage is another contraindication. VADs are not indicated for dysrhythmias. Other indications for a VAD include cardiogenic shock and inability to wean from cardiopulmonary bypass. Always be aware of the possibility of device failure.

79. **Correct answer: D**
The fourth heart sound, S_4, is always pathologic after the first 24 hours of life and indicates a decreased ventricular compliance. The S_4 is produced when an atrial contraction fills up the ventricle. S_4 is rarely heard in the newborn and occurs just before the S_1 heart sound. During the first 24 hours of life, the S_4 may be heard just after the first heart sound and sounds like a clicking noise.

80. **Correct answer: A**
It is important to explain that this patient needs a pacemaker or AICD that can deliver a more powerful impulse when needed (demand). The asynchronous mode will override her internal pacemaker.

81. **Correct answer: A**
This patient's pulse is very irregular and he is complaining of getting "zapped" often. The patient says he is exhausted from the repeated shocks and asks for pain medication. His EKG shows sinus bradycardia with numerous pacemaker spikes. The AICD has a faulty lead; a lead was probably dislodged or the lead was damaged on insertion. Either way, he needs a new AICD or new leads.

82. **Correct answer: A**
Pacemaker syndrome is due to a loss of atrial kick or regurgitation against a closed A-V valve. Fatigue, agitation, and forgetfulness are primary symptoms of this condition. It would be possible this patient's atrial lead was damaged or has failed.

83. **Correct answer: C**
Pneumonia secondary to immobility is the primary reason for infection with VADs. Some type of ventilatory support may also be needed. Just the fact that tubes are placed into the body is a potential source of infection, but this is usually minimized by good hand washing and aseptic technique. Newer VADs are smaller and lighter, enabling the patient more mobility, but pneumonia continues to be the most common infection noted.

84. **Correct answer: C**
Patients who have aortic insufficiency often exhibit Quincke's sign. This sign is elicited by pressing upward from underneath the nail bed on the fingertip. A visible pulsation is seen in the nail bed. This results from a pulse with a rapid initial hard pulsation followed by a sudden collapse as blood flows back through an incompetent valve.

85. **Correct answer: C**
In a patient with a cardiac tamponade, stroke volume decreases. Because the heart cannot adequately fill or eject its contents adequately, stroke volume decreases and causes a decreased cardiac output. Contractility decreases because the muscle cannot adequately stretch and contract effectively.

86. **Correct answer: D**
Beck's triad consists of distended neck veins, muffled heart sounds, and hypotension. In tamponade, tachycardia is an early sign. A narrowed pulse pressure occurs; fluid cannot be ejected from the heart. The muffled heart sounds occur because the fluid in the sac minimizes the transmission of sound waves.

87. **Correct answer: B**
Phentolamine (Regitine) 1 mg/ml solution should be injected into the affected area if dopamine infiltrates. It may take as much as 5 ml to treat the area.

88. **Correct answer: A**
A dilated superior vena cava would appear on X-ray if a patient had a cardiac tamponade. The vena cava is dilated because blood cannot empty into the right atrium. The mediastinum would be widened. A CXR will not show delineation of the pericardium or epicardium. A pneumothorax may exist, but would not be an expected finding on X-ray.

89. **Correct answer: B**
Early signs of left ventricular failure are tachypnea and tachycardia. Severe left ventricular failure also causes dyspnea and retractions.

90. **Correct answer: B**
A popliteal blood pressure at least 40 mmHg higher than a brachial blood pressure is known as Hill's sign. Hill's sign reflects the rapid rise in pulsation found in patients with aortic insufficiency. DeMusset's sign is also found in aortic insufficiency (the bobbing of the head in time with the forceful pulse).

91. **Correct answer: B**
This patient is probably suffering from pericarditis. The CXR will probably show a pericardial effusion. The elevated sed. rate and WBCs indicate infection. In pericarditis, leaning forward often relieves chest pain and laying supine makes it worse. If the pain worsens on inspiration, it is because the lungs expand and come in contact with the pericardium. The patient will probably also have a fever. One of the things to monitor is any sign of a cardiac tamponade and to make certain anticoagulants are discontinued.

92. **Correct answer: A**
The purpose of treating a patient who has CHF with vasoactive and inotropic medications is to decrease the workload of the heart by vasodilation (reduce preload and afterload) and improve contractility. These medications will decrease preload and afterload and increase contractility.

93. **Correct answer: D**
Your next priority is to defibrillate the patient with 200 Joules with a biphasic defibrillator.

94. **Correct answer: B**
Digoxin is classified as both a negative chronotrope and a positive inotrope.

95. **Correct answer: C**
Pacemaker spikes are not followed by p waves. The pacemaker is not capturing. The first thing the nurse should do is increase the milliamperes. The nurse should also check the pacemaker connections and try turning the patient on the side if tolerated.

96. **Correct answer: B**
Type I aneurysms are the most common type of aortic aneurysms. Tears begin in the ascending aorta, and the dissection extends beyond the aortic arch.

97. **Correct answer: D**
A type III aneurysm involves a tear in the descending aorta, with distal dissection only. They are not the rarest form of aneurysm, occurring in 20–30% of cases.

98. **Correct answer: C**
A risk factor for an aortic aneurysm would not include hypotension. Risk factors include connective tissue disorders, medial necrosis of the aorta, coarctation of the aorta, blunt chest trauma, pregnancy, family history of aortic aneurysm, and hypertension.

99. **Correct answer: B**
This patient most likely has an abdominal aortic aneurysm that could dissect at any moment. Make the patient comfortable with a minimum of movement and inform the physician immediately.

100. **Correct answer: C**
Avoid grapefruit when taking colchicine.

101. **Correct answer: D**
If a patient becomes tachycardic, the QT and the RR intervals shorten.

102. **Correct answer: A**
Bronchospasms are an adverse drug reaction to Plavix administration. Some asthmatics are prone to bronchospasms and should be advised to report an increase in frequency and/or severity while taking Plavix. Pneumonia is an adverse reaction to enoxaparin

sodium (Lovenox) administration. Apnea may be seen with fentanyl administration. Hemoptysis is an adverse reaction to prasugrel (Effient) administration.

103. Correct answer: B

The right ventricle infarction is often seen in the patient with an inferior wall MI and ST elevation in leads V_1 and V_2. A right side 12-lead EKG should be done to verify the right ventricular infarction.

104. Correct answer: C

Potassium and magnesium levels should be monitored closely for any patient on dofetilide. This drug blocks potassium channels to delay QT interval. Hypokalemia and hypomagnesemia may increase the risk of drug induced Torsade de pointes.

105. Correct answer: C

Headache and hallucinations are symptoms of an adverse reaction to clopidogrel bisulfate (Plavix). Additional CNS symptoms would include confusion, depression, dizziness, and fatigue. These findings should be reported to the physician immediately; Plavix administration should be discontinued and alternative anticoagulation therapy started. Aspirin, Angiomax, and Lovenox adverse reactions do not include hallucinations.

106. Correct answer: D

Dofetilide is contraindicated until amiodarone serum levels drop below 0.3 mcg/ml. Since amiodarone's half-life is around 60 days, probable recent administration during the patient's resuscitation would place the patient at risk for profoundly widened QT interval and risk for another cardiac event.

107. Correct answer: A

Upright QRS in leads V_1, and V_2 show right bundle branch blocks. A simple way to remember which type of bundle branch block with a QRS wider than 0.12 seconds is to think of the turn signals on your car. For a right turn you must push the lever up, for a left turn the lever must go down. So, looking at V_1 and V_2, if the QRS is upright, then there is a right bundle branch block. If V_1 and V_2 are downward in force, then it is a left bundle branch block.

108. Correct answer: A

Using ICHD nomenclature, the first V is the chamber paced.

Chamber Paced	**Chamber Sensed**	**Mode of Response**	**Programmability, Rate modulation**	**Antiatachy-arrhythmia Function**
V = Ventricle	V = Ventricle	I = Inhibit	P = Simple programmable	P = Pacing
A = Atrium	A = Atrium	T = Triggered	M = Multiprogrammable	S = Shock
D = Dual chamber	D = Dual chamber	D = Dual (T & I)	R = Rate modulation	Dual = Dual (P & S)

109. Correct answer: C

Using ICHD nomenclature, the second V is the chamber sensed.

110. Correct answer: B

Quinidine and hypomagnesemia can lead to Torsade de pointes (also known as polymorphic ventricular tachycardia), a recurrent ventricular tachycardia that turns on its axis every 6–8 beats, giving the EKG a twisting or "turning on point" look. Hypomagnesemia may occur when the patient receives total parenteral nutrition.

111. Correct answer: B

Esmolol is incompatible with furosemide. Furosemide administration requires alternative venous access or oral administration. Esmolol is compatible with cimetidine, penicillin, and midazolam.

112. Correct answer: B

The most common cause of idiopathic dilated cardiomyopathy is alcohol. Even though the exact causes are unknown, a large number of alcoholics develop dilated cardiomyopathy. Three possible reasons have been identified:

1. The alcohol itself, or the metabolites, have a toxic effect
2. Alcohol sometimes contains additives, such as cobalt
3. The cause may be nutritional in origin, such as a thiamine deficiency

New research shows a possible viral link to the chronic alcoholism.
It is interesting that this type of cardiomyopathy might reverse itself if the drinking is stopped. Other types of cardiomyopathy are not reversible.

113. Correct answer: D

The maximum daily dose of Ofirmev is 4,000 mg for a patient weighing >50 kg. Ofirmev is the parenteral form of acetaminophen. Dosing should be watched very closely to avoid toxic acetaminophen levels. For patients weighing <50 kg, dosing should be calculated at 12.5 mg/kg. Preparation of Ofirmev should not be diluted and should not be administered any faster than over 15 minutes. Caution patients not to take any over-the-counter (OTC) medications without speaking with his/her primary care physician first as many OTCs contain acetaminophen and may lead to toxic levels.

114. Correct answer: D

Congestive heart failure results in a systemic venous engorgement because blood does not flow forward and is allowed to pool in organs and peripheral circulation. Tissues become hypoxic and further diminish function until complete failure and death.

115. Correct answer: C

The type of cardiomyopathy characterized by replacement of normal cells by fatty tissue is known as arrhythmogenic cardiomyopathy. This is a relatively new classification of cardiomyopathy. The normal myocardial cells are replaced by fatty tissue and fibrous tissue. The right ventricle is primarily affected. Conduction cannot occur normally, and the patient will have multiple ventricular arrhythmias and right ventricular failure. Young people are at risk for sudden death. The cause of this condition is unknown, but some research has shown a possible link to an autosomal dominant gene.

116. Correct answer: B

Leads V_2, V_3, V_4, I, and AVL are indicative of an anterolateral MI. The MI could also include V_5, and V_6, which are also lateral leads.

117. Correct answer: A
Life-threatening side effects of propranolol include laryngospasms and bronchospasms in addition to bradycardia, bone marrow suppression, and hypotension. Complete heart block and dizziness are side effects of propaferone (Rythmol). Lidocaine may cause respiratory depression and cardiovascular collapse. Polymorphic VT and dyspnea are life-threatening side effects of sotalol (Betapace).

118. Correct answer: C
Regurgitation systolic murmurs are associated with VSD, tricuspid regurgitation, and mitral valve regurgitation. Regurgitation systolic murmurs are caused by blood flow from an area of higher pressure throughout systole to an area of lower pressure.

119. Correct answer: D
When administering nitroglycerin, it is important to have normal saline or other volume expander at bedside in case of vascular collapse. The potential collapse is related to peripheral venous and arterial dilation (relative hypovolemia). Only non-polyvinyl chloride tubing may be used for infusion because PVC may be absorbed by the nitroglycerin. Filtration is not required before infusion. Nitroglycerin is only compatible with D5W, normal saline, lactated ringers, D5NS, and half normal saline for infusion.

120. Correct answer: B
Abnormal Q waves on an EKG signify a complete thickness infarction of myocardium. When the tissue dies due to myocardial infarction, it becomes electrically dead, causing the opposing energy to become the dominant feature. Partial thickness myocardial death would be a non-Q wave MI.

121. Correct answer: D
The most common new-onset dysrhythmia seen in a patient with a diagnosis of pulmonary edema is atrial fibrillation. Atrial fibrillation is the result of the constant stretching and disruption of normal pathways in the atrium due to increased preload from the pulmonary congestion.

122. Correct answer: B
There are multiple reasons for pacemaker insertion, including symptomatic bradycardia, bradycardia with escape beats, overdrive pacing, bradycardia/arrest, and acute MI with sinus dysfunction. In addition, Mobitz type II, complete heart block, and development of a new bundle branch block are reasons for pacemaker insertion.

123. Correct answer: C
Right ventricular afterload may be reduced by inhaled nitric oxide. Use of inhaled nitric oxide, nitroglycerin, nitroprusside, PGE1, or hyperventilation reduces right ventricular afterload. Epinephrine increases systemic afterload due to vasoconstriction and promotes increased PVR because of the increased left heart pressures. Hypoventilation and subsequent hypoxia also increase right heart afterload.

124. Correct answer: A
Mr. C. has endocarditis. Janeway lesions are flat and painless erythematous areas found predominantly on palms and soles of the feet. Osler's nodes are small, painful nodules also associated with endocarditis and found on fingers and toes. Roth spots are seen when examining the retina. They are rounded and white and associated with endocarditis. It is thought that microvascular clots form in the heart and pass through the

microcirculation and impede peripheral circulation, sometimes causing necrosis. Pella's sign is not a medical term.

125. **Correct answer: D**
The only definitive way to diagnose myocarditis is via an endomyocardial biopsy.

126. **Correct answer: D**
Procainamide's adverse effects include severe hypotension (usually because of a rapid infusion) and A-V block. Procainamide may also widen the QRS complex due to slow impulse conduction through the Purkinje fibers and ventricular myocardium. If the QRS widens more than 35–50%, the drug should be discontinued. Adverse effects usually disappear when the drug is discontinued. Two of the actions of procainamide are depression of the excitability of cardiac muscle and slowing the conduction in the atria.

127. **Correct answer: A**
The antagonist for morphine or other opioids is Narcan (naloxone). Generally, the naloxone dose is 0.4 mg IV. This dose can be repeated about every 3 to 4 minutes three times. When giving Narcan, you must always be alert for the patient to relapse once the dose wears off. Administering multiple follow-up doses is not uncommon.

128. **Correct answer: B**
This patient has dilated cardiomyopathy that is causing systolic dysfunction. Patients with this type of cardiomyopathy will have S_3 and S_4 gallops, and the EKG may show atrial fibrillation, ventricular dysrhythmias, or a sinus tachycardia most of the time. The patient may have a systolic murmur of the AV valves. The patient will probably also have peripheral edema or ascites, hepatomegaly, and pale, cool extremities. It is possible to have changes in mentation. Hypertrophic and restrictive cardiomyopathies are diastolic dysfunctions.

129. **Correct answer: A**
Motion of cardiac valves and detection of pericardial fluid is done with M-mode echocardiography. M-mode echocardiography enables evaluation of anatomic relationships and the relative sizes of each.

130. **Correct answer: B**
The type of echocardiography that shows the quantity of flow across an obstruction is known as continuous-wave Doppler echocardiography. This type of echocardiography is used to detect direction of shunting, estimating cardiac output, and assessing ventricular diastolic function. This type of echocardiography provides a good estimate of pressure gradients.

131. **Correct answer: C**
Dobutamine is used to improve cardiac output by acting on beta1 adrenergic receptors in the heart. It may cause minimal peripheral vasodilation but primarily acts to increase contractility, coronary blood flow, and heart rate to improve cardiac output. Dopamine acts on alpha-adrenergic receptors in the heart. Norepinephrine is a catecholamine that acts on both alpha-and beta-adrenergic receptors in the cardiovascular tissue.

132. **Correct answer: B**
Alpha-adrenergic effects of norepinephrine include peripheral arteriolar vasoconstriction. Increased force of myocardial contraction and increased AV conduction time are the effects of beta adrenergic sympathetic stimulation.

133. **Correct answer: A**
Epinephrine 1:1,000 is kept at the bedside of a patient beginning lisinopril administration should the patient exhibit angioedema. Angioedema of the face, glottis, larynx, and tongue may lead to upper airway obstruction. Treatment with 0.3–0.5 ml of epinephrine 1:1,000 SQ is used to treat the anaphylactic reaction.

134. **Correct answer: A**
Nifedipine is a calcium channel blocker.

135. **Correct answer: C**
It is important that adenosine be given rapidly because if adenosine is given slowly, it may cause systemic vasodilation and reflex tachycardia, further compromising cardiac output. Blurred vision is an expected adverse reaction. The patient should be monitored for development of atrial fibrillation, bradycardia, and heart blocks. Withhold adenosine if the patient is in atrial fibrillation, atrial flutter, and second-degree type II or complete heart block. Adenosine slows conduction via the AV node, and these rhythms may degrade to ventricular fibrillation

136. **Correct answer: D**
A heart murmur associated with acute valvular regurgitation is called S_4. S_1 and S_2 are normal sounds. S_3 is associated with fluid status. S_4 is associated with ventricular compliance.

137. **Correct answer: B**
Radio-frequency waves destroy myocardial tissue with heat. These waves actually heat the tissue around the active sites and prevent reentry looping. Once the temperature reaches 50° C, cell damage and death occur. The continuing heat creates a lesion about 2–5 mm in diameter. This "burned" area causes necrosis and will not conduct electricity.

138. **Correct answer: D**
A high CVP reading may indicate LV, RV or biventricular failure, tricuspid regurgitation or stenosis, hypertension, hypervolemia, or cardiac tamponade. A low CVP reading may represent increased contractility or hypovolemia.

139. **Correct answer: A**
New-onset atrial fibrillation frequently develops as sequelae to pulmonary edema.

140. **Correct answer: A**
Hydralazine is incompatible with furosemide, phenobarbital, aminophylline, and ampicillin. Hydralazine is compatible with heparin, dobutamine, hydrocortisone, potassium chloride, prostaglandin E1, and Dex/AA.

141. **Correct answer: B**
Nesiritide is an appropriate drug for heart patients with acute decompensated congestive heart failure. The action of nesiritide is to cause arterial and venous smooth muscle relaxation to decrease cardiac afterload. This relieves pulmonary congestion and cardiac workload. Constrictive pericarditis, obstructive cardiomyopathy, and pericardial tamponade are all examples of preload dependent heart diseases and nesiritide should never be administered. The dilative effects of nesiritide would diminish venous blood to the heart, worsening cardiac function.

142. **Correct answer: B**
Dofetilide (Tikosyn) should not be administered to any patient with a prolonged QT interval. Since Tikosyn blocks potassium channels to widen the QT interval, preexisting prolonged QT syndrome and could develop into life-threatening arrhythmias.

143. **Correct answer: A**
Tikosyn is the brand name for dofetilide, a methanesulfonanilide used as an antiarrhythmic to specifically treat atrial fibrillation. Mexiletine hydrochloride is also known as Mexitil, a lidocaide analogue administered for ventricular arrhythmias. Sotalol is more commonly known as Betapace and is also used to treat ventricular arrhythmias. Flecainide, Tambocar, is used to treat ventricular tachycardia.

144. **Correct answer: C**
Under the new 2010 American Heart Association guidelines for chest compressions, the rescuer should compress the sternum of an adult to a depth of 2 inches.

145. **Correct answer: B**
The sequence for adults receiving basic life support is CAB. The 2010 American Heart Association Guidelines for CPR and Emergency Cardiovascular Care have changed the BLS sequence to compressions, airway, and breathing.

146. **Correct answer: A**
The 2010 American Heart Association Guidelines for CPR and Emergency Cardiovascular Care do not recommend routine use of cricoid pressure during cardiac arrest. There is some evidence that the use of cricoid pressure impedes the airway when performed incorrectly.

147. **Correct answer: D**
Continuous wave capnography is the most reliable method of confirming and monitoring correct placement of an ETT. Capnography can monitor the effectiveness of chest compressions and detect the return of spontaneous circulation. Use of capnography is a recommendation of the 2010 American Heart Association Guidelines for CPR and Emergency Cardiovascular Care.

148. **Correct answer: D**
According to the 2010 American Heart Association Guidelines for CPR and Emergency Cardiovascular Care, high quality CPR is the single most important component of a successful outcome for a patient requiring advanced cardiac life support.

149. **Correct answer: C**
According to the 2010 American Heart Association Guidelines for CPR and Emergency Cardiovascular Care, atropine is no longer recommended for routine use in the management of PEA or asystole.

150. **Correct answer: C**
If an adult post cardiac arrest patient is treated with therapeutic hypothermia, the patient should be evaluated via neurologic signs, biomarkers, electrophysiologic studies, and imaging where available at 72 hours (3 days) after cardiac arrest.

151. **Correct answer: A**
There is no evidence that water acts as an obstructive foreign body, so it is not necessary to try and remove it prior to proceeding with BLS. The new BLS starts with

compressions, not airway. CPR cannot be performed effectively in water because compressions require a firm surface. Actually, spinal cord injuries are not common among drowning victims.

152. Correct answer: C
The right side 12-lead EKG looks at the right ventricle and the posterior heart. Some facilities have the capability of performing 16-lead EKGs, which look at the entire heart without having to move the precordial leads. This complete view of the heart's vasculature status allows for pinpointing the site of the myocardial infarction.

153. Correct answer: B
Although the patient may want to be compliant with his plan of care, financial limitations may prohibit him from receiving expensive treatments, medications, and support services. If the patient is to start an antiplatelet medication, request from the physician that over-the-counter medications be considered before the use of more expensive brand-name drugs if the patient cannot afford to continue drugs that are started while he is in the hospital. The patient may be better able to afford and continue "baby aspirin" therapy versus Plavix. If brand-name and generic drugs are required, attempt to contact the drug manufacturer and ask about discounts or special programs for low-income patients. Home visits would be paid for by the patient. Follow-up phone calls by the unit staff or case management may prove cost-effective in verifying patient compliance and in answering any questions that the patient has. A cardiology appointment would likely be scheduled earlier than 3 months after discharge to ensure that the patient's plan of care is effective and appropriate for his needs. Although exercise is beneficial, the cost of a gym membership might be prohibitive. Instead, suggest starting a walking club with other friends or neighbors to slowly increase activity while limiting costs. The companionship will improve the patient's physical, psychological, and social health.

154. Correct answer: D
The exercise stress test requires that the patient walk on a treadmill or ride a stationary bike for at least 30 to 60 minutes. For this patient, that level of activity would be difficult, if not impossible, owing to his decreased mobility and pain. The best choice is to first inform the physician of the patient's stated limitations and request an alternative test. The stress echocardiography uses dobutamine to stress the cardiac tissues without requiring the patient to walk or ride. The Weight-lift test does not exist.

155. Correct answer: C
Anginal pain usually occurs when approximately 75% of the artery's diameter becomes occluded. Pain is more pronounced with exertion or emotional distress, when oxygen demand by cardiac tissue cannot be met by oxygen supply via the occluded arteries. The severity of pain may be compounded with vasospasms that further restrict blood flow through the coronary arteries.

156. Correct answer: C
Lead V_1 is the best lead to monitor for RBBB.

157. Correct answer: C
Treadmill stress testing may miss as many as 40% of cases of single-vessel disease. LV dysfunction may be diagnosed via a thallium test (myocardial scintigraphy). A positive treadmill test may not be positive for CAD.

158. Correct answer: D

Ms. M. is presenting with chest wall pain, most likely as the result of her having undergone open-heart surgery. Although the pain is expected, to support recovery and ensure the best possible outcome, the nurse will need to address pain and discomfort. If left untreated, Ms. M. may not perform deep-breathing exercises or participate fully in physical therapy, placing her at risk for other postoperative complications. Morphine and diazepam will treat both pain and muscle spasms. There is no indication of infection to the wound site, and the pain described by the patient is not consistent with another infarction. EKG changes would most likely be seen. The physician should be contacted if the pain and spasms do not resolve with morphine and diazepam administration or if the pain should present differently with EKG changes.

159. Correct answer: D

The drug of choice to treat AV nodal and atrioventricular re-entrant arrhythmias is adenosine. Adenosine is a naturally occurring substance in the body and has a very short half-life (only a few seconds). Adenosine slows AV nodal conduction or can stop the conduction process altogether, potentially causing a transient AV block (seen as asystole). The patient may experience mild to moderate chest discomfort, slight hypotension, bradycardia, and possibly flushing. Amiodarone and quinidine are antiarrhythmics. Clonidine is an antihypertensive.

160. Correct answer: C

Systemic lupus erythematosus (SLE) is a chronic inflammatory autoimmune disease that affects the vascular and connective tissues within any body system and organ. As a result of the disease, inflammation may be increased and the stress of injury would further exacerbate the SLE. Symptoms and conditions to monitor closely for include pericarditis, hypertension, diarrhea, thrombocytopenia, anemia, leucopenia, joint and muscle pain, vasculitis, proteinurea, seizures, depression, pneumonia, pleural effusions, nausea, and ulcers.

161. Correct answer: C

A drug that can cause a significant rise in the INR is amiodarone, as do aspirin and sulfomamides. Statins, ethacrinic acid, and penicillin cause only a moderate rise in INR.

162. Correct answer: B

A drug that will significantly decrease the INR would be vitamin K. Vitamin K is widely used as an antidote for warfarin, but can actually decrease the INR too much and increase warfarin resistance, so careful monitoring is critical. Warfarin breakdown is also accelerated by barbiturates. Nafcillin, high-dose vitamin C, and cyclosporine decrease the INR only moderately. Other drugs that significantly decrease the INR include rifampin, phenobarbital, and glutethimide.

163. Correct answer: D

This patient has probably developed cardiogenic shock. The MI has impaired the heart's ability to pump effectively. The cardiac output falls and the body reacts by vasoconstricting peripheral circulation and increasing the heart rate. Tachycardia is also the result of catecholamine release, and the myocardial oxygen consumption increases. The left ventricle works harder, but has been compromised by the MI. Preload increases because fluid cannot be pumped out of the chambers effectively. The S_3 is a signal of increased preload. Pulmonary congestion occurs due to increased left heart pressures.

164. Correct answer: C
A new holosystolic murmur at the lower left sternal border means that turbulent blood flow is occurring there. The turbulence is caused by a hole that is allowing blood to flow through a previously closed area. The SvO_2 will increase due to the mixing of blood. This condition must be corrected surgically.

165. Correct answer: B
Acute pericarditis is usually self-limiting within 2 to 6 weeks after its onset. Treatment includes bed rest, oxygen therapy, antiviral, antifungal, or antibacterial agents. In addition, drainage and management of cardiac tamponade may be necessary. The classic presentation of chronic pericarditis (also known as constrictive pericarditis) demonstrates fibrous pericardial thickening. Treatment may include the extreme measure of pericardiotomy (removal of the pericardium).

166. Correct answer: B
An infarct in the left main coronary artery is an ominous sign. Sudden death may occur, along with heart blocks and atrial and ventricular dysrhythmias.

167. Correct answer: C
A coronary perfusion pressure of at least 50 mmHg is required to maintain auto-regulatory control.

168. Correct answer: C
Pulsus paradoxus may be present in conjunction with asthma, emphysema, cardiac tamponade, restrictive pericarditis, or hemorrhagic shock. Pulse pressure is the difference between systolic and diastolic blood pressure. Pulsus parvus means a small or weak pulse. Pulsus alternans means the upstroke is more powerful than the down-stroke—that is, the stroke alternates in strength.

169. Correct answer: D
Prophylactic administration of nitroglycerine translingual spray should be taken 5 to 10 minutes before activity. Each metered dose of nitroglycerine spray is 0.4 mg and has a duration of 30–60 minutes. The spray may be administered under or on the tongue and still be effective.

170. Correct answer: B
If your patient receiving transdermal nitroglycerin states intent to use a hot tub, sauna, electric blankets, or magnetic therapy, then as his nurse you should notify the physician and request a change from transdermal to an extended release tablet or capsule. Transdermal NTG, either by patch or ointment plus an external heat source, is dangerous. More nitroglycerin is increased in the presence of high and/or prolonged exposure to heat. The medication will not rub off in water or sweat and normal bathing will not have the same effect. As a nurse, you should never advise a patient to change the medication amount ordered. The physician should be notified for any intent by the patient to change medication dosing or administration route. The better advice for the patient is to use the hot tub with caution and for short periods with the heat turned down and to never use the hot tub alone in case of emergency.

171. Correct answer: B
Visitation policies vary by institution. However, it is best to identify one person as the point of contact. HIPAA regulations require limitations on the release of any medical information be set by the patient if the patient is able to communicate his or

her wishes. If the patient is unable to make this decision, the next of kin can act as a contact person.

172. Correct answer: A
The best response would be to respond collaboratively and interact with other professionals. Ideally, this conference should occur ASAP.

173. Correct answer: C
Utilizing the internal mammary artery means grafts do not have to come from the saphenous veins in the leg, minimizing the risk for infection from another site. In the graft procedure, the internal mammary artery is separated at only one end and reanastomosed to the affected coronary artery distal to the affected area. The patency of the resulting graft is generally quite good. After 10 years, approximately 90% of grafts are still patent.

174. Correct answer: A
Your patient just underwent a percutaneous intervention for stent placement, after which he was returned to your telemetry unit. You note a rash over the patient's trunk and arms. This is probably due to an allergic reaction to the contrast dye. Iodine dye is used and will cause a rash, itching, swelling, and can also lead to laryngospasm and anaphylaxis in some patients. It is imperative to determine whether the patient is allergic to iodine, shellfish, or horses prior to initiating the procedure.

175. Correct answer: A
Along with acute ST elevation, another indicator of necrosis would be an abnormal Q wave. If the Q wave appears within about six hours of a transmural MI, it is an ominous sign. If the Q wave is more than 0.04 seconds long, it is a sign of necrosis. In an inferior MI, the Q wave should not exceed 0.03 seconds or it is indicative of necrosis.

176. Correct answer: C
Quite often, the patient develops cardiogenic shock and requires emergent placement of a VAD. If the nurse is able to at least explain the function of the device, it can be a great relief to the family.

177. Correct answer: B
The patient is approaching crisis and may feel hopeless. The nurse should take the time to fully explore and validate the patient's feelings, then decide on the appropriate course of action.

178. Correct answer: D
If the patient is bleeding, the blood may settle into the lumbar area. Blood is heavy and will flow into the retroperitoneal area because of gravity. More than an hour may pass and several hundred milliliters of blood may be lost before vital signs are affected.

179. Correct answer: D
The aortogram is the established standard for definitive diagnosis of aortic dissection and is the only invasive procedure listed as an option for this question. This test is sometimes called an aortic angiogram with (radiopaque) contrast dye.

180. Correct answer: C
The P wave represents depolarization of the atrium and the QRS the depolarization of the ventricles; the size difference is related to the muscle mass involved in the polarization. The P wave's amplitude represents the amount or size of the muscle mass involved in the

depolarization of the atrium. The QRS wave represents the amount or size of the muscle mass involved in the depolarization of the ventricles. The greater the muscle mass, the greater the change in amplitude. Non-patient-related factors that may affect these waves' amplitude include gain setting, lead placement, and interference. Patient-related factors may include electrolyte imbalances, hypertrophy, and cardiac injury.

181. Correct answer: A

Your patient with obstructive jaundice has no prior history of cardiac arrhythmias. He asks why he is on a cardiac monitor. Your best response is, "You may develop a slower heart rate. This monitor will alert staff to any dangerous drop in your heart rate." Obstructive jaundice may lead to cardiac changes. The other options use medical terminology and may further frighten the patient.

182. Correct answer: B

Patients with heart transplants do not feel cardiac pain because the heart has been denervated when removed from the donor.

183. Correct answer: B

When the heart is denervated, it has no connection to the autonomic nervous system, so a reflexive response does not occur. A sympathetic stimulant must be used to provide this response. If no other complications occur, the ventricle will eventually adjust to not receiving autonomic input.

184. Correct answer: A

Pain is a cardinal sign of an arterial obstruction. The nurse should check for pallor, other signs of an arterial blockage, sensation, and quality of pulses. If the obstruction is venous, the limb may exhibit cyanosis.

185. Correct answer: B

Your patient received streptokinase about 30 minutes ago for a lateral wall STEMI. You would expect reperfusion rhythms to occur. Reperfusion rhythms such as ventricular tachycardia, sinus bradycardia, accelerated idioventricular rhythm, and underlying sinus rhythms with ventricular ectopy may occur. The patient should experience less chest pain. The CPK isoenzymes may temporarily become elevated as blood flows freely through newly opened arteries. CHF is not a result of this therapy.

186. Correct answer: C

Family members are probably quite used to providing care for this patient because of his quadriplegia. Explain the rationale for the procedure, and then demonstrate it. Do not ignore the patient. There is no point in speaking slowly unless the caregiver or the patient has difficulty understanding your instructions. Teaching quickly is counterproductive and may be considered rude and unprofessional. Allow time for a return demonstration of skills and allow for questions.

187. Correct answer: C

You should feel only a mild tingling sensation. You should not fear this device to the point of not performing CPR, and CPR should not be delayed in any event. If the ICD fires, anyone touching the patient at that moment may feel the tingling sensation.

188. Correct answer: B

The magnet is used to inhibit the shocking (tachy) feature of the ICD. It can shut down a malfunctioning ICD. Patient teaching includes letting the patient know the dangers of being in proximity to large magnets. Most ICDs have a warning tone built in so that if the patient comes too near a magnet, the tone is emitted. The type of tone produced varies with the device's manufacturer.

189. **Correct answer: B**
Radio ablation uses waves that actually heat the tissue around the active sites and prevent reentry loop. Once the temperature reaches 50° C, cell damage and death occur. The continuing heat creates a lesion approximately 2–5 mm in diameter. This "burned" area causes necrosis and will not conduct electricity.

190. **Correct answer: D**
Ibutilide is a relatively new Class III/IV medication. It must be used at the time of the cardioversion and will be ineffective if used prior to the cardioversion.

191. **Correct answer: C**
If the CVP catheter is in the right ventricle and touches the myocardium, PVCs can result. Occasionally, the physician will insert the catheter a bit too far, causing PVCs. In this case, the catheter simply has to be withdrawn to a better position in the right atrium. This is a rare occurrence. If the patient's catheter was left in the right ventricle, the V-tach might continue and the patient might suffer cardiac arrest.

192. **Correct answer: A**
The circumflex coronary artery feeds the left atrium and left ventricle. Infarctions as a result of occlusion of this artery result in lateral or left-sided heart damage. The left anterior descending artery and the circumflex artery both branch off from the left coronary artery.

193. **Correct answer: B**
New-onset or acute mitral valve regurgitation is often a result of myocardial infarction of the left anterior descending and circumflex arteries. These arteries feed the papillary muscles, which in turn support mitral valve function. Prolonged ischemia causes the papillary and/or chordae tendinae of the mitral valve to rupture and prevent full closure of the mitral valve during systole. As the blood flows back into the left atrium, the murmur can be auscultated.

194. **Correct answer: C**
Patients with peripheral vascular disease are often hypothermic because of poor circulation. Healing is also slowed because of the decrease in circulation. The nurse should provide proper alignment without impeding circulation and monitor the patient's peripheral pulses for presence and quality. The color and temperature of the extremity should be monitored and results charted.

195. **Correct answer: A**
The injuries to the patient's chest may have caused a pulmonary artery laceration or a cardiac contusion (the latter condition is more likely). His blood pressure is low and the EKG shows ST-segment elevation in the anterior leads. If the myocardium is contused, it will react the same way as if an MI had occurred. The ST elevation may be the result of a physiologic insult to a coronary artery, and an area of the myocardium may be ischemic. If so, the pumping function of the myocardium will be compromised and may need additional support with inotropes. The patient may undergo angiography and/or surgery. Volume replacement may be necessary. This patient is probably in the first stage of cardiogenic shock.

196. Correct answer: D
Approximately 24 hours after a surgical procedure, the release of inflammatory cell mediators can lead to vasodilation. This patient has a permanent pacemaker, but apparently her heart rate cannot compensate for the drop in blood pressure. The cardiac output did not increase as a result of the reduced systemic resistance. Her pacemaker did not allow the heart rate to climb above 70. The dobutamine acted on the pump and increased the heart's contractility. This patient also has a history of a previous MI.

197. Correct answer: C
A carotid bruit is the significant physical finding associated with carotid stenosis. Heberden's nodules and Broussard's nodules are both seen with arthritis. The systolic murmur is an indication of a valvular problem.

198. Correct answer: C
COPD causes changes in the 12-lead EKG due to the workload for the right side of the heart. Changes commonly seen in patients with COPD include tall, peaked P waves, right axis deviation, right ventricular hypertrophy, and low-voltage QRS.

199. Correct answer: A
The progressive care nurse should immediately report any BUN/creatinine ratio >20 in the presence of decreased urine output to the physician for a patient on nesiritide. The increased creatinine level and decreased urine output are indicators of compromised/diminished blood flow to the kidneys with impending development of prerenal azotemia. Azotemia is an adverse reaction to nesiritide administration. With prerenal azotemia, other lab results to monitor and report include a urine osmolality of <500 mOsm/L and a urine specific gravity >1.015.

200. Correct answer: C
Integrilin (eptifbatide) is used primarily for patients with acute coronary syndrome to inhibit platelet aggregation.

201. Correct answer: D
If the conversation is not hushed and you overhear the statement as part of your regular duties, it would be appropriate to clarify or correct misinformation if it would not involve diagnosing the patient's disease process. In this case, the patient provides you an opportunity to teach him about his cardiac murmur. Aortic stenosis will cause a murmur, but the harshness or degree of auscultation is not directly correlated with the degree of severity or risk to the patient. Based on his statement, he may not understand what a diagnosis of aortic stenosis entails. By asking about his comprehension, you will be able to determine what his degree of understanding is, which knowledge you may correct or clarify, and to what degree his physician may need to discuss his prognosis or plan of care.

202. Correct answer: B
Mr. B. would exhibit signs and symptoms of hypercalcemia, confirmed by his calcium level of 13.5 mg/dL. Signs and symptoms would include smooth-muscle relaxation, lethargy, confusion, shortened QT interval, bradycardia, heart blocks, bundle branch blocks, and hypertension. Symptoms can be further compounded by the effects of digitalis and, possibly, digitalis toxicity.

203. Correct answer: A
Due to the decreased availability of calcium essential to the coagulation phase (used within the intrinsic, extrinsic, and common pathways), the patient will not have

formed permanent clots. The platelet plugs formed over damaged vessels initially after surgery may be dislodged by blood flow, leading to recurrent bleeding at postoperative days 7 to 10.

204. Correct answer: D
Peripartum cardiomyopathy develops during the first 3 to 4 months after completion of pregnancy. Sometimes the cause is myocarditis.

205. Correct answer: A
Dilated cardiomyopathy causes systolic dysfunction. As a result, you will hear S_3 and S_4 gallops and the EKG may show atrial fibrillation, ventricular dysrhythmias, or sinus tachycardia most of the time. The patient may have a systolic murmur of the AV valves. In addition, the patient will probably have peripheral edema or ascites, hepatomegaly, and pale, cool extremities. Changes in mentation are possible as well. Hypertrophic and restrictive cardiomyopathies are diastolic dysfunctions.

206. Correct answer: C
The correct dosing for ticagrelor (Brilinta) is to give 180 mg PO once then 90 mg PO BID to begin in 5 days. To avoid severe bleeding risks, hold administration of Brilinta at least 5 days before and after an invasive procedure, such as stent placement, oral surgery, and elective surgery.

207. Correct answer: A
Ticagrelor (Brilinta) was designed to always be taken concurrently with aspirin. Maximum benefit was found to be maintained with aspirin dosing at 75–100 mg PO daily. Ticagrelor effectiveness decreases when aspirin dosing exceeds 100 mg per day. Patients should be counseled to avoid over-the-counter medications containing aspirin.

208. Correct answer: D
Coumadin (warfarin) blocks vitamin K coagulation factors of II, VII, IX, X, and XI of the extrinsic pathway. Normal PT is in the range of 11.2 to 13.2 seconds. A PT of 28 seconds indicates severe risk of bleeding and the Coumadin dose should be held and the physician notified immediately. Many laboratories and physicians will use the INR value for purposes of Coumadin titration, as it is more reliable and standardized. The PT value must still be obtained to determine the INR calculation. The INR target is 2 to 3.5. INR values >4.5 indicate that the patient is at increased risk for bleeding, and a value >6 indicates the need for vitamin K administration.

209. Correct answer: D
This patient has increased exercise intolerance, edema, and dyspnea, all of which are signs of left ventricular failure. The crackles are probably the result of fluid buildup in the lungs. Because the left heart cannot pump effectively, the fluid backs up.

210. Correct answer: B
The pH is normal (compensated), the CO_2 level is high (respiratory acidosis), and the HCO_3 level is normal. As you were reading along, you probably expected a question about a cardiac issue, not ABGs. Read each question carefully as you could easily misinterpret what a question is asking.

211. Correct answer: D
Mrs. N.'s intolerance for activity and crackles indicate pulmonary congestion. Edema indicates third spacing. All of these symptoms are cardinal signs of CHF.

212. **Correct answer: C**
This patient's heart cannot pump the fluid out and the lungs are congested (dyspnea). Edema is a sign of pump failure. The patient will probably develop ascites and hepatomegaly.

213. **Correct answer: C**
The type of myocardial infarction that involves the entire thickness of myocardium in a region is called transmural. "Transmural" describes the full thickness of the myocardial wall. "Subendocardial" indicates that the infarction has not affected the full thickness of the myocardium. The anterioseptal and inferior walls are potential locations of the myocardial infarction.

214. **Correct answer: A**
Your patient with an implanted cardiac defibrillator should have thresholds checked frequently during administration of amiodarone. Amiodarone may affect the pacing threshold of implanted cardiac defibrillators, so the pacing settings should be verified prior to and during amiodarone administration. Anisindione is an anticoagulant and administration is contraindicated for a patient with an invasive device such as an implanted cardiac defibrillator.

215. **Correct answer: C**
Increased preload may be caused by renal problems. An overload of fluid is present in the intravascular space. Preload may also be increased in cases where resistance is increased, such as in valve dysfunctions or vasoconstriction. Anything that blocks fluid from progressing forward or prevents elimination of fluids is a potential cause of increased preload. If the heart fails and the myocardium cannot pump fluid out, such as in damage from surgery, cardiomyopathies, or decreased stretch following heart surgery, preload increases.

CARDIOVASCULAR REFERENCES

Adam, A., Nicholson, C., & Owens, L. (2008). Alcoholic dilated cardiomyopathy. *Nursing Standard, 22*(38), 42–47.

Ahmed, S., Van Gelder, I. C., Wiesfeld, A. C., Van Veldhuisen, D. J., & Links, T. P. (2011). Determinants and outcome of amiodarone-associated thyroid dysfunction. *Clinical Endocrinology, 75*(3), 388–394.

Ahrens, T., Prentice, D., & Kleinpell, R. M. (2011). *Progressive care nursing certification: Preparation, review, and practice exams.* St. Louis, MO: McGraw-Hill.

Alba, A. C., McDonald, M., Rao, V., Ross, H. J., & Delgado, D. H. (2011). The effect of ventricular assist devices on long-term post-transplant outcomes: A systematic review of observational studies. *European Journal of Heart Failure, 13*(7), 785–795.

Aldous, S. J., Florkowski, C. M., Crozier, I. G., & Than, M. P. (2012). The performance of high sensitivity troponin for the diagnosis of acute myocardial infarction is underestimated. *Clinical Chemistry & Laboratory Medicine, 50*(4), 727–729.

Aldous, S. J., Richards, M., Cullen, L., Troughton, R., & Than, M. (2012). Diagnostic and prognostic utility of early measurement with high-sensitivity troponin T assay in patients presenting with chest pain. *Canadian Medical Association Journal, 184*(5), E260–E268.

Alpendurada, F., Guha, K., Sharma, R., Ismail, T. F., Clifford, A., Banya, W., . . . Prasad, S. K. (2011). Right ventricular dysfunction is a predictor of non-response and clinical outcome following cardiac resynchronization therapy. *Journal of Cardiovascular Magnetic Resonance, 13*, 68.

Alspach, J. G. (2012). Acute myocardial infarction without chest pain: A life-threatening variant? *Critical Care Nurse, 32*(4), 10–13.

American Association of Critical-Care Nurses. (2006). *AACN core curriculum for critical care nursing.* St. Louis, MO: Saunders.

American Journal of Critical Care. (2012). RS28 novice critical care nurse performance of defibrillation, cardioversion, and transcutaneous pacing. *American Journal of Critical Care, 21*(3), e83.

Andersson, H., Sejersten, M., Clemmensen, P., & Grande, P. (2010). Prognosis and high-risk complication identification in unselected patients with ST-segment elevation myocardial infarction treated with primary percutaneous coronary intervention. *Acute Cardiac Care, 12*(3), 102–108.

Appenzeller, S., Pineau, C. A., & Clarke, A. E. (2011). Acute lupus myocarditis: Clinical features and outcome. *Lupus, 20*(9), 981–988.

Azabagic, S., Cickusic, A. J., & Zukic, E. (2012). Effects of short-term octreotide therapy on TSH adenoma with atrial fibrillation: Case report. *HealthMed, 6*(3), 1081–1086.

Bae, S., Ke, Q., Koh, Y. Y., Lee, W., Choi, J. H., Kang, P. M., & Morgan, J. P. (2010). Exacerbation of acute viral myocarditis by tobacco smoke is associated with increased viral load and cardiac apoptosis. *Canadian Journal of Physiology and Pharmacology, 88*(5), 568–575.

Bar-Yishay, I., Gilutz, H., Cafri, C., Ilia, R., & Zahger, D. (2010). Isolated inferior wall ST segment depression as an early sign of acute anterior wall myocardial infarction. *Acute Cardiac Care, 12*(4), 119–123.

Benoit-Marand, M., Ballion, B., Borrelli, E., Boraud, T., & Gonon, F. (2011). Inhibition of dopamine uptake by D2 antagonists: An in vivo study. *Journal of Neurochemistry, 116*(3), 449–458.

Berkowitz, R., Alhaj, E., Manchikalapudi, R. B., Satya, K., Dadfarmay, S., & Zakir, R. (2010). Determinants of right ventricular failure in patients admitted with acute left heart failure. *Congestive Heart Failure, 16*(6), 243–248.

Bhatt, A. G., & Monahan, K. M. (2011). Nonreentrant supraventricular tachycardia misdiagnosed as inappropriate sinus tachycardia. *Pacing and Clinical Electrophysiology, 34*(8), e70–e73.

Borders, C. W., Bennett, S., Mount, C., & Claassen, S. L. (2012). A rare case of acute diffuse alveolar hemorrhage following initiation of amiodarone: A case report. *Military Medicine, 177*(1), 118–120.

Boyce, B. A., Brady, Y., & Homer, B. (2012). Incidence and severity of phlebitis in patients receiving peripherally infused amiodarone. *Critical Care Nurse, 32*(4), 27–71.

Brady, W., & Truwit, J. (Eds). (2009). *Critical decisions in emergency and acute care electrocardiology.* St. Louis, MO: Saunders.

Braunwald, E. (2011). Clinical efforts to reduce myocardial infarct size: The next step. *Journal of Cardiovascular Pharmacology and Therapeutics, 16*(3–4), 349–353.

Brorsen, A. (2012). *CEN examination review*, MA: Jones & Bartlett Learning.

Brorsen, A., & Rogelet, K. (2009). *PCCN certification review.* Sudbury, MA: Jones & Bartlett.

Buchner, S., Debl, K., Barlage, S., Griese, D., Fredersdorf, S., Jeron, A., . . . Luchner, A. (2010). Dynamic changes in N-terminal pro-brain natriuretic peptide in acute coronary syndromes treated with percutaneous coronary intervention: A marker of ischemic burden, reperfusion and outcome. *Clinical Chemistry & Laboratory Medicine, 48*(6), 875–881.

Buckley, R. (2011). ISAR-REACT 4-bivalirudin similar to abciximab/heparin in reducing ischemic outcomes in NSTEMI and has significantly less bleeding. *MD Conference Express*, 14–15.

Bueltmann, M., Kong, X., Mertens, M., Yin, N., Yin, J., Liu, Z., . . . Kuebler, W. M. (2009). Inhaled milrinone attenuates experimental acute lung injury. *Intensive Care Medicine, 35*(1), 171–178.

Buerke, M., Lemm, H., Dietz, S., & Werdan, K. (2011). Pathophysiology, diagnosis, and treatment of infarction-related cardiogenic shock. *Herz, 36*(2), 73–83.

Chabot, A., Jiang, B. H., Shi, Y., Tardif, J. C., & Dupuis, J. (2011). Role of aldosterone on lung structural remodelling and right ventricular function in congestive heart failure. *BMC Cardiovascular Disorders, 11*, 72.

Chestovich, P. J., Kwon, M. H., Cryer, H. G., Tillous, A., & Hiatt, J. R. (2011). Surgical procedures for patients receiving mechanical cardiac support. *American Surgeon, 77*(10), 1314–1317.

Chulay, M., & Burns, S. (2010). *Essentials of Progressive care nursing* (2nd ed). St. Louis, MO: McGraw-Hill.

Cooper, L. T. (2009). Myocarditis. *The New England Journal of Medicine, 360*(15), 1526–1538.

Correia, E., Rodrigues, B., Santos, L. F., Moreira, D., Gama, P., Cabral, C., & Santos, O. (2011). Longitudinal left ventricular strain in hypertrophic cardiomyopathy: Correlation with non-sustained ventricular tachycardia. *Echocardiography, 28*(7), 709–714.

Cowie, M. R. (2012). Recent developments in the management of heart failure. *The Practitioner, 256*(1752), 25–29.

Curley, M. A. Q. (2007). *Synergy: The unique relationship between nurses and patients.* St. Louis, MO: Saunders.

Dande, A. S., Pandit, A. S., & Galin, I. D. (2011). Takotsubo cardiomyopathy followed by neurogenic stunned myocardium in the same patient: Gradations of the same disease? *Cardiology, 118*(3), 175–178.

Donohoe-Dennison, R. (2007). *Pass CCRN* (3rd ed). St. Louis, MO: Mosby.

Dunlay, S. M., Weston, S. A., Killian, J. M., Bell, M. R., Jaffe, A. S., & Roger, V. L. (2012). Thirty-day rehospitalizations after acute myocardial infarction: A cohort study. *Annals of Internal Medicine, 157*(1), 11–18.

Dziewierz, A., Siudak, Z., Rakowski, T., Dubiel, J. S., & Dudek, D. (2010). Predictors and in-hospital outcomes of cardiogenic shock on admission in patients with acute coronary syndromes admitted to hospitals without on-site invasive facilities. *Acute Cardiac Care, 12*(1), 3–9.

Elliot, K. (2010). Hypertrophic cardiomyopathy: An inherited cardiac condition. *British Journal of Cardiac Nursing, 5*(10), 486–491.

Fontana, P., Boutellier, U., & Toigo, M. (2010). Non-invasive haemodynamic assessments using Innocor during standard graded exercise tests. *European Journal of Applied Physiology, 108*(3), 573–580.

Gandy, W. E., & Grayson, S. (2012). Cardiac zebras: Diagnosing Wellens and Brugada syndromes on 12-lead ECGs. *EMS World, 41*(9), 24–28.

Grothe, C., Belasco, A., Bettencourt, A., Diccini, S., Vianna, L., Pignatari, A., . . . Barbosa, D. (2009). Lethality of endocarditis due to *S. aureus* among patients on hemodialysis. *Nephrology Nursing Journal, 36*(6), 613–619, 632.

Halawa, A., Henry, P. D., & Sarubbi, F. A. (2011). Candida endocarditis associated with cardiac rhythm management devices: Review with current treatment guidelines. *Mycoses, 54*(4), e168–174.

Hardin, S., & Kaplow, R. (2005). *Synergy for clinical excellence: The AACN synergy model for patient care.* St. Louis, MO: Saunders.

Heggemann, F., Hamm, K., Kaelsch, T., Sueselbeck, T., Papavassiliu, T., Borggrefe, M., & Haghi, D. (2011). Global and regional myocardial function quantification in Takotsubo cardiomyopathy in comparison to acute anterior myocardial infarction using two-dimensional (2D) strain echocardiography. *Echocardiography, 28*(7), 715–719.

Herman, D. S., Lam, L., Taylor, M. R., Wang, L., Teekakirikul, P., Christodoulou, D., . . . Seidman, C. E. (2012, February 16). Truncations of titin causing dilated cardiomyopathy. *The New England Journal of Medicine, 366*(7), 619–628.

Huang, Z. L., Urade, Y., & Hayaishi, O. (2011). The role of adenosine in the regulation of sleep. *Current Topics in Medicinal Chemistry, 11*(8), 1047–1057.

Hwang, E. S., & Pak, H. N. (2012). Mid-septal hypertrophy and apical ballooning, potential mechanism of ventricular tachycardia storm in patients with hypertrophic cardiomyopathy. *Yonsei Medical Journal, 53*(1), 221–223.

Johnson-Coyle, L., Jensen, L., & Sobey, A. (2012). Peripartum cardiomyopathy: Review and practice guidelines. *American Journal of Critical Care, 21*(2), 89–98.

Jois, P. (2011). NSTEMI and STEMI: Therapeutic Updates 2011. *Emergency Medicine Reports, 32*(1), 1–7.

Jones & Bartlett Learning. (2011). *2012 Nurse's drug handbook. (*11th ed). Sudbury, MA: Jones & Bartlett Learning.

Kaneko, Y., Nakajima, T., Irie, T., Ota, M., Kato, T., Iijima, T., . . . Kurabayashi, M. (2011). Differential diagnosis of supraventricular tachycardia with ventriculoatrial dissociation during ventricular overdrive pacing. *Pacing & Clinical Electrophysiology, 34*(8), 1028–1030.

Kang, D. H., Kim, Y. J., Kim, S. H., Sun, B. J., Kim, D. H., Yun, S. C., . . . Sohn, D. W. (2012). Early surgery versus conventional treatment for infective endocarditis. *The New England Journal of Medicine, 366*(26), 2466–2473.

Karaca, M. A., Ozucelik, D. N., Cobanoglu, M., Kabakci, G., Sivri, B., & Karcioglu, O. (2011). Is this heart attack worse than the other? Use of D-dimer levels in non-ST elevation myocardial infarction. *HealthMed, 5*(4), 789–793.

Khan, A. H., Khadem, A., Basta, M. M., Magdy, N., Gardner, M. J., Parkash, R., . . . Sapp, J. L. (2010). Differential entrainment distinguishes atrioventricular nodal reentry tachycardia from atrioventricular reentrant tachycardia. *Pacing & Clinical Electrophysiology, 33*(11), 1335–1341.

Kilicgedik, A., Karabay, C., Aung, S., Guler, A., Kalayci, A., Tasar, O., & Kirma, C. (2012). A successful percutaneous closure of ventricular septal defect following septal myectomy in patients with hypertrophic obstructive cardiomyopathy. *Perfusion, 27*(3), 253–255.

Kirchberger, I., Meisinger, C., Heier, M., Kling, B., Wende, R., Greschik, C., . . . Kuch, B. (2011). Patient-reported symptoms in acute myocardial infarction: Differences related to ST-segment elevation. *Journal of Internal Medicine, 270*(1), 58–64.

Kurt, I. H., Batur, M. K., & Unal, I. (2011). The effect of streptokinase therapy in STEMI and conventional therapy in NSTEMI patients on TIMI risk index, B-type natriuretic peptide and high-sensitive C-reactive protein. *The Anatolian Journal of Cardiology, 11*(6), 530–535.

Lampert, R., Salberg, L., & Burg, M. (2010). Emotional stress triggers symptoms in hypertrophic cardiomyopathy: A survey of the Hypertrophic Cardiomyopathy Association. *Pacing & Clinical Electrophysiology, 33*(9), 1047–1053.

Leggieri, N., Gouriet, F., Thuny, F., Habib, G., Raoult, D., & Casalta, J. P. (2012). Legionella longbeachae and endocarditis. *Emerging Infectious Diseases, 18*(1), 95–97.

Lidegaard, Ø., Løkkegaard, E., Jensen, A., Skovlund, C. W., & Keiding, N. (2012). Thrombotic stroke and myocardial infarction with hormonal contraception. *The New England Journal of Medicine, 366*(24), 2257–2266.

Loughran, S., Kealy, J., Shook, A., & Kaan, A. (2012). The development and evaluation of a competency-based program for patients with a ventricular assist device. *Canadian Journal of Cardiovascular Nursing, 22*(3), 18–23.

Lynn, J. S., Singh, A., & Snoey, E. R. (2011). Can we exclude the diagnosis of non-ST segment myocardial infarction on the basis of a single troponin I and a symptom duration ≥8 hours? *ISRN Cardiology,* Special section, 1–7.

Lynn-McHale Wiegand, D. J. (Ed). (2011). *AACN procedure manual for critical care* (6th ed). St. Louis, MO: Saunders.

Malasana, G., Day, J. D., Weiss, J. P., Crandall, B. G., Bair, T. L., May, H. T., . . . Bunch, T. J. (2011). Strategy of rapid cardioversion minimizes the significance of early recurrent atrial tachyarrhythmias after ablation for atrial fibrillation. *Journal of Cardiovascular Electrophysiology, 22*(7), 761–766.

Marian, A. J. (2010). Update on hypertrophic cardiomyopathy. *Texas Heart Institute Journal, 37*(3), 322–323.

Marino, R., Magrini, L., Ferri, E., Gagliano, G., & Di Somma, S. (2010). B-type natriuretic peptide and non-invasive haemodynamics and hydration status assessments in the management of patients with acute heart failure in the emergency department. *High Blood Pressure & Cardiovascular Prevention, 17*(4), 219–225.

Mathias, W., Kowatsch, I., Saroute, A. N., Osório, A. F. F., Sbano, J. C. N., Dourado, P. M. M., . . . Tsutsui, J. M. (2011). Dynamic changes in microcirculatory blood flow during dobutamine stress assessed by quantitative myocardial contrast echocardiography. *Echocardiography, 28*(9), 993–1001.

Mavrogeni, S., Bratis, K., Kitsiou, A., & Kolovou, G. (2012). Streptococcal tonsillitis and acute streptococcal myocarditis: An unusual combination assessed by cardiac magnetic resonance imaging and endomyocardial biopsy. *Annals of Otology, Rhinology & Laryngology, 121*(9), 604–608.

McIntosh, V. J., & Lasley, R. D. (2012). Adenosine receptor-mediated cardioprotection: Are all 4 subtypes required or redundant? *Journal of Cardiovascular Pharmacology and Therapeutics, 17*(1), 21–33.

Mead, N. E., & O'Keefe, K. P. (2009). Wellen's syndrome: An ominous EKG pattern. *Journal of Emergencies, Trauma & Shock, 2*(3), 206–208.

Meyer, S., Todd, D., Wright, I., Gortner, L., & Reynolds, G. (2008). Non-invasive assessment of cardiac output with portable continuous-wave Doppler ultrasound. [Review article.] *Emergency Medicine Australasia, 20*(3), 201–208.

Moore, A. D., & Hill, J. (2012). Myocardial infarction and pregnancy: A case report. *AANA Journal, 80*(1), 32–36.

Movahed, M. R., Ramaraj, R., Hashemzadeh, M., & Hashemzadeh, M. (2010). Nationwide trends in the age adjusted prevalence of non-ST elevation myocardial infarction (NSTEMI) across various races and gender in the USA. *Acute Cardiac Care, 12*(2), 58–62.

Natarajan, A., Hindocha, D., Kular, N., Fergey, S., & Davis, J. R. (2012). Vasculitic rash: Do not jump to conclusions. *Clinical Medicine, 12*(2), 179–180.

Ng, T. M., Ackerbauer, K. A., Hyderi, A. F., Hshieh, S., & Elkayam, U. (2012). Comparative effects of nesiritide and nitroglycerin on renal function, and incidence of renal injury by traditional and RIFLE criteria in acute heart failure. *Journal of Cardiovascular Pharmacology and Therapeutics, 17*(1), 79–85.

Noureldin, R. A., Liu, S., Nacif, M. S., Judge, D. P., Halushka, M. K., Abraham, T. P., ... Bluemke, D. A. (2012). The diagnosis of hypertrophic cardiomyopathy by cardiovascular magnetic resonance. *Journal of Cardiovascular Magnetic Resonance, 14*, 17.

O'Donovan, K. (2012). Acute management of right ventricular infarction. *British Journal of Cardiac Nursing, 7*(3), 118–123.

O'Donovan, K. (2012). Amiodarone and its role in arrhythmia. *Nurse Prescribing, 10*(5), 241–246.

Oliver, J. (2011). Hypertrophic cardiomyopathy and inherited heart conditions. *British Journal of Healthcare Assistants, 5*(4), 163–167.

Oliver, J., & Skirton, H. (2010). Familial dilated cardiomyopathy: Effective management of the family to improve prognosis. *British Journal of Cardiac Nursing, 5*(5), 224–228.

Paolucci, H., Nutter, B., & Albert, N. M. (2011). RN knowledge of vascular access devices management. *Journal of the Association for Vascular Access, 16*(4), 221–225.

Paraskevas, K. I., Mikhailidis, D. P., Oikonomou, K., & Verhoeven, E. L. (2012). Local versus general anesthesia for carotid endarterectomy: Issues beyond stroke, myocardial infarction, and death rates. *Angiology, 63*(6), 405–408.

Patel, P. A., Lowe, E., Baig, W., & Sandoe, J. (2011). Hepatorenal syndrome precipitated by infective endocarditis. *British Journal of Hospital Medicine, 72*(9), 532–533.

Pere, K. (2012). Developing nursing expertise in caring for older advanced stage heart failure patients and their families: Palliative and end-of-life care. *Canadian Journal of Cardiovascular Nursing, 22*(3), 12–17.

Pernicova, I., Garg, S., Bourantas, C. V., Alamgir, F., & Hoye, A. (2010). Takotsubo cardiomyopathy: A review of the literature. *Angiology, 61*(2), 166–173.

Pierce, D., Calkins, B. C., & Thornton, K. (2012). Infectious endocarditis: Diagnosis and treatment. *American Family Physician, 85*(10), 981–986.

Planinc, D. (2011). Echocardiography in non-invasive assessment of hemodynamics. *Kardio List, 6*(12), 433–435.

Powner, D. J., & Truong, H. (2011). Takotsubo cardiomyopathy: Its possible impact during adult donor care. *Progress in Transplantation, 21*(4), 344–350.

Quin, E. M., Cuoco, F. A., Forcina, M. S., Coker, J. B., Yoe, R. H., Spencer, W. H., . . . Gold, M. R. (2011). Defibrillation thresholds in hypertrophic cardiomyopathy. *Journal of Cardiovascular Electrophysiology, 22*(5), 569–572.

Rezkalla, S. H., & Kloner, R. A. (2010). Influenza-related viral myocarditis. *WMJ: Official Publication of the State Medical Society of Wisconsin, 109*(4), 209–213.

Rubenstein, J. C., & Roth, J. A. (2011). Atrioventricular junction ablation and pacemaker implantation for heart failure associated with atrial fibrillation: Potential issues and therapies in the setting of acute heart failure syndrome. *Heart Failure Reviews, 16*(5), 457–465.

Samara, M. A., & Tang, W. H. (2011). Device monitoring strategies in acute heart failure syndromes. *Heart Failure Reviews, 16*(5), 491–502.

Schultz, J. C., Hilliard, A. A., Cooper, L. T., & Rihal, C. S. (2009). Diagnosis and treatment of viral myocarditis. *Mayo Clinic Proceedings, 84*(11), 1001–1009.

Sheikh-Taha, M., & Zeitoun, A. (2012). Effect of intermittent nesiritide administration on kidney function. *Journal of Cardiovascular Pharmacology and Therapeutics, 17*(2), 229–230.

Suzuki, M., Enomoto, D., Seike, F., Fujita, S., & Honda, K. (2012). Clinical features of early myocardial rupture of acute myocardial infarction. *Angiology, 63*(6), 453–456.

Szabo, S., Oikonomopoulos, T., & Hoffmeister, H. M. (2009). Myocarditis. *The New England Journal of Medicine, 361*(4), 423.

Topal, F. E., Oguzturk, H., Topal, F., Turtay, M. G., & Yildirim, B. (2012). Relations of the congestive cardiac failure with troponin I and CK-MB. *HealthMed, 6*(2), 643–647.

Wang, N. C., Bhattacharya, S., & Gheorghiade, M. (2011). The potential role of cardiac resynchronization therapy in acute heart failure syndromes. *Heart Failure Reviews, 16*(5), 481–490.

Wang, N. C., Fonarow, G. C., & Gheorghiade, M. (2011). The potential application of electrophysiology diagnostics and therapeutics in acute heart failure syndromes. *Heart Failure Reviews, 16*(5), 437–439.

Wang, N. C., Piccini, J. P., & Gheorghiade, M. (2011). Implantable cardioverter-defibrillator implementation in acute heart failure syndromes: Unanswered questions. *Heart Failure Reviews, 16*(5), 477–480.

Wang, W., Zhu, W. H., Qi, Y. Q., Fu, S. L., & Gong, F. Q. (2012). Cardiogenic shock: Do not forget the possibility of Kawasaki disease. *The Turkish Journal of Pediatrics, 54*(1), 86–89.

Watanabe, K., Sukumaran, V., Veeraveedu, P. T., Thandavarayan, R. A., Gurusamy, N., Ma, M., . . . Suzuki, K. (2011). Regulation of inflammation and myocardial fibrosis in experimental autoimmune myocarditis. *Inflammation & Allergy Drug Targets, 10*(3), 218–225.

Watcher, R. (2012). *Understanding patient safety* (2nd ed). Los Altos, CA: Lange.

Wehrens, X. H., Vos, M. A., Doevendans, P. A., & Wellens, H. J. (2002). Novel insights in the congenital long QT syndrome. *Annals of Internal Medicine, 137*(12), 981–992.

Weng, C., Chen, Q., Ma, Y., & He, Q. (2009). A meta-analysis of the effects of atrial overdrive pacing on sleep apnea syndrome. *Pacing & Clinical Electrophysiology, 32*(11), 1434–1443.

Werdan, K., Ruß, M., Buerke, M., Delle-Karth, G., Geppert, A., & Schöndube, F. A. (2012). Cardiogenic shock due to myocardial infarction: Diagnosis, monitoring and treatment. *Deutsches Aerzteblatt International, 109*(19), 343–351.

Westphal, N., Plicht, B., & Naber, C. (2009). Infective endocarditis—prophylaxis, diagnostic criteria, and treatment. *Deutsches Aerzteblatt International, 106*(28–29), 481–490.

Whitlock, A., & MacInnes, J. (2011). Acute heart failure: Patient assessment and management. *British Journal of Cardiac Nursing, 6*(11), 516–525.

Wilker, E. H., Yeh, G., Wellenius, G. A., Davis, R. B., Phillips, R. S., & Mittleman, M. A. (2012). Ambient temperature and biomarkers of heart failure: A repeated measures analysis. *Environmental Health Perspectives, 120*(8), 1083–1087.

Wilson, M. G., Chandra, N., Papadakis, M., O'Hanlon, R., Prasad, S. K., & Sharma, S. (2011). Hypertrophic cardiomyopathy and ultra-endurance running—two incompatible entities? *Journal of Cardiovascular Magnetic Resonance, 13*, 77.

Wilson, V. (2012). Myocardial infarction symptoms and appropriate action: Awareness in people with diabetes. *British Journal of Cardiac Nursing, 7*(6), 287–292.

Wozakowska-Kaplon, B., Bartkowiak, R., & Janiszewska, G. (2010). A decrease in serum aldosterone level is associated with maintenance of sinus rhythm after successful cardioversion of atrial fibrillation. *Pacing & Clinical Electrophysiology, 33*(5), 561–565.

Yeh, R. W., Sidney, S., Chandra, M., Sorel, M., Selby, J. V., & Go, A. S. (2010). Population trends in the incidence and outcomes of acute myocardial infarction. *The New England Journal of Medicine, 362*(23), 2155–2165.

Yue, A. M., & Foster, W. M. (2011). Repetitive nonsustained supraventricular tachycardia: What is the mechanism? *Pacing & Clinical Electrophysiology, 34*(10), 1297–1300.

Zhao, Q., Wu, T. G., Lin, Y., Li, B., Luo, J. Y., & Wang, L. X. (2010). Low-dose nesiritide improves renal function in heart failure patients following acute myocardial infarction. *Heart and Vessels, 25*(2), 97–103.

Section 5

Pulmonary

SECTION 5: PULMONARY QUESTIONS

1. **The volume of gas remaining in the lungs at the end of one normal expiration is called**
   A. Residual volume
   B. Capacitance
   C. Total lung capacity
   D. Functional residual capacity

2. **The volume of gas left in the lungs following a maximal respiratory effort is known as the**
   A. Vital capacity
   B. Total lung capacity
   C. Residual volume
   D. Dead airspace

3. **Which of the following conditions is most likely to lead to inaccurate oxygen saturation values on a pulse oximeter?**
   A. Probe placement on an earlobe
   B. Hyperthermia
   C. Decreased peripheral perfusion
   D. Cyanotic heart disease

4. **The functional residual capacity is defined as**
   A. The amount of air in lungs after normal expiration
   B. The amount of gas that can be forcefully exhaled after maximum inspiration
   C. The amount of gas normally exhaled after a maximum inhalation
   D. The amount of gas left in the lungs after a maximum exhalation

5. **Gas exchange in the lungs requires movement of gas between the atmosphere, alveoli, and pulmonary vasculature. This movement of gasses is via**
   A. Passive diffusion
   B. Osmotic pressure
   C. Airway resistance
   D. Hydrostatic pressure

6. **Your patient was admitted from the ED and is septic. The respiratory therapist who has just drawn an ABG sample asks you if the patient has a fever. The possibility of fever will have what effect on the sample he just collected?**
   A. The PO_2 will be falsely elevated
   B. The pH will rise

C. Fever has no effect
D. The HCO_3 will be elevated

7. **The cells responsible for forming a barrier for alveoli are**
   A. Histocytes
   B. Type II alveolar epithelial cells
   C. Macrophages
   D. Type I alveolar epithelial cells

8. **In the lungs, communicating channels through holes in the alveolar wall allowing gas movement between alveoli are called**
   A. Preacinar arteries
   B. Alveolar pores of Kohn
   C. Canae of Smolder
   D. The palmar arteries

9. **Type II alveolar cells produce**
   A. Surfactant
   B. Phagocytes
   C. Macrocytes
   D. Carbon dioxide

10. **A diagnosis of asthma may be made by**
    A. A PEFR of 100–125
    B. A FiO_2 of 80%
    C. A decreased FEV_1
    D. Wheezing

11. **The FIO_2 for a nasal cannula set at a flow rate of 6 L/min is**
    A. 21%
    B. 24%
    C. 30%
    D. 40%

12. **Your patient has been on a nasal cannula and now requires a non-rebreather mask to maintain his oxygenation saturation at acceptable levels. A non-rebreather mask can deliver what percentage of oxygen when the O_2 flow rate is set at 10–15 L/min?**
    A. 24–40%
    B. 30–40%
    C. 60–80%
    D. 50–60%

13. **Your patient required placement of chest tube after aspiration of a pleural effusion. When assessing a patient with a chest tube drainage system, which of the following statements is correct?**
    A. Check for subcutaneous emphysema around the insertion site by auscultation
    B. If using a Pleur-Evac with autotransfusion connection, make certain all clamps are open

C. The average chest tube size for an adult is 20 French
D. If using a chest tube drainage system with a one-way valve and suction, water is required to maintain a seal

14. **The patient you are caring for will require oxygen therapy at home, so it is important that the patient is taught**
A. To secure oxygen tanks in a vertical position
B. To wear synthetic clothing to reduce the risk of static electricity
C. To use alcohol-based swabs to reduce oral dryness
D. To use only a nasal cannula and not a mask

15. **Your elderly male patient has been diagnosed with end-stage mesothelioma. He came to the ED because of severe respiratory distress. He is now in your PCU receiving palliative care. Which of the following occupations is more likely to be associated with a diagnosis of mesothelioma?**
A. Bricklayer
B. Gardener
C. Office manager
D. Shipbuilder

16. **Pulse oximetry readings are considered unreliable when oxygen saturation levels fall below**
A. 55%
B. 60%
C. 80%
D. 70%

17. **The nursing student assigned to you for the day asks you to explain the oxyhemoglobin dissociation curve. You reply that the oxyhemoglobin dissociation curve is**
A. A relationship between dissolved oxygen and the affinity for oxygen by the hemoglobin molecule
B. A graphic representation of carbon dioxide content versus oxygen content in arterial blood
C. A measure of methemoglobin
D. A way to calculate gas transport across the alveoli

18. **Your patient with COPD has been receiving 600 mg of theophylline daily in divided doses. Which of the following assessment findings should be reported to the physician immediately, as these findings represent potential theophylline toxicity?**
A. The patient is lethargic
B. Atrial tachycardia with occasional PVCs has developed
C. The patient's blood glucose is 50
D. The patient has a systolic blood pressure of 160 mmHg

19. **The respiratory therapist has just drawn an arterial blood gas sample. The syringe contains a small amount of heparin. What effect will too much heparin have on the sample, if any?**
A. Increase the $PaCO_2$
B. No effect

C. Decrease the bicarbonate
D. Totally prevent clotting

20. **You are preparing to administer a loading dose of theophylline to your patient with COPD. For every 0.5 mg/kg given, you would expect a ___ increase in blood theophylline levels.**
A. 0.25 mcg/ml
B. 0.5 mg/ml
C. 0.75 mg/ml
D. 1 mcg/ml

21. **Your patient is currently taking theophylline. As a progressive care nurse, you know this patient should be taught to**
A. Stop smoking while taking this medication because smoking decreases medication clearance, leading to toxicity
B. Avoid current alcohol consumption while on theophylline as alcohol increases medication clearance
C. Notify the physician of any huge change in weight to adjust dosing
D. Avoid a high-protein, low carbohydrate diet, as it will increase theophylline elimination

22. **A measurement of total oxygen consumption is**
A. SvO_2
B. $ETCO_2$
C. $PtCO_2$
D. SjO_2

23. **Your patient required endotracheal intubation. Which of the following statements is true regarding the use of capnography to verify endotracheal tube placement?**
A. Placement of the device can be difficult to learn initially
B. It is not necessary to auscultate lung sounds when this device is used
C. $ETCO_2$ is a moderately reliable indicator of correct tube placement
D. It is not a substitute for pulse oximetry

24. **Your patient had 1,350 ml of pleural effusion removed via thoracentesis and immediately began coughing and was dyspneic. You believe he has developed**
A. Re-expansion pulmonary edema
B. A pneumothorax
C. A cardiac tamponade
D. A hemothorax

25. **Your patient has a confirmed flail chest. What alteration in acid–base balance would you expect with this condition?**
A. Metabolic alkalosis
B. Metabolic acidosis
C. Respiratory acidosis
D. Respiratory alkalosis

26. Your 45 year old patient was admitted to the PCU for a severe cough. She states that the cough has lasted 3 weeks. She also reports the coughing comes in long episodes that continue until she vomits. When you attempt to obtain a sputum specimen, what little sputum she produces is very thick and white. What condition do you suspect this patient has developed?

A. Asthma
B. Gastroesophageal reflux
C. Pertussis
D. Pneumonia

27. The driving pressure of air divided by airflow rate determined by airway diameter is known as

A. A V-Q mismatch
B. A compliance curve
C. Airway resistance
D. Driving force curve

28. What is the drug of choice for treating pertussis?

A. Penicillin VK
B. Amoxicillin
C. Azithromycin
D. Doxycycline

29. Patients with uncontrolled asthma may receive steroids and neuromuscular blocking agents in an attempt to mitigate their symptoms. These patients are at increased risk for

A. Hypertension
B. Prolonged muscle weakness
C. Renal failure
D. Hepatic failure

30. Your patient contracted a wound infection secondary to an appendix removal 6 days ago. She presented to the ED complaining of incisional pain and elevated temperature. She was started on intravenous gentamicin, then transferred to your PCU. As a progressive care nurse, you know gentamicin is also useful in the treatment of

A. Otitis media
B. Gram-positive rods
C. *Pseudomonas aeruginosa*
D. Bacillus

31. You suspect your patient is developing a pulmonary embolism. Signs and symptoms of a pulmonary embolus can include

A. Sinus bradycardia or a normal EKG
B. Pleuritic chest pain, decreased cardiac output
C. ABGs show respiratory acidosis, increased respiratory rate
D. Decreased PAS pressure

32. **Which of the following statements is true when a patient has a pulmonary embolism?**
    A. Respiratory acidosis occurs
    B. Heparin is used to dissolve clots
    C. Normal D-dimer results can rule out a pulmonary embolism
    D. Metabolic alkalosis develops

33. **Pulmonary embolism is actually considered a complication of deep venous thrombosis. To assess for deep venous thrombosis, which of the following signs should be assessed?**
    A. Moses'
    B. Davis'
    C. Corrigan's
    D. Hamman's

34. **Your new patient was admitted directly from her physician's office to the PCU. The patient fell from a tree. She now complains of stabbing substernal pain each time she changes her position. Her chest X-ray results were just relayed to your unit by the radiologist. The patient has been diagnosed with a pneumomediastinum. A common significant finding in a patient with a pneumomediastinum is**
    A. Cullen's sign
    B. Grey–Turner's sign
    C. Hamman's sign
    D. Handes' sign

35. **Which of the following drugs is classified as a methylxanthine?**
    A. Morphine
    B. Theophylline
    C. Prednisone
    D. Atropine

36. **Your patient has been slightly hypoxic since admission to the PCU. She sustained a tension pneumothorax following an automobile accident and had a chest tube placed in the ED. What potential imbalance would be expected with her hypoxic state?**
    A. Hypochloremia
    B. Respiratory alkalosis
    C. Decreased bicarbonate levels
    D. Hypokalemia

37. **A student nurse asks you to explain the concept of hypoxemia. Hypoxemia is best defined as**
    A. A decrease in oxygen at the cellular level
    B. A decrease in oxygen at the alveolar level
    C. A decrease in oxygen levels in venous blood
    D. A decrease in oxygen levels in arterial blood

38. **Which of the following conditions is the most probable cause of the acid–base imbalance of uncompensated respiratory alkalosis?**
    A. Kidney failure
    B. A side effect of theophylline
    C. Hyperventilation
    D. Hypoventilation

39. **A possible treatment to best improve airflow in status asthmaticus is the use of**
    A. PEEP
    B. Heliox
    C. Norepinephrine
    D. Nebulizer treatments

40. **If you hear faint breath sounds on the left side of the chest and normal sounds on the right side immediately after your patient has been intubated, most likely**
    A. The ETT has an air leak
    B. The physician has intubated the esophagus
    C. The ETT is at the carina
    D. The right main stem bronchus has been intubated

41. **Analyze the following arterial blood gas results from a patient on 2 L O_2 via a nasal cannula:**
    pH 7.47
    CO_2 33
    HCO_3 21
    A. Normal
    B. Compensated respiratory acidosis
    C. Uncompensated respiratory alkalosis
    D. Uncompensated metabolic alkalosis

42. **Analyze the following arterial blood gas values**
    pH 7.39
    CO_2 28
    HCO_3 19
    A. Compensated metabolic acidosis
    B. Compensated respiratory acidosis
    C. Uncompensated metabolic acidosis
    D. Uncompensated respiratory acidosis

43. **Analyze the following capillary blood gas results for a patient on 21% oxygen**
    pH 7.42
    CO_2 41
    HCO_3 23
    A. Compensated respiratory acidosis
    B. Compensated respiratory alkalosis

C. Normal
D. Compensated metabolic acidosis

44. Analyze the following arterial blood gas results from a patient with a ventricular septal injury from a stab wound

pH 7.57
CO_2 22
HCO_3 31

A. Uncompensated (mixed) respiratory/metabolic alkalosis
B. Compensated respiratory acidosis
C. Compensated metabolic alkalosis
D. Uncompensated respiratory alkalosis

45. Analyze the following arterial blood gas values

pH 7.38
CO_2 65
HCO_3 36

A. Uncompensated metabolic alkalosis
B. Compensated respiratory acidosis
C. Compensated metabolic acidosis
D. Uncompensated respiratory acidosis

46. Analyze the following arterial blood gas values from an adult patient with tetralogy of Fallot

pH 7.17
CO_2 41
HCO_3 14

A. Normal
B. Compensated respiratory acidosis
C. Uncompensated respiratory acidosis
D. Uncompensated metabolic acidosis

47. Interpret the following arterial blood gas results from a victim of a gunshot wound to the chest

pH 7.23
CO_2 61
HCO_3 23

A. Compensated respiratory acidosis
B. Uncompensated metabolic acidosis
C. Uncompensated respiratory acidosis
D. Normal

48. One cause of decreased SvO_2 in a patient is

A. An increased metabolic rate
B. Sedation
C. A decreased metabolic rate
D. Increased cardiac output

49. **Your new patient has severe bronchitis. She has been treated at her extended care facility with a non-rebreather mask for 5 days. Today, she is exhibiting increased distress with chest discomfort, restlessness, a dry hacking cough with dyspnea, and numbness in her extremities. Pulmonary function tests (PFTs) indicate a decreased vital capacity (VC), decreased compliance, and decreased functional residual capacity (FRC). As the nurse caring for this patient, you should anticipate orders to**
    A. Administer Lasix 40 mg IV
    B. Prepare for intubation with 100% FiO_2
    C. Take the patient for a CT scan and prepare to give tPA
    D. Check the pulse oximeter correlation with an arterial blood gas and decrease the FiO_2

50. **As patients age from birth through old age, chest wall compliance decreases. One of the reasons for this change is**
    A. Arterial oxygen tension increases
    B. Total lung capacity decreases
    C. Costal cartilage degeneration
    D. Decreased residual volume

51. **Which medication listed below is both an analgesic and an amnestic?**
    A. Barbiturates
    B. Propofol
    C. Atropine
    D. Ketamine

52. **Which of the following statements about cyanosis is true?**
    A. Cyanosis is directly related to increased $PaCO_2$
    B. Fingertip clubbing is an indication of chronic hypoxia
    C. Cyanosis may be observed when 1 to 3 grams of Hgb is desaturated
    D. Cyanosis may be easily observed in cases of anemia and polycythemia

53. **The respiratory therapist tells you he is covering too many patients and cannot perform postural drainage on your patient. He says your patient needs the left upper lobes drained if possible. The correct position to help this patient is**
    A. Flat on left side
    B. Flat with hips elevated
    C. Supine
    D. Semi-reclining

54. **Your patient has a hemothorax. What is the proper location of a chest tube for evacuation of a hemothorax?**
    A. Second intercostal space, midclavicular line
    B. Second intercostal space, midaxillary line
    C. Fifth intercostal space, midaxillary line
    D. Fifth intercostal space, midclavicular line

55. **An example of the hypoxemic type of respiratory failure is**
    A. Increased dead air space
    B. ARDS

C. PaO_2 <60 mmHg while person is at rest, at sea level, on room air
D. Right heart failure

56. **Where does the hypoxemic drive to breathe originate?**
A. The cerebellum
B. The aortic and carotid arteries
C. The hypothalamus
D. The medulla

57. **Severe carbon monoxide poisoning occurs when carboxyhemoglobin levels are higher than which of the following percentages?**
A. 10–15%
B. 20–40%
C. 40–50%
D. 50–60%

58. **Carbon monoxide has an affinity for hemoglobin thought to be 200–300 times greater than oxygen. Elimination of carbon monoxide from the body is via the**
A. Kidneys
B. Liver
C. Spleen
D. Lungs

59. **The nurse reporting to you on a new patient states that the patient has developed subcutaneous emphysema. Subcutaneous emphysema usually occurs in the area of the**
A. Head
B. Neck
C. Abdomen
D. Thorax

60. **Pulse oximetry should never be used**
A. To determine oxygen saturation values
B. During a cardiac arrest
C. As a determinant for predicting hemoglobin affinity for oxygen
D. To help determine a patient's activity tolerance

61. **A SpO_2 value of 95% correlates with which of the following PaO_2 values?**
A. 75
B. 80
C. 90
D. 98

62. **To prevent complications with a chest tube drainage system, the suction level should not be higher than**
A. –20 cm/H_2O
B. –30 cm/H_2O
C. –40 cm/H_2O
D. –50 cm/H_2O

63. **Which of the following statements is true regarding chest tube drainage systems?**
    A. Drainage of frank blood in amounts >100 ml/hour is not significant
    B. Drainage tubing should be placed horizontally on the bed, then down to the collection chamber
    C. All drainage tubing should be dependent to the insertion site
    D. Chest tube drainage from a mediastinal tube should bubble in the water seal chamber

64. **Which of the following drugs is considered to be a mucolytic agent?**
    A. Atropine
    B. Terbutaline
    C. Acetylcysteine
    D. Albuterol

65. **Side effects of acetylcysteine include**
    A. Red urine
    B. Headache
    C. Hypertension
    D. Bronchospasms

66. **Patients often have decreases in lung compliance simply from the effects of aging. Which of the following conditions actually increases lung compliance?**
    A. Pulmonary edema
    B. Pleural effusions
    C. Obesity
    D. Emphysema

67. **One of the most effective ways to relieve bronchospasms is**
    A. To use adrenalin
    B. Use of an antihistamine
    C. Use prednisone
    D. To use a B2 receptor agonist

68. **When the resident attempts to place a central line, air is accidentally introduced into the line when the IV tubing becomes disconnected. The best position in which to place this patient to minimize a venous air embolism is**
    A. Reverse Trendelenburg
    B. Right side
    C. Trendelenburg with left decubitus tilt
    D. Left side

69. **A venous air embolism may be caused by**
    A. Hemodialysis
    B. Pulmonary artery catheters
    C. Radial arterial catheters
    D. Peritoneal dialysis

70. **A risk factor for thrombolic emboli includes**
    A. A patient who is 1 week postpartum
    B. Carcinoma

C. Long bone fractures
D. Heparin administration

71. **You are caring for a patient with an acute exacerbation of reactive airway disease. The patient has a history of asthma. Which of the following signs indicates this patient is suffering from acute respiratory distress?**
A. Expiratory wheezes
B. Grunting
C. Sternocleodomastoid retractions
D. Inspiratory wheezes

72. **Your patient has ceased wheezing during his asthma attack. This change in his condition**
A. Indicates the patient is improving
B. Only means the nebulizer treatment is working
C. Indicates the patient is in complete respiratory failure
D. Means the patient's anxiety has decreased

73. **Wheezing is present in a number of medical conditions. In which of the following conditions is wheezing usually not present?**
A. Smoke inhalation
B. Pneumonia
C. Near drowning
D. Bronchitis

74. **Your patient tells you he has been taking Slo-Bid for his asthma. Side effects of this medication include**
A. Lethargy
B. Flaccidity
C. Bradycardia
D. Muscle cramps

75. **Long-acting forms of B2 agonists used in the treatment of asthma include**
A. Salmeterol (Serevent®)
B. Albuterol (Proventil® HFA, Ventolin® HFA, Accuneb®, ProAir®)
C. Metaproterenol (Alupent®)
D. Levalbuterol (Xoponex® HFA, Xoponex® nebulizer solution)

76. **Which of the following are symptoms of active tuberculosis?**
A. Dry cough, weight loss, night sweats
B. Hemoptysis, fever, night sweats, weight loss
C. Chest pain, wheezing, hemoptysis
D. Weight loss, hemoptysis, wheezing

77. **Your patient has a 14-mm induration at the site of his PPD. What does this mean?**
A. He has a positive PPD
B. He has latent TB
C. His results are indeterminate
D. He has a false-positive result

78. **Which of the following medications is not used to treat TB?**
    A. Isoniazid
    B. Pyrazidamide
    C. Rimantadine
    D. Rifampin

79. **A patient recently admitted from the ED requires immediate intubation. The physician orders succinylcholine. Which of the following conditions is not a side effect of succinylcholine?**
    A. Hypotension
    B. Malignant hypothermia
    C. Hypokalemia
    D. Smooth muscle contraction

80. **Accessory pathways connecting a small airway to an airspace normally supplied by another pathway is called**
    A. A cartilaginous bronchus
    B. A membranous bronchiole
    C. A canal of Lambert
    D. The portal of Menifer

81. **Falsely low readings on a pulse oximeter may be due to**
    A. Vasodilation
    B. Vascular dyes
    C. Patient motion
    D. Fever

82. **Which of the following considerations should the PCU nurse know prior to the administration of vancomycin?**
    A. Vancomycin is nephrotoxic
    B. Vancomycin must be administered intramuscularly
    C. Vancomycin should always be given with an aminoglycoside
    D. Vancomycin is specific for *Staphylococcus aureus*

83. **Precautions used when handling respiratory equipment or providing respiratory treatments in the PCU include**
    A. Using an alcohol-based antiseptic agent if your hands are visibly soiled before, during, and after patient care
    B. Using an alcohol-based antiseptic solution only if you have worn gloves during contact with the patient
    C. Using an antimicrobial soap and water before and after providing patient care
    D. Only decontaminating your hands after providing care if gloves are worn

84. **The ED nurse who transferred your patient reported that your patient had been previously intubated by paramedics with an LMA. The patient is now conscious and is on a nasal cannula at 2 L/min. Which of the following statements is true regarding the use of laryngeal mask airways (LMAs)?**
    A. Nurses routinely insert these airways
    B. There is a low risk of aspiration

C. It is a temporary airway
D. The vocal cords must be visualized

85. Your patient was finally released from the hospital two weeks ago after a difficult course of treatment for sepsis. She was seen in the ED for follow-up for a small laceration. Today she is visiting staff in the PCU and says she plans to visit her family in Colorado Springs. Part of the teaching for this patient should include information on the effects of high altitude on her ability to oxygenate effectively. Which of the following changes would be expected on her blood gas results?

A. The PaO_2 increases
B. No effect would occur
C. O_2 saturation would decrease
D. The pH would decrease

86. Which of the following pulmonary dilators is used for the treatment of pulmonary hypertension?

A. Dobutamine
B. Dopamine
C. Inhaled nitric oxide
D. Epinephrine

87. An action of nitric oxide includes which of the following effects?

A. Vascular smooth muscle relaxation
B. To augment prostaglandin synthesis
C. To release macrophages
D. To increase pulmonary vascular resistance

88. Which of the following statements is true regarding the administration of CPAP?

A. CPAP cannot be delivered via an endotracheal tube
B. CPAP allows for a decrease in functional residual capacity
C. CPAP provides decreased pressure to the posterior pharynx
D. CPAP may be administered via nasal prongs

89. An adverse effect of excessive CPAP is

A. Continuous need to increase oxygen over time
B. A rise in intrathoracic pressure
C. Intraventricular hemorrhage
D. A sudden change in cerebral blood flow

90. Your new patient requires mechanical ventilation via a tracheostomy. If positive inspiratory pressure (PIP) is increased on a mechanical ventilator, what effect should this have on your patient's blood gases?

A. It increases the $PaCO_2$ and decreases the PaO_2
B. It decreases the $PaCO_2$ and decreases the PaO_2

C. It decreases the $PaCO_2$ and increases the PaO_2
D. It decreases the pH and decreases the $PaCO_2$

91. **Fluid therapy in ARDS is directed toward**
A. Keeping a high CO state
B. Maintaining a low protein content
C. Maintaining hyponatremia
D. Maintaining a low circulating fluid volume

92. **The nurse just coming on shift to care for your patient brought several ampules of normal saline to the bedside in preparation for suctioning your patient. Research has shown that use of normal saline does not thin secretions and may cause which of the following adverse effects?**
A. Decreased mean arterial pressure
B. Decreased intrathoracic pressure
C. Anxiety
D. Bronchodilation

93. **In the PCU, patients may be mechanically ventilated by a variety of ventilator modes. Which of the following ventilator modes allows the patient to breathe spontaneously?**
A. HFV
B. SIMV
C. CMV
D. Oscillator

94. **Many of the ventilator circuits used in a PCU utilize a closed catheter suction system. Which of the following is a disadvantage of closed catheter suctioning of a mechanically ventilated patient?**
A. The patient does receive oxygen during the procedure
B. The extra weight of the inline tubing
C. Cost is higher with a single-use catheter
D. Cost is effective if used sporadically

95. **Your patient will require long-term ventilatory support via a tracheostomy. A disadvantage of using a tracheostomy tube is**
A. Subcutaneous emphysema
B. It increases airway resistance
C. The airway is less stable
D. It allows for right mainstem intubation

96. **Your patient requires a stoma stent. The function of a stoma stent is**
A. To prevent aspiration
B. To avoid translaryngeal intubation
C. To provide the ability for the patient to speak
D. To keep the stoma tract open

97. **Which of the following statements about silicone or plastic tracheostomy tubes is true?**
   A. Silicone holds up to repeated cleaning
   B. Wire-reinforced tubes cannot be used in MRI imaging
   C. A one-way speaking valve is easy to use
   D. The tubes offer a lower cost to the facility

98. **Mask continuous positive airway pressure (CPAP) should be used with caution if a patient has**
   A. Low functional residual capacity (FRC)
   B. A basilar skull fracture
   C. Sinusitis
   D. Pneumonia

99. **Analyze the following arterial blood gas values**
   pH 7.52
   CO_2 42
   HCO_3 37
   A. Uncompensated metabolic alkalosis
   B. Compensated metabolic acidosis
   C. Uncompensated respiratory alkalosis
   D. Uncompensated mixed respiratory/metabolic alkalosis

100. **Analyze the following arterial blood gas values**
   pH 7.43
   CO_2 36
   HCO_3 25
   A. Compensated respiratory acidosis
   B. Normal
   C. Compensated metabolic acidosis
   D. Compensated metabolic alkalosis

101. **Analyze the following arterial blood gas values**
   pH 7.11
   CO_2 67
   HCO_3 15
   A. Uncompensated respiratory acidosis
   B. Uncompensated metabolic alkalosis
   C. Compensated metabolic acidosis
   D. Uncompensated (mixed) respiratory/metabolic acidosis

102. **Analyze the following arterial blood gas values**
   pH 7.38
   CO_2 25
   HCO_3 16
   A. Compensated respiratory alkalosis
   B. Compensated metabolic acidosis

C. Uncompensated metabolic acidosis
D. Uncompensated respiratory acidosis

103. Analyze the following blood gas values
pH 7.49
CO_2 29
HCO_3 23
A. Uncompensated respiratory alkalosis
B. Compensated respiratory acidosis
C. Compensated metabolic alkalosis
D. Uncompensated metabolic acidosis

104. Analyze the following arterial blood gas values
pH 7.43
CO_2 29
HCO_3 22
A. Uncompensated metabolic alkalosis
B. Uncompensated respiratory alkalosis
C. Compensated respiratory alkalosis
D. Compensated metabolic alkalosis

105. Analyze the following arterial blood gas values
pH 7.32
CO_2 67
HCO_3 25
A. Uncompensated metabolic alkalosis
B. Uncompensated respiratory acidosis
C. Compensated metabolic acidosis
D. Compensated respiratory acidosis

106. Analyze the following arterial blood gas values
pH 7.37
CO_2 36
HCO_3 24
A. Normal
B. Compensated respiratory acidosis
C. Compensated metabolic acidosis
D. Compensated respiratory alkalosis

107. Analyze the following arterial blood gas values from a patient on room air
pH 7.16
CO_2 54
HCO_3 21
A. Uncompensated metabolic alkalosis
B. Uncompensated (mixed) respiratory/metabolic acidosis
C. Compensated metabolic acidosis
D. Uncompensated respiratory acidosis

108. Which of the following medications is given orally to inhibit rapid rise in pulmonary artery pressure secondary to hypoxia?

A. Calcium channel blockers
B. Nitric oxide
C. Sidenafil
D. Plavix

109. Which of the following statements about laryngeal mask airways is true?

A. It may be inserted by any nurse
B. It may cause hoarseness after removal
C. The patient must have an absent gag reflex
D. The laryngeal mask airway (LMA) eliminates the risk of aspiration

110. During a cardiac arrest, your patient aspirated gastric contents. Which of the following statements is true regarding this type of aspiration?

A. If the pH of the material is <2.5, necrosis will be minimal
B. The patient always develops ARDS
C. Onset of symptoms is gradual
D. There is little danger of atelectasis

111. The best position for a patient with ARDS is

A. Prone
B. On right side
C. On left side
D. Supine

112. You are receiving report on a patient with pulmonary hypertension. Which of the following symptoms is consistent with presentation of pulmonary hypertension?

A. A prominent S_4
B. Decreased respiratory rate
C. Dyspnea with exertion
D. Left-side heart failure

113. Your patient is suffering from primary pulmonary hypertension. Which of the following medication groups would be used to treat this condition?

A. Beta-blockers
B. Calcium channel blockers
C. MAO-inhibitors
D. Catecholamine

114. If left untreated, pulmonary hypertension may result in which of the following sequelae?

A. Increased left atrium pressures
B. Irreversible thinning of the medial smooth muscles in the arterioles
C. Reversible thickening of the lateral smooth muscle in the arterioles
D. Increased right ventricular pressures

115. What is the purpose of screening for collagen vascular disease and coagulation disorders in a patient with suspected pulmonary hypertension?

A. Hypoxemia triggers a decrease in collagen creation
B. Hypoxia results in decreased elastin production
C. Decreased blood flow results in blood pooling
D. Hypoxemia destroys collagen

116. An absolute contraindication for use of rapid sequence intubation is

A. Total loss of facial and/or oropharyngeal landmarks, which requires a surgical airway
B. An airway where intubation may not be successful
C. A "crash" airway where the patient is in arrest
D. There is no absolute contraindication for the use of rapid sequence intubation

117. Which of the following situations is not an indication for the use of rapid sequence intubation?

A. Prolonged respiratory effort that results in fatigue or failure
B. Uncooperative trauma patient with life-threatening injuries
C. Stab wound to neck with expanding hematoma
D. All cervical spine injuries

118. During rapid sequence intubation, cricoid cartilage pressure is often used to help prevent vomiting and aspiration of gastric contents. The esophagus is obstructed by the pressure to the anterior neck. This maneuver is known as the

A. Hamman's maneuver
B. King maneuver
C. Sellick maneuver
D. Pitt maneuver

SECTION 5: PULMONARY ANSWERS

1. **Correct answer: D**
   Functional residual capacity is the volume of gas remaining in the lungs at the end of one normal expiration.

2. **Correct answer: C**
   Residual volume is the volume of gas left in the lungs following a maximal respiratory effort.

3. **Correct answer: C**
   Inaccurate oxygen saturation values on a pulse oximeter are likely due to decreased peripheral perfusion. Adequate perfusion must exist for the probe on a pulse oximeter to register an accurate evaluation of hemoglobin saturation. If the patient is hypothermic or has decreased peripheral perfusion, the results will be inaccurate. Vasoconstriction, position of the probe, and patient motion can also cause inaccurate readings on a pulse oximeter.

4. **Correct answer: A**
   The functional residual capacity is defined as the amount of air in lungs after normal expiration. The formula for functional residual capacity is FRC = ERV (expired residual volume) + the RV (residual volume). The normal FRC in healthy lungs is about 2,000–3,000 ml.

5. **Correct answer: A**
   Gas exchange in the lungs requires passive diffusion of gas between the atmosphere, alveoli, and pulmonary vasculature.

6. **Correct answer: B**
   Fever causes the pH to rise. Most ABG machines are calibrated to 37° C. If the patient has a fever, the oxyhemoglobin curve will be shifted to the right. More oxygen will be given off to the tissues, so the machine has to be calibrated to account for the temperature.

7. **Correct answer: D**
   The cells that are responsible for forming a barrier for alveoli are type I epithelial cells. Type I cells line the outside of the alveoli and are easily inflamed by inhaled toxins or heated air. In addition, type I cells maintain the blood–gas interface. Type II cells produce surfactant.

8. **Correct answer: B**
   In the lungs, communicating channels through holes in the alveolar wall allowing gas movement between alveoli are called alveolar pores of Kohn.

9. **Correct answer: A**
   Type II alveolar cells produce surfactant. Surfactant is a lipoprotein and functions by increasing surface tension of alveoli and allowing alveoli to expand and contract. We should have some residual pressure in the alveoli at the end of respiration to keep the alveoli open (physiologic PEEP). If surfactant production is impaired, the alveoli's ability to exchange O_2 is compromised. Type I cells line the outside of the alveoli.

10. **Correct answer: C**
A diagnosis of asthma may be made by a decreased FEV_1. The forced expiratory volume (FEV) is how much air is exhaled during the first second of effort. This amount should be ≥75% of the predicted normal value(s). In asthmatics, this value is decreased because of obstruction. The forced vital capacity (FVC) is the total amount of gas exhaled as forcefully and rapidly as possible after taking a maximal inspiration. The result should be above 80%.

11. **Correct answer: D**
The FIO_2 for a nasal cannula set at a flow rate of 6 L/min is 40%. The nasal cannula is generally considered a low-flow oxygen device unless connected to a high-flow system. If using a flow >4 L/min., the oxygen should be humidified to prevent drying the mucosal membranes.

12. **Correct answer: C**
A non-rebreather mask can deliver 60–80% of oxygen when the O_2 flow rate is 10–15 L/min. If both exhalation ports have one-way valves, then near-100% oxygen may be reached. To prevent suffocation in patients where the oxygen is disconnected, non-rebreathing masks now have only one one-way valve to prevent/limit inhalation of room air. Limiting the inhalation of room air results in decreasing the highest concentration of actual inspired oxygen to 60–80%.

13. **Correct answer: B**
If using a Pleur-Evac with autotransfusion connection, make certain all clamps are open. When using any autotransfusion drainage system, make sure to connect the system per the manufacturer's recommendations. Most connections are color coded for easy connecting. Clamps must remain open to allow for blood collection and prevent increased intrathoracic pressures. Subcutaneous air should be checked by palpation and borders marked for further monitoring. If a one-way valve system and suction is used, water is not required to maintain a seal because the valve meets this function.

14. **Correct answer: A**
It is important that the patient and any family members be taught to store oxygen tanks in the upright position. Synthetic materials often cause static electricity. Only lemon-glycerin swabs and not alcohol-based swabs should be used if the patient has dry lips. In this case we do not know if this patient will use O_2 via a mask or cannula.

15. **Correct answer: D**
Mesothelioma is a cancer of the mesothelium. Most cases begin in the pleura or peritoneum.

Mesothelioma is a relatively rare cancer, with approximately 2,000 new cases diagnosed in the United States each year. It occurs more often in men than in women, and the risk of developing this disease increases with age. Symptoms of mesothelioma may not appear until 30 to 50 years after exposure to asbestos. An increased risk of developing mesothelioma has been found among shipyard workers, people who work in asbestos mines and mills, producers of asbestos products, workers in the heating and construction industries, and other trades people.

Symptoms of mesothelioma include dyspnea, pleural effusions, weight loss, and abdominal pain and swelling due to an excess of fluid in the abdomen. Other symptoms of peritoneal mesothelioma may include bowel obstruction, clotting disorders, anemia, and fever. Symptoms with metastases may include pain, dysphagia, or swelling of the neck or face.

Asbestos has been widely used in many industrial products, including cement, duct linings, sound insulation, brake linings, roof shingles, flooring products, textiles, and thermal insulation. If tiny asbestos particles float in the air, especially during the manufacturing process, they may be inhaled or swallowed and can cause serious health problems. In addition to mesothelioma, exposure to asbestos increases the risk of lung cancer, asbestosis, and cancers of the trachea, larynx, and kidney. Smoking does not appear to increase the risk of mesothelioma, but the combination of smoking and exposure increases a person's risk of developing bronchial cancer.

16. **Correct answer: D**
Pulse oximetry readings are considered unreliable when oxygen saturation levels fall below 70%. Pulse oximetry accuracy is impacted by patient motion, low perfusion, venous pulsation, light, poor probe positioning, edema, anemia, and carbon monoxide levels. It is important to compare pulse oximetry values against arterial blood gases to validate values below 70% on the pulse oximeter.

17. **Correct answer: A**
The oxyhemoglobin dissociation curve is a curve that reflects the relationship between dissolved oxygen and the affinity for oxygen by the hemoglobin molecule.

18. **Correct answer: B**
Atrial tachycardia with occasional PVCs is an assessment finding that should be reported to the physician immediately as potential theophylline toxicity. Dosing at 600 mg per day is a high dose and places the patient at risk for toxicity. If diet and/or medications are taken that decrease normal theophylline excretion, the patient may quickly become toxic from the theophylline. Other symptoms to report include insomnia, anxiety, confusion, disorientation, headaches, hypotension, hyperglycemia, and abdominal pain with diarrhea, nausea and vomiting. Diligently monitor electrolytes.

19. **Correct answer: C**
Too much heparin in a glass syringe has dilutional effects and decreases the bicarbonate and the $PaCO_2$.

20. **Correct answer: D**
For every 0.5 mg/kg of theophylline given, there should be a 1 mcg/ml increase in blood levels. Study question note: When given a question with numbers, pay close attention to the type of measurement used. If you know that theophylline level is measured in mcg/ml, then you would be able to automatically rule out 0.5 and 0.75 mg/ml as answers.

21. **Correct answer: D**
Patients taking theophylline should be advised to avoid a high-protein, low carbohydrate diet as it will increase theophylline elimination, leading to low serum levels. Smoking also will cause an increase in medication clearance with resultant low serum levels. Alcohol consumption while on theophylline may result in toxicity due to a

decrease in clearance. Dosing is based on ideal weight, not actual weight, as theophylline does not bind well in the presence of body fat.

22. **Correct answer:** A
    SvO_2 is a measurement of total oxygen consumption.

23. **Correct answer:** D
    Capnography ($PetCO_2$) is not a substitute for pulse oximetry. **Capnography** monitors the concentration or partial pressure of carbon dioxide (CO_2) in the respiratory gases. A pulse oximeter measures the availability of sites on the hemoglobin molecule for oxygen transport versus how many sites are occupied.

24. **Correct answer:** A
    This patient has developed re-expansion pulmonary edema. Removal of large amounts of pleural fluid increases negative intrapleural pressure. Edema occurs when the lung does not re-expand. The patient then develops a severe cough and dyspnea. If the symptoms occur during a thoracentesis, the procedure should be stopped.

25. **Correct answer:** C
    A flail chest is a very painful condition that limits respiratory effort because of the pain. Analgesia and sedation that may be required may also depress respiratory drive and excursion. The CO_2 will increase, PaO_2 will decrease, and the pH will be below 7.35. The patient will develop respiratory acidosis.

26. **Correct answer:** C
    This patient's symptoms are indicative of pertussis. She reports the coughing comes in long episodes that continue until she vomits. What little sputum she produces is very thick and white. A PCR nasal probe should be done as soon as possible. Her family should be examined for signs of pertussis, especially if there are infants or children under the age of 2 or those who have not had a TDaP booster in the past 5 years.

27. **Correct answer:** C
    The driving pressure of air divided by airflow rate determined by airway diameter is known as airway resistance.

28. **Correct answer:** C
    Macrolide antibiotics such as azithromycin, clarithromycin, and erythromycin are recommended treatments for pertussis. Penicillins and tetracyclines are ineffective in treating pertussis.

29. **Correct answer:** B
    Patients with uncontrolled asthma may receive steroids and neuromuscular blocking agents in an attempt to mitigate their symptoms. These patients are at increased risk for prolonged muscle weakness. Uncontrolled asthma symptoms during an attack may lead to prolonged and extensive muscle use to maintain independent respirations. Prolonged effort may result in respiratory failure due to respiratory muscle fatigue. Administration of a neuromuscular blocking agent further inhibits the smooth muscle retractions. Long-term steroid use has been linked to muscle wasting. Ventilatory weaning may be prolonged as respiratory muscles recover from both the disease process and pharmacologic intervention.

30. **Correct answer: C**
Gentamicin is effective against gram-negative rods and penicillin-resistant staphylococci, *Escherichia coli* strains, and *Pseudomonas aeruginosa*. Gentamicin may cause ototoxicity and nephrotoxicity. Gentamicin must never be given as IV push—only as a drip over at least 30–60 minutes. If the patient has oliguria or anuria, the dose must be decreased or discontinued.

31. **Correct answer: B**
Signs and symptoms of a pulmonary embolus can include pleuritic chest pain and decreased cardiac output. An acute pulmonary embolism can be associated with right heart failure. The patient may suffer from nonspecific chest pain, dyspnea, tachycardia, hypotension, shock, and possibly coma.

32. **Correct answer: C**
A normal D-dimer rules out a pulmonary embolism. If the D-dimer is elevated, it may be caused by multiple other conditions. Hyperventilation occurs subsequent to hypoxemia caused by the PE, so respiratory alkalosis will be present, not metabolic alkalosis. Heparin does not dissolve existing clots.

33. **Correct answer: A**
Use Moses' sign to assess for deep venous thrombosis (DVT). Moses' sign is elicited by pressing the calf toward the tibia. This may also elicit pain. These results are not exclusive to DVT but may complement a diagnosis. Traditionally, we were taught to assess Homan's sign: dorsiflexion of the ankle while bending the knee. If that elicited pain, the patient had a problem with circulation and possibly DVT.

34. **Correct answer: C**
A very common and significant finding in a patient with a pneumomediastinum is Hamman's sign. Hamman's sign is a "crunching" sound or a slight clicking sound with each heart sound auscultated over the apex of the heart.

35. **Correct answer: B**
Methylxanthines are an important classification of drugs. In addition to theophylline, caffeine and theobromine are also methylxanthines. Methylxanthines can be found in coffee, tea, and cocoa. Low doses of drugs in this classification can stimulate cortical arousal and in higher doses cause insomnia. They can cause tachycardias and increase production of gastric acid and digestive enzymes. Methylxanthines also inhibit histamine release.

36. **Correct answer: A**
Your patient is probably hypochloremic. Chronic hypoxia leads to chronic respiratory acidosis. The kidneys then retain bicarbonate in the form of sodium bicarbonate. The bicarbonate is exchanged for sodium chloride. Ammonia is weak acid, and excess amounts must be removed from the body. This is done by releasing ammonium chloride. In chronic hypoxia there is an increase in bicarbonate levels and a decrease in chloride levels. Other causes of hypochloremia are NG suction, vomiting, and diarrhea.

37. **Correct answer: D**
Hypoxemia is a decreased oxygen level in the arterial blood or a PaO_2 <80 mmHg. Hypoxia is a decreased oxygen level at the cellular level.

38. **Correct answer: C**
Hyperventilating causes respiratory alkalosis because the patient is unable to get enough oxygen, often due to bronchial constriction. Hypoventilation causes a buildup of CO_2, causing respiratory acidosis, not respiratory alkalosis.

39. **Correct answer: B**
Airflow in a patient with status asthmaticus may be improved by the use of heliox. Heliox is a helium–oxygen mixture that can help with delivery of inhaled medications to decrease the work of breathing. The PEEP must be carefully regulated so as not to cause barotrauma or a dynamic hyperinflation, and it might improve airflow. Norepinephrine is a vasoconstrictor. Nebulizers may also work, but if the patient is compromised the effectiveness is minimal at best.

40. **Correct answer: D**
If you hear faint breath sounds on the left side of the chest and normal sounds on the right side immediately after your patient has been intubated, most likely the right main stem bronchus has been intubated. The right main stem bronchus is somewhat wider and has less of an angle off the main stem bronchus, so it is much more readily intubated.

41. **Correct answer: C**
This result is uncompensated respiratory alkalosis. The pH is greater than 7.45, so the value is an uncompensated alkalosis. To determine whether the alkalosis is respiratory or metabolic, find the value that represents alkalosis: in this case, the CO_2 at <35 mmHg.

42. **Correct answer: A**
This result is compensated metabolic acidosis. The pH is between 7.35 and 7.45, so the value is compensated, but because it is closer to 7.35, the value is considered acidotic. To determine whether the acidosis is respiratory or metabolic, find the value that represents acidosis: in this case, the HCO_3 at <22 mEq/L.

43. **Correct answer: C**
The pH is between 7.35 and 7.45, the CO_2 is between 35 and 45 mmHg, and the HCO_3 is between 22 and 26 mEq/L. All the results are within normal ranges, so this ABG is considered normal.

44. **Correct answer: A**
This result is an uncompensated (mixed) respiratory/metabolic alkalosis. The pH is greater than 7.45, so the value is uncompensated. To determine whether the acidosis is respiratory or metabolic, find the value that represents alkalosis. This would be both the HCO_3 at >26 mEq/L and the CO_2 <35 mmHg, meaning the cause of the alkalosis is both respiratory and metabolic in nature.

45. **Correct answer: B**
This ABG result indicates a compensated respiratory acidosis. The pH is between 7.35 and 7.45, so the value is compensated, but because it is closer to 7.35 the value is considered acidotic. To determine whether the acidosis is respiratory or metabolic, find the value that represents acidosis: in this case, the CO_2 at >45 mmHg.

46. **Correct answer: D**
The result of this blood gas analysis is an uncompensated metabolic acidosis. The pH is less than 7.35, so the value is uncompensated acidosis. To determine whether the acidosis is respiratory or metabolic, find the value that represents acidosis. In this case, the $HCO_3 < 22$ mEq/L.

47. **Correct answer: C**
This blood gas result indicates an uncompensated respiratory acidosis. The pH is <7.35, so the value indicates an uncompensated acidosis. Next, determine which respiratory or metabolic value represents acidosis: in this case, the CO_2 at >45 mmHg.

48. **Correct answer: A**
One cause of decreased SvO_2 is an increased metabolic rate. An increased metabolic rate would increase the O_2 uptake by tissues, resulting in a lower value measured by venous blood gases. The other answers result in a lower tissue oxygen requirement, and thus higher values of oxygen remain in the bloodstream.

49. **Correct answer: D**
This patient is exhibiting signs and symptoms of oxygen toxicity after 5 days of oxygen therapy at >50% FiO_2. Non-rebreather masks provide a minimum of 60% FiO_2 at 6 Lpm. An arterial blood gas would show an increased PaO_2 >100 mmHg, ruling out respiratory failure (PaO_2 <60) that would require intubation. The dry, hacking cough rules out pulmonary edema and the need for Lasix. Numbness in the extremities is from the oxygen radicals in the blood, not a neurologic impairment that would indicate the need for a CT scan with possible tPA administration.

50. **Correct answer: C**
From birth, chest wall compliance decreases. Much of the decrease is due to degeneration and calcification of the costal cartilage; the elasticity decreases as well. Vertebrae develop osteoporosis and a degree of kyphosis can occur. Weight gain is common and posture is affected. Children are more commonly suffering from obesity and frequently develop back problems early in life. The chest wall compliance decreases as does vital capacity. Residual volume increases, PaO_2 decreases, and $PaCO_2$ increases.

51. **Correct answer: D**
Ketamine is both an analgesic and an amnestic.

52. **Correct answer: B**
Fingertip clubbing is an indication of chronic hypoxia.

53. **Correct answer: D**
A semi-reclining or upright position promotes upper lobe drainage. Fluid or secretions will collect if the patient is flat.

54. **Correct answer: C**
To evacuate hemothorax, the tube is placed in the fifth intercostal space, midaxillary line. The chest tube will be low in the thoracic cavity and uses gravity to help clear the fluid. If a hemothorax is not completely removed, there is a possibility an infection will result, which can lead to empyema. When assessing a patient, it is a good idea to

ask (if possible) the origin of any small scars on the thoracic area, as the patient may have had previous problems requiring a chest tube.

55. **Correct answer: B**
ARDS is a type of hypoxemic respiratory failure; the $PaCO_2$ may be decreased or normal. There may be a ventilation/perfusion mismatch (pneumonia, atelectasis) due to an intrapulmonary shunt, or there is increased alveolar dead space (shock, pulmonary embolism). Pulmonary fibrosis may reduce diffusion capacity (COPD, ARDS).

56. **Correct answer: B**
The hypoxemic drive to breathe originates in the aortic and carotid arteries. In the bifurcation of the internal and external carotid arteries, carotid bodies, and aortic bodies (in the carotid arch) are chemoreceptors. When the supply of oxygen decreases, stimulation of the aortic and/or carotid bodies occurs and, in turn, stimulates cortical activity. The result is adrenal gland secretions (epinephrine, norepinephrine), tachycardia, tachypnea, increased respiratory rate, and increased blood pressure.

57. **Correct answer: B**
Severe carbon monoxide poisoning occurs when carboxyhemoglobin levels are higher than 20–40%. If carbon monoxide levels are above 60%, the patient will be comatose and probably die. Smokers often have carboxyhemoglobin levels of 5–10%. Normal levels in nonsmokers are less than 2%.

58. **Correct answer: D**
Elimination of carbon monoxide from the body is via the lungs. In cases of severe carbon monoxide (CO) poisoning, hyperbaric therapy must be utilized to force the CO molecule off the hemoglobin, but it is eliminated by the lungs.

59. **Correct answer: D**
Subcutaneous emphysema usually occurs in the thorax as a result of a pulmonary air leak. This air leak may be secondary to the patient receiving positive pressure ventilation or from alveolar rupture from a pneumothorax. The air travels along under the skin, may be easily palpated, and may feel like a crackling sensation. Patients who have chest tubes often have at least a small amount of subcutaneous emphysema at the tube insertion site. Sometimes the patient feels pain when palpation is performed because the air tears the tissue. The free air must be reabsorbed, and this may take several days.

60. **Correct answer: B**
Pulse oximetry should never be used during a cardiac arrest. During resuscitation, blood pressure and blood flow may vary. The pharmacologic effects of medications such as vasoactive drugs used during resuscitation will compromise SpO_2 values.

61. **Correct answer: B**
Pulse oximetry values do not directly correlate with PaO_2. You must use ABGs to determine the PaO_2, the amount of oxygen available to the tissues. SpO_2 only measures the number of hemoglobin binding sites that are occupied compared with the number of hemoglobin binding sites available. The columns listed below show the probable correlation.

Interpretation of Pulse Oximetry Values (SpO_2)

Value of Pulse Oximeter (%)	Probable PaO_2
97	100
95	80
94	70
90	60
85	50
75	40
57	30
32	20
10	10

62. **Correct answer: C**
To prevent complications with chest tube drainage systems, the suction level should not be higher than –40 cm/H_2O. Maintaining suction levels at higher than –40 cm/H_2O may cause re-expansion pulmonary edema, pleural air leaks, and lung tissue entrapment. The lung may not be able to expand properly.

63. **Correct answer: B**
Chest tube drainage tubing should be placed horizontally on the bed then down to the collection chamber. If a mediastinal chest tube is in place, bubbling in the water seal chamber may indicate a communication between the mediastinal space and the pleural space. The physician should be notified immediately. However, some sporadic bubbling will occur when suction is first turned on because fluid has to displace air in the collection chamber. Chest tube tubing that is dependent or coiled will allow for the accumulation of drainage. This obstruction may increase pressure in the lung.

64. **Correct answer: C**
Acetylcysteine is considered to be a mucolytic agent. Acetylcysteine has a sulfide group that effectively splits disulfine bonds in mucin molecules. The viscosity of the mucus is reduced. Atropine is an anticholinergic. Terbutaline and albuterol are B2 agonists.

65. **Correct answer: D**
Side effects of acetylcysteine include bronchospasms. Thinning the mucus may promote excessive coughing with resultant brochospasms. Additional side effects include rhinorrhea, stomatitus, nausea, and vomiting.

66. **Correct answer: D**
Emphysema actually increases lung compliance. Pulmonary edema, pleural effusions, and obesity decrease lung compliance. Other factors that decrease compliance are atelectasis, fibrotic changes, abdominal distension, pain (causes splinting), and flail chest (pain and loss of structure).

67. **Correct answer: D**
One of the most effective ways to relieve bronchospasms is to use a B2 receptor agonist. The B2 receptor agonists lower cellular calcium levels and relax bronchial smooth muscle. The selective B2 receptor agonists do not produce cardiac stimulation. The cardiac stimulation can result in tachycardia and reduced cardiac output.

68. **Correct answer: C**
The best position to place this patient to minimize the venous air embolism is Trendelenburg with left decubitus tilt. This position minimizes any air from migrating through the heart and into the lungs.

69. **Correct answer: A**
A venous air embolism may be caused by hemodialysis. Other potential causes are central and pulmonary artery catheters, endoscopy, and automatic pressure-driven injectors.

70. **Correct answer: B**
A risk factor for thrombolic emboli includes carcinoma. Neoplasms, obesity, trauma, dysrhythmias, congestive heart failure (CHF), and prolonged immobility are also factors.

71. **Correct answer: C**
Sternocleodomastoid retractions indicate that an asthmatic patient is using accessory muscles to facilitate ventilation. Air is trapped in the air passages, so the patient has to create a higher negative pleural pressure by elevating the rib cage.

72. **Correct answer: C**
Your patient ceased wheezing during his asthma attack. This change in his condition means respiratory failure and intubation are imminent. If the patient is wheezing, it means air is getting through a narrowed opening. Asthmatics undergo air trapping when the inspired air must exit through a narrowed air passage. If the patient stops wheezing, it means no air is able to enter or exit the air passages.

73. **Correct answer: B**
Wheezing would not usually be present if the patient had pneumonia. There is an old mnemonic for asthma that can assist the acute care nurse with determining a possible cause of a patient's distress. This mnemonic is ASTHMATIC:

A Asthma: Precipitating factor or event
S Stasis: DVT, pulmonary embolus
T Toxins: Smoke, chemical irritants, insecticides, perfumes, cleaning agents
H Heart: CHF, noncardiogenic pulmonary edema
M Mechanical: Foreign body aspiration
A Allergy: Anaphylaxis, aspiration (gastric contents), near drowning
T Trauma: Upper airway, possible lower airway
I Infection: Bronchitis, bronchiolitis, croup, pneumonia
C Congenital: Cystic fibrosis, chronic COPD

74. **Correct answer: D**
Slo-Bid is a form of theophylline. Side effects of theophylline include muscle cramps, jitteryness, headache, nausea, vomiting, dysrhythmias, and gastrointestinal issues.

75. **Correct answer: A**
Long-acting forms of B2 agonists used in the treatment of asthma include salmeterol (Serevent®) and formoterol (Foradil®). Short-acting beta2 agonists used for emergency treatment of asthma include albuterol (Proventil® HFA, Ventolin® HFA, Accuneb®, ProAir®), metaproterenol (Alupent®), levalbuterol (Xoponex® HFA, Xoponex® nebulizer solution), and pirbuterol (Maxair®).

76. **Correct answer: B**
The most common symptoms seen with active TB are night sweats, fever, fatigue, hemoptysis, weight loss, and chest pain. The cough would not be dry, and there would not be wheezing.

77. **Correct answer: A**
The patient has a positive PPD. Until a chest X-ray and AFB sputum culture are done, this patient is highly suspicious for TB. It is important to find out if the patient received BCG if they were born outside the United States. Once TB is confirmed, treatment should start right away for this patient and he should be placed in a room with a laminar airflow system.

78. **Correct answer: C**
Rimantadine is used to shorten the length and severity of influenza. It is not used to treat TB. Isoniazid, rifampin, and pyrazidamide are all medications used to treat latent TB infections.

79. **Correct answer: D**
Succinylcholine combines with acetylcholine to cause smooth muscle relaxation, not contraction. Prolonged use may cause a change in blocking action and result in potassium-regulated alterations in electrical activity. Side effects of succinylcholine include malignant hyperthermia and hypertension or hypotension, hyperkalemia, anaphylaxis, and increased intraocular pressure.

80. **Correct answer: C**
Accessory pathways connecting a small airway to an airspace normally supplied by other pathways are called canals of Lambert.

81. **Correct answer: C**
Falsely low readings on a pulse oximeter may be due to patient motion. If the patient is hypothermic or has decreased peripheral perfusion, the results will be inaccurate. Position of the probe can also cause inaccurate readings on a pulse oximeter.

82. **Correct answer: A**
Prior to the administration of vancomycin, the PCU nurse should know that vancomycin is nephrotoxic, especially if used in combination with aminoglycosides. Vancomycin is used in the treatment of methicillin-resistant strains (*Staphylococcus epidermidis*) and must be administered by slow intravenous drip.

83. **Correct answer: C**
Antimicrobial soap and water may be used to decontaminate hands before, during, and after patient care regardless of glove use, visible soiling, or no apparent soiling. Hands should always be decontaminated using soap and water, waterless soap, or alcohol-based antiseptic agent before and after patient care to prevent the spread of organisms from patient to patient or from surfaces. Alcohol-based antiseptic agents should only be used if no visible soiling is observed.

84. Correct answer: C
The laryngeal mask airway was intended as a temporary airway. It requires minimal training to insert, but cannot be placed by RNs as a matter of course. The patient must be unconscious and/or without gag reflex. The seal around the mask is a low pressure seal, so it cannot be used on patients with high peak ventilator pressures. The LMA has a significant risk of aspiration. Advantages with use of this airway are that it is simply blindly inserted into the hypopharynx, does not require visualization of the vocal cords, and does not traumatize the trachea. Patients will not have hoarseness or lose their voice altogether. At best, patients will complain of a mild sore throat.

85. Correct answer: C
At higher altitudes there is decreasing atmospheric pressure to force oxygen into the lungs, and therefore the O_2 saturation would decrease. To compensate, the person must breathe faster. The percentage of oxygen remains the same and the partial pressure of the oxygen decreases. Arterial PaO_2 decreases, and the O_2 saturation decreases as well. The rapid breathing will result in hyperventilation, lowering the pH and raising the $PaCO_2$ levels.

86. Correct answer: C
Inhaled nitric oxide (iNO) is a selective pulmonary vasodilator to treat pulmonary hypertension. iNO reduces death or the need for extracorporeal membrane oxygenation (ECMO), but the positive effect is in reducing the ECMO requirement. Do not use iNO on patients who are dependent on a right-to-left shunt.

87. Correct answer: A
An action of nitric oxide is to cause vascular smooth muscle relaxation. Nitric oxide is the molecule released from the endothelium that enables smooth muscle relaxation. Nitric oxide inhibits platelet aggregation and adherence and is thought to alter vascular permeability. It may also participate in nonspecific immunity because it is generated when macrophages are activated.

88. Correct answer: D
CPAP, or continuous positive airway pressure, may be delivered by nasal prongs, nasopharyngeal tubes, or endotracheal tubes. CPAP provides increased pressure to the posterior pharynx and increases transpulmonary pressure. It can prevent alveolar collapse and helps prevent obstructive apnea.

89. Correct answer: B
Excessive CPAP may increase intrathoracic pressure to the point of compressing the right atrium and vena cava. The preload will be decreased and cardiac output will be reduced.

90. Correct answer: C
If positive inspiratory pressure (PIP) is increased on a mechanical ventilator, the result is a decrease in the $PaCO_2$ and an increase in the PaO_2.

91. Correct answer: D
Fluid therapy in ARDS is directed toward maintaining a low circulating fluid volume. The fluid volume is kept low to keep the intracardiac and intrapleural pressures at minimal levels. If too much fluid is present, there may be leakage through damaged capillaries into the interstitial space.

92. **Correct answer: C**
Research on normal saline use in tracheal suctioning has proven that normal saline causes anxiety, increased risk for hospital-acquired pneumonia, and bronchoconstriction. Current recommendations focus on dry suctioning, frequent oral care, balanced hydration, and position changes prevent complications associated with intubation and mechanical ventilation.

93. **Correct answer: B**
SIMV, or synchronized intermittent mandatory ventilation, still provides a set frequency of breaths and either volume or pressure. The patient is permitted to breathe spontaneously at their own volume between mandatory ventilations. If the spontaneous breath occurs at the same time as a mandatory breath, the ventilator will synchronize with the patient, thus preventing "stacked" breaths. The other modes of ventilation listed (CMV, HFV, and oscillation) represent full control of setting by an operator and not the patient's responses.

94. **Correct answer: B**
When a closed system is used, there is extra weight that can increase tension on the catheter or tubing. This may cause the ET or trach to move. Lack of available oxygen and cost effectiveness are characteristics of open catheter suctioning. The inline system is multi-use and is cost effective. Many manufacturers make the inline tubing for both ET tubes and tracheostomy tubes. Nurses must make certain they are using the correct tube for suctioning. Another problem with the inline catheters is the extra tubing that hangs out when the catheter is not in use. The patient may easily reach this tubing and extubate themselves or push the catheter down the airway and obstruct airflow.

95. **Correct answer: A**
A disadvantage of using a tracheostomy tube is subcutaneous emphysema. There are a large number of potential complications with the use of a tracheostomy tube. Some of these complications include tracheal stenosis, tracheal malacia, aspiration, infection, hemorrhage, and pneumothorax.

96. **Correct answer: D**
The function of a stoma stent is to keep the stoma tract open. The stents can be manufactured in either the straight or curved configuration. The stent rests against the anterior wall of the trachea and allows for freer passage of air and the patient can breathe spontaneously around the tube. Because of the differing nature of air passages, the stents are made straight and curved.

97. **Correct answer: B**
Silicone or plastic tracheostomy tubes contain wires, so the magnet in the MRI will attract the wires in the tube. The silicone or plastic tubes cannot tolerate repeated cleanings. Use of a one-way speaking valve is contraindicated when using a foam cuff because the cuff may lie at an angle to the valve due to its orientation in the airway. Cost is actually higher to facilities because the tubes are difficult to keep clean and are labor intensive.

98. **Correct answer: B**
CPAP should be used with caution in patients with basilar skull fractures. Research has shown that pneumocephalus may occur if a basilar skull fracture exists. CPAP helps by

increasing the functional residual capacity by helping to re-expand the alveoli. Patients that have acute cardiogenic pulmonary edema may also benefit from the use of CPAP.

99. **Correct answer: A**
This result is an uncompensated metabolic alkalosis. The pH is greater than 7.45, so the value is uncompensated. To determine whether the alkalosis is respiratory or metabolic, find the value that represents alkalosis: in this case, the HCO_3 at >26 mEq/L.

100. **Correct answer: B**
The pH is between 7.35 and 7.45, the CO_2 is between 35 and 45 mmHg, and the HCO_3 is between 22 and 26 mEq/L. All the results are within normal ranges, so this ABG is considered normal.

101. **Correct answer: D**
This is an uncompensated (mixed) respiratory/metabolic acidosis. The pH is less than 7.35, so the value is uncompensated acidosis. To determine whether the acidosis is respiratory or metabolic, find the value that represents acidosis. This would be both the HCO_3 at <22 mEq/L and the CO_2 > 45 mmHg, meaning the cause of the acidosis is both respiratory and metabolic in nature.

102. **Correct answer: B**
This blood gas result indicates a compensated metabolic acidosis. The pH is between 7.35 and 7.45, so the gas is compensated, but the value is closer to acidosis, making the value compensated acidosis. Determine which respiratory or metabolic value is acidotic: in this case, the HCO_3 at <22 mEq/L.

103. **Correct answer: A**
This result signifies an uncompensated respiratory alkalosis. The pH is greater than 7.45, so the value is uncompensated alkalosis. To determine whether the alkalosis is respiratory or metabolic, find the value that represents alkalosis: in this case, the CO_2 at <35 mmHg.

104. **Correct answer: C**
This result demonstrates a compensated respiratory alkalosis. The pH is between 7.35 and 7.45, so the value is compensated, but because it is closer to 7.45, the value is considered alkalotic. To determine whether the alkalosis is respiratory or metabolic, find the value that represents alkalosis: in this case, the CO_2 at <35 mmHg.

105. **Correct answer: B**
This result is an uncompensated respiratory acidosis. The pH is less than 7.35, so the value is uncompensated. To determine whether the acidosis is respiratory or metabolic, find the value that represents acidosis: in this case, the CO_2 at >45 mmHg.

106. **Correct answer: A**
The pH (between 7.35 and 7.45), the CO_2 (between 35 and 45 mmHg), and the HCO_3 (22 and 26 mEq/L) are within normal ranges, so the ABG is considered normal.

107. **Correct answer: B**
This result is an uncompensated (mixed) respiratory/metabolic acidosis. The pH is less than 7.35, so the value is uncompensated acidosis. To determine whether the acidosis is respiratory or metabolic, find the value that represents acidosis. This would be both the HCO_3 at <22 mEq/L and the CO_2 >45 mmHg, meaning the cause of the acidosis is both respiratory and metabolic in nature.

108. **Correct answer:** C
Sidenafil is given orally to inhibit rapid rise in pulmonary artery pressure secondary to hypoxia.

109. **Correct answer:** C
Prior to insertion of an LMA, the patient must have an absent gag reflex. The laryngeal mask airway cannot be inserted by nurses unless they have specialized training. The LMA does not usually cause hoarseness because it does not pass through the vocal cords. There is a high risk of aspiration with LMA usage.

110. **Correct answer:** C
Symptoms from aspirated gastric contents have a gradual onset. The patient may develop ARDS, but not always. If the pH is >2.5, very little necrosis will occur. If the pH is <2.5, there is probability of pulmonary edema, necrosis, bleeding, and atelectasis.

111. **Correct answer:** A
Prone positioning is the best position to promote drainage and oxygenation for a patient with ARDS. It is often the most difficult position to achieve without proper lifting and safety devices.

112. **Correct answer:** C
Patients with pulmonary hypertension present with dyspnea during exertion, right-sided heart failure, increased respiratory and heart rates, and a prominent S_2. Additional signs of pulmonary hypertension include fatigue and lethargy, enlarged liver, and pulmonary congestion. Cyanosis is a late sign of pulmonary hypertension.

113. **Correct answer:** B
Calcium channel blockers are used to treat primary pulmonary hypertension. Patients treated with nitric oxide improve faster when also treated with calcium channel blockers due to abnormalities in the membrane function.

114. **Correct answer:** D
Without initial, aggressive treatment of pulmonary hypertension, the medial smooth muscles in arterioles irreversibly thicken. This is due to development of high right-sided ventricular pressures and heart failure.

115. **Correct answer:** C
Pulmonary hypertension results in hypoxia and hypoxemia, leading to vasoconstriction. As vasoconstriction continues, the vessel walls begin to alter with increases in elastin and collagen. Prolonged vasoconstriction leads to increased shunting and blood pooling. Serum testing for abnormalities further increases the risks and progression of irreversible epithelial changes.

116. **Correct answer:** A
An absolute contraindication for use of rapid sequence intubation (RSI) is a total loss of facial and/or oropharyngeal landmarks, which requires a surgical airway. Another absolute contraindication is a total upper airway obstruction that requires surgical intervention. Relative contraindications for RSI include an airway where intubation may not be successful or an arrest "crash" intubation when there is no time for preoxygenation, pretreatment, or induction and paralysis.

117. Correct answer: D

Rapid sequence intubation (RSI) is not necessary to use for all cervical spine-injured patients. It would be appropriate for use if there is edema and loss of airway patency. Prolonged respiratory effort that results in fatigue or failure, a stab wound to neck with an expanding hematoma, and an uncooperative trauma patient with life-threatening injuries are indications for use of RSI.

118. Correct answer: C

During rapid sequence intubation, cricoid cartilage pressure is often used to help prevent vomiting and aspiration of gastric contents. The esophagus is obstructed by the pressure to the anterior neck. This maneuver is known as the Sellick maneuver. The American Heart Association takes the position that the Sellick maneuver not be routinely used unless the person performing the maneuver is well trained and experienced.

PULMONARY REFERENCES

Abunasser, J., Tejada, J. P., & Foley, R. J. (2012). The diagnosis and management of pulmonary embolism. *Connecticut Medicine, 76*(1), 5–14.

Agarwal, R., Aggarwal, A. N., & Gupta, D. (2010). Role of noninvasive ventilation in acute lung injury/acute respiratory distress syndrome: A proportion meta-analysis. *Respiratory Care, 55*(12), 1653–1660.

Ahrens, T., Prentice, D., & Kleinpell, R. M. (2011). *Progressive care nursing certification: Preparation, review and practice exams*. St. Louis, MO: McGraw-Hill.

Allan, P. F., Amjadi, D. K., & Haynes, R. L. (2011). Diffuse alveolar hemorrhage: A rare manifestation of trauma. *Military Medicine, 176*(9), 1071–1076.

Almond, M. H., McAuley, D. F., Wise, M. P., & Griffiths, M. J. (2012). Influenza-related pneumonia. *Clinical Medicine, 12*(1), 67–70.

American Association of Critical-Care Nurses. (2006). *AACN core curriculum for critical care nursing*. St. Louis, MO: Saunders.

Anand, R. J., Whelan, J. F., Ferrada, P., Duane, T. M., Malhotra, A. K., Aboutanos, M. B., & Ivatury, R. R. (2012). Thin chest wall is an independent risk factor for the development of pneumothorax after chest tube removal. *American Surgeon, 78*(4), 478–480.

Azemi, T., Almahasneh, F., Elbash, F., Cheema, M., Divinagracia, T., Dougherty, J., . . . Sadiq, I. (2012). Ultrasound-assisted catheter-directed thrombolytic therapy for management of acute pulmonary embolism. *Connecticut Medicine, 76*(4), 197–200.

Ballantine, M., Bhimani, M., & Milne, W. K. (2012). Diagnostic approach to pulmonary embolism in a rural emergency department. *Canadian Journal of Rural Medicine, 17*(1), 17–20.

Blaiss, M. S., Nathan, R. A., Stoloff, S. W., Meltzer, E. O., Murphy, K. R., & Doherty, D. E. (2012). Patient and physician asthma deterioration terminology: Results from the 2009 Asthma Insight and Management survey. *Allergy and Asthma Proceedings, 33*(1), 47–53.

Borba Monteiro, M., Cortozi Berton, D., Fontoura Moreira, M.Â., Saldanha Menna-Barreto, S., & Zimermann Teixeira, P. J. (2012). Effects of expiratory positive airway pressure on dynamic hyperinflation during exercise in patients with COPD. *Respiratory Care, 57*(9), 1405–1412.

Boulet, L. P. (2011). Asthma control, education, and the role of the respiratory therapist. *Canadian Journal of Respiratory Therapy, 47*(4), 15–21.

Boutou, A. K., Pitsiou, G. G., Trigonis, I., Papakosta, D., Kontou, P. K., Chavouzis, N., ... Stanopoulos, I. (2011). Exercise capacity in idiopathic pulmonary fibrosis: The effect of pulmonary hypertension. *Respirology, 16*(3), 451–458.

Boyer, L., Plantier, L., Dagouassat, M., Lanone, S., Goven, D., Caramelle, P., . . . Boczkowski, J. (2011). Role of nitric oxide synthases in elastase-induced emphysema. *Laboratory Investigation, 91*(3), 353–362.

Brandão, D. C., Britto, M. C., Pessoa, M. F., de Sá, R. B., Alcoforado, L., Matos, L. O., . . . de Andrade, A. D. (2011). Heliox and forward-leaning posture improve the efficacy of nebulized bronchodilator in acute asthma: A randomized trial. *Respiratory Care, 56*(7), 947–952.

Brorsen, A. (2012). *CEN examination review*. Burlington, MA: Jones & Bartlett Learning.

Brorsen, A., & Rogelet, K. (2009). *PCCN certification review*. Sudbury, MA: Jones and Bartlett.

Cantón, R., & del Campo, R. (2010). Cystic fibrosis: Deciphering the complexity. *Clinical Microbiology and Infection, 16*(7), 793–797.

Cao, B., Ren, L. L., Zhao, F., Gonzalez, R., Song, S. F., Bai, L., . . . Wang, C. (2010). Viral and *Mycoplasma pneumoniae* community-acquired pneumonia and novel clinical outcome evaluation in ambulatory adult patients in China. *European Journal of Clinical Microbiology & Infectious Diseases, 29*(11), 1443–1448.

Caramori, G., Lasagna, L., Casalini, A. G., Adcock, I. M., Casolari, P., Contoli, M., . . . Bertorelli, G. (2011). Immune response to Mycobacterium tuberculosis infection in the parietal pleura of patients with tuberculous pleurisy. *PLoS ONE, 6*(7), 1–17.

Castor, J. M., Wood, R. K., Muir, A. J., Palmer, S. M., & Shimpi, R. A. (2010). Gastroesophageal reflux and altered motility in lung transplant rejection. *Neurogastroenterology and Motility, 22*(8), 841–850.

Choi, J. H., Kim, E. J., Kim, Y. S., Kim, T. H., Choi, J., Kwon, S. Y., . . . Lee, S. H. (2011). Effectiveness of nasal surgery alone on sleep quality, architecture, position, and sleep-disordered breathing in obstructive sleep apnea syndrome with nasal obstruction. *American Journal of Rhinology & Allergy, 25*(5), 338–341.

Chulay, M., & Burns, S. (2010). *Essentials of progressive care nursing* (2nd ed.). St. Louis, MO: McGraw-Hill.

Conese, M. (2011). Cystic fibrosis and the innate immune system: Therapeutic implications. *Endocrine, Metabolic & Immune Disorders Drug Targets, 11*(1), 8–22.

Curley, M. A. Q. (2007). *Synergy: The unique relationship between nurses and patients*. St. Louis, MO: Saunders.

DeBonville, D. (2012). Is atypical pneumonia becoming... more typical? *Medical Laboratory Observer, 44*(9), 14–18.

Dhaked, R. K., Singh, M. K., Singh, P., & Gupta, P. (2010). Botulinum toxin: Bioweapon & magic drug. *Indian Journal of Medical Research, 132*(5), 489–503.

Ding, Q., Luckhardt, T., Hecker, L., Zhou, Y., Liu, G., Antony, V. B., . . . Thannickal, V. J. (2011). New insights into the pathogenesis and treatment of idiopathic pulmonary fibrosis. *Drugs, 71*(8), 981–1001.

Donohoe-Dennison, R. (2007). *Pass CCRN (*3rd ed.). St. Louis, MO: Mosby.

dos Santos, V. M., Zembrzuski, M. M., Gouvea, I. P., Nery, N. S., & dos Santos, L. A. (2011). Massive pleural effusion due to metastasis of prostate cancer. *The West Indian Medical Journal, 60*(6), 690–693.

Driver, C. (2012). Pneumonia part 1: Pathology, presentation and prevention. *British Journal of Nursing, 21*(2), 103–106.

Driver, C. (2012). Pneumonia part 2: Signs, symptoms and vaccinations. *British Journal of Nursing, 21*(4), 245–249.

Echevarría, I. M., & Schwoebel, A. (2012). Development of an intervention model for the prevention of aspiration pneumonia in high-risk patients on a medical-surgical unit. *MEDSURG Nursing, 21*(5), 303–308.

Eisenstadt, E. S. (2010). Dysphagia and aspiration pneumonia in older adults. *Journal of the American Academy of Nurse Practitioners, 22*(1), 17–22.

Fadda, G. (2012). Tuberculosis: Novel approaches to an old disease. *Journal of Infection In Developing Countries, 6*(1), 4–5.

Fink, J. B., & Ari, A. (2011). Posture perfect: The role of positioning during bronchodilator administration with oxygen or heliox. *Respiratory Care, 56*(7), 1056–1057.

Freeman, S. (2011). Care of adult patients with a temporary tracheostomy. *Nursing Standard, 26*(2), 49–56.

Fujioka, M., & Yakabe, A. (2009). Does inhalation injury increase the mortality rate in burn patients? Investigation of relationship between inhalation injury and severity of burn surface. *Signa Vitae, 4*(2), 20–22.

Gaguski, M. E., Brandsema, M., Gernalin, L., Martinez, E. , & Steele-Moses, S. K. (2010). Assessing dyspnea in patients with non-small cell lung cancer in the acute care setting. *Clinical Journal of Oncology Nursing, 14*(4), 509–513.

Galloway, M. (2012). Improving long-term outcomes in asthma. *Practice Nurse, 42*(2), 19–21.

Griffiths, K. (2011). Cystic fibrosis and the role of support workers. *British Journal of Healthcare Assistants, 5*(7), 326–330.

Gul, E. E., Abdulhalikov, T., Aslan, R., & Aydogdu, I. (2011). A rare and undesirable complication of heparin-induced thrombocytopenia: Acute massive pulmonary embolism. *Clinical and Applied Thrombosis/Hemostasis, 17*(5), 546–548.

Gunta, S., & Kamath, S. (2012). A case of pulmonary embolism and stroke in a 16-year-old girl. *WMJ, 111*(2), 58–60.

Hallowell, R. W., Reed, R. M., Fraig, M., Horton, M. R., & Girgis, R. E. (2012). Severe pulmonary hypertension in idiopathic nonspecific interstitial pneumonia. *Pulmonary Circulation, 2*(1), 101–106.

Hardin, S., & Kaplow, R. (2005). *Synergy for clinical excellence: The AACN synergy model for patient care*. St. Louis, MO: Saunders.

Hawley, P. C., & Hawley, M. P. (2011). Difficulties in diagnosing pulmonary embolism in the obese patient: A literature review. *Vascular Medicine, 16*(6), 444–451.

Headley, C. M., & Melander, S. (2011). When it may be a pulmonary embolism. *Nephrology Nursing Journal, 38*(2), 127–152.

Hebeda, C. B., Teixeira, S. A., Tamura, E. K., Muscará, M. N., de Mello, S. B., Markus, R. P., & Farsky, S. H. (2011). Nitric oxide modulates lipopolysaccharide-induced endothelial platelet endothelial cell adhesion molecule expression via interleukin-10. *Clinical and Experimental Immunology, 165*(2), 172–179.

Hira, H. S., & Ranjan, R. (2011). Role of percutaneous closed needle pleural biopsy among patients of undiagnosed exudative pleural effusion. *Lung India, 28*(2), 101–104.

Hirst, D., & Robson, T. (2010). Nitric oxide in cancer therapeutics: Interaction with cytotoxic chemotherapy. *Current Pharmaceutical Design, 16*(4), 411–420.

Homer, R. J., Elias, J. A., Lee, C. G., & Herzog, E. (2011). Modern concepts on the role of inflammation in pulmonary fibrosis. *Archives of Pathology & Laboratory Medicine, 135*(6), 780–788.

Hu, X. H., Duan, Y. Y., Li, Y., & Xue, Z. Q. (2010). Early responses of VEGF during acute lung injury induced by seawater immersion after open chest trauma. *Respiration, 79*(6), 490–496.

Husain, L. F., Hagopian, L., Wayman, D., Baker, W. E., & Carmody, K. A. (2012). Sonographic diagnosis of pneumothorax. *Journal of Emergencies, Trauma & Shock, 5*(1), 76–81.

Hutchinson, A., Brand, C., Irving, L., Roberts, C., Thompson, P., & Campbell, D. (2010, May). Acute care costs of patients admitted for management of chronic obstructive pulmonary disease exacerbations: Contribution of disease severity, infection and chronic heart failure. *Internal Medicine Journal, 40*(5), 364–371.

Idla, A., Kivistik, T., Põder, K., Malikov, V., Annus, R., Pulges, A., & Põder, P. (2012). Blunt injury of descending thoracic aorta: Complicated but successful endovascular treatment. *Acta Angiologica, 18*(1), 35–39.

Inonu, H., Doruk, S., Sahin, S., Erkorkmaz, U., Celik, D., Celikel, S., & Seyfikli, Z. (2012). Oxidative stress levels in exhaled breath condensate associated with COPD and smoking. *Respiratory Care, 57*(3), 413–419.

Jankowich, M. D., & Rounds, S. (2010). Combined pulmonary fibrosis and emphysema alters physiology but has similar mortality to pulmonary fibrosis without emphysema. *Lung, 188*(5), 365–373.

Jiayun, X., Adeboyejo, O., Wagley, E., Aubrecht, J., Mi-Kyung, S., Thiry, L., & DeVito-Dabbs, A. (2012). Daily burdens of recipients and family caregivers after lung transplant. *Progress in Transplantation, 22*(1), 41–48.

Jones & Bartlett Learning. (2011.) *2012 nurse's drug handbook. (*11th ed.). Sudbury, MA: Jones & Bartlett Learning.

Kadaria, D., Long, A., Spencer, J., Pant, N., Bankole, O., & Sprabery, L. (2011). Catamenial pneumothorax: A rare cause of primary spontaneous pneumothorax. *Tennessee Medicine, 104*(3), 35–36.

Kaufman, G. (2011). Asthma: Pathophysiology, diagnosis and management. *Nursing Standard, 26*(5), 48–56.

Kaufman, G. (2012). Asthma update: Recommendations for diagnosis, treatment and management. *Primary Health Care, 22*(5), 32–39.

Keal, J. L., & Davies, P. D. (2011). Tuberculosis: A forgotten plague? *Journal of the Royal Society of Medicine, 104*(5), 182–184.

Kirschbaum, C., & Peeples, C. (2011). Donation after cardiac death for lung transplant: A case study. *Progress in Transplantation, 21*(2), 156–160.

Koç, U., Karnak, D., Güzin Ö. K., & Kayacan, O. (2012). Trace elements (copper, zinc and selenium) in acute COPD exacerbation. *Trace Elements & Electrolytes, 29*(1), 59–64.

Kopcke, D., Harryman, O., Benbow, E. W., Hay, C., & Chalmers, N. (2011). Mortality from pulmonary embolism is decreasing in hospital patients. *Journal of the Royal Society of Medicine, 104*(8), 327–331.

Korkmaz, A., Ozlu, T., Ozsu, S., Kazaz, Z., & Bulbul, Y. (2012). Long-term outcomes in acute pulmonary thromboembolism: The incidence of chronic thromboembolic pulmonary hypertension and associated risk factors. *Clinical and Applied Thrombosis/Hemostasis, 18*(3), 281–288.

Kosciuch, J., Krenke, R., Gorska, K., Baran, W., Kujawa, M., Hildebrand, K., & Chazan, R. (2012). Comparison of airway wall remodeling in asthma and COPD: Biopsy findings. *Respiratory Care, 57*(4), 557–564.

Leder, S. B., Suiter, D. M., & Green, B. G. (2011). Silent aspiration risk is volume-dependent. *Dysphagia, 26*(3), 304–309.

Legare, C., & Sawatzky, J. V. (2010). Dyspnea in the thoracic trauma patient: A human response to illness. *Journal of Trauma Nursing, 17*(1), 36–44.

Light, R. W. (2011). Pleural controversy: Optimal chest tube size for drainage. *Respirology, 16*(2), 244–248.

Lo, D., & Shapiro, M. L. (2010). Extrathoracic lung herniation from blunt trauma: A review. *Journal of Surgical Radiology, 1*, 20–31.

Luisetti, M., Bruno, P., Kadija, Z., Suzuki, T., Raffa, S., Torrisi, M. R., . . . Mariotta, S. (2011). Relationship between diffuse pulmonary fibrosis, alveolar proteinosis, and granulocyte-macrophage colony stimulating factor autoantibodies. *Respiratory Care, 56*(10), 1608–1610.

Lynn-McHale Wiegand, D. J. (Ed.). (2011). *AACN procedure manual for critical care* (6th ed.). St. Louis, MO: Saunders.

MacKenzie, M. (2011). An alternative to the standard tracheostomy tube: One clinic's experience with stoma stents. *Canadian Journal of Respiratory Therapy, 47*(3), 24–28.

Mailhot, G. (2012). Vitamin D bioavailability in cystic fibrosis: A cause for concern? *Nutrition Reviews, 70*(5), 280–293.

Manno, E. (Ed). (2012). *Emergency management in neurocritical care.* Hoboken, NJ: Wiley-Blackwell.

Matura, L. A. (2011). Pulmonary arterial hypertension: An overview. *British Journal of Cardiac Nursing, 6*(6), 268–277.

McCutcheon, L., & Yelland, M. (2011). Iatrogenic pneumothorax: Safety concerns when using acupuncture or dry needling in the thoracic region. *Physical Therapy Reviews, 16*(2), 126–132.

McGrath, E. E., & Anderson, P. B. (2011). Diagnosis of pleural effusion: A systematic approach. *American Journal of Critical Care, 20*(2), 119–128.

McManus, R., Fitzmaurice, D., Murray, E., & Taylor, C. (2012). Thromboembolism. *American Family Physician, 85*(2), 188–190.

Meyer, G., Roy, P. M., Gilberg, S., & Perrier, A. (2011). Pulmonary embolism. *Praxis, 100*(4), 237–239.

Milian, A., Nierenberg, K., Fleming, L. E., Bean, J. A., Wanner, A., Reich, A., . . . Kirkpatrick, B. (2007). Reported respiratory symptom intensity in asthmatics during exposure to aerosolized Florida red tide toxins. *Journal of Asthma, 44*(7), 583–587.

Mirmohammad-Sadeghi, M., Etesampour, A., Gharipour, M., Shariat, Z., Nilforoush, P., Saeidi, M., . . . Sadeghi, F. M. (2009). Early chest tube removal after coronary artery bypass graft surgery. *North American Journal of Medical Sciences, 1*(7), 333–337.

Mooi, F. R., van Loo, I. H., van Gent, M., He, Q., Bart, M. J., Heuvelman, K. J., . . . Mertsola, J. (2009). *Bordetella pertussis* strains with increased toxin production associated with pertussis resurgence. *Emerging Infectious Diseases, 15*(8), 1206–1213.

Murphy, K. R., Meltzer, E. O., Blaiss, M. S., Nathan, R. A., Stoloff, S. W., & Doherty, D. E. (2012). Asthma management and control in the United States: Results of the 2009 Asthma Insight and Management survey. *Allergy and Asthma Proceedings, 33*(1), 54–64.

Murphy, K. R., Uryniak, T., Martin, U. J., & Zangrilli, J. (2012). The effect of budesonide/formoterol pressurized metered-dose inhaler on predefined criteria for worsening asthma in four different patient populations with asthma. *Drugs in R&D, 12*(1), 9–14.

Musani, M. H. (2011). Asymptomatic saddle pulmonary embolism: Case report and literature review. *Clinical and Applied Thrombosis/Hemostasis, 17*(4), 337–339.

Myatt, R. (2011). Reducing length of stay through the use of ambulatory chest drains and nurse-led follow-up. *British Journal of Cardiac Nursing, 6*(11), 549–552.

Nagarsheth, K., & Kurek, S. (2011). Ultrasound detection of pneumothorax compared with chest X-ray and computed tomography scan. *The American Surgeon, 77*(4), 480–484.

Namazy, J. A., & Schatz, M. (2011). Asthma and rhinitis during pregnancy. *The Mount Sinai Journal of Medicine, 78*(5), 661–670.

Nathan, R. A., Meltzer, E. O., Blaiss, M. S., Murphy, K. R., Doherty, D. E., & Stoloff, S. W. (2012). Comparison of the Asthma in America and Asthma Insight and Management surveys: Did asthma burden and care improve in the United States between 1998 and 2009? *Allergy and Asthma Proceedings, 33*(1), 65–76.

Nishino, T. (2011). Dyspnea and its interaction with pain. *Journal of Anesthesia, 25*(1), 157–161.

Nosotti, M., Mendogni, P., Rosso, L., Tosi, D., Palleschi, A., Basciu, M., . . . Ferrero, S. (2012). Alveolar adenoma of the lung: Unusual diagnosis of a lesion positive on PET scan: A case report. *Journal of Cardiothoracic Surgery, 7*(1), 1–4.

Nuccio, P. F. (2011). Inhalation injuries. *The Journal for Respiratory Care Practitioners, 24*(10), 34–36.

Pai, R. P., Kangath, R. V., & Brown, T. A. (2011). Saddle pulmonary thromboembolism with zero Wells' score. *Connecticut Medicine, 75*(2), 89–91.

Parent, F., Bachir, D., Inamo, J., Lionnet, F., Driss, F., Loko, G., . . . Simonneau, G. (2011, July 7). A hemodynamic study of pulmonary hypertension in sickle cell disease. *The New England Journal of Medicine, 365*(1), 44–53.

Pathak, V., Hurtado Rendon, I. S., & Smina, M. (2012). Necrotizing pneumonia caused by group C streptococci in a young adult. *Respiratory Care, 57*(3), 454–456.

Perry, M. (2008). Knowing the early signs of pulmonary embolism. *Practice Nursing, 19*(12), 620–623.

Phillips, K. M., Burker, E. J., & White, H. C. (2011t). The roles of social support and psychological distress in lung transplant candidacy. *Progress in Transplantation, 21*(3), 200–226.

Piazza, G., & Goldhaber, S. Z. (2011). Chronic thromboembolic pulmonary hypertension. *The New England Journal of Medicine, 364*(4), 351–360.

Pierson, D. J. (2011). Saddle pulmonary embolism: Is it the same as "massive" PE? *Critical Care Alert, 19*(8), 58–60.

Poms, A., & Kingman, M. (2011). Inhaled treprostinil for the treatment of pulmonary arterial hypertension. *Critical Care Nurse, 31*(6), e1–e10.

Richter, T., & Ragaller, M. (2011). Ventilation in chest trauma. *Journal of Emergencies, Trauma & Shock, 4*(2), 251–259.

Robinson, T. (2011). Identification, assessment and management of pleurisy. *Nursing Standard, 25*(31), 6–12.

Roman, M., Weinstein, A., & Macaluso, S. (2003). Primary spontaneous pneumothorax. *MEDSURG Nursing, 12*(3), 161–169.

Salzman, S. H. (2012). Which pulmonary function tests best differentiate between COPD phenotypes? *Respiratory Care, 57*(1), 50–60.

Sanz, F., Restrepo, M. I., Fernández, E., Mortensen, E. M., Aguar, M. C., Cervera, Á., . . . Blanquer, J. (2011). Hypoxemia adds to the CURB-65 pneumonia severity score in hospitalized patients with mild pneumonia. *Respiratory Care, 56*(5), 612–618.

Seliman, A. M. A., El-Soussi, A. H., Sultan, M. A. A., & Othman, S. Y. (2011). Effect of implementing nursing guidelines for tube feeding on the occurrence of aspiration among critically ill patients. *Nature & Science, 9*(11), 164–175.

Shah, K. J., Scileppi, R. M., & Franz, R. W. (2011). Treatment of pulmonary embolism using ultrasound-accelerated thrombolysis directly into pulmonary arteries. *Vascular and Endovascular Surgery, 45*(6), 541–548.

Shalli, S., Saeed, D., Fukamachi, K., Gillinov, A. M., Cohn, W. E., Perrault, L. P., & Boyle, E. M. (2009). Chest tube selection in cardiac and thoracic surgery: A survey of chest tube-related complications and their management. *Journal of Cardiac Surgery, 24*(5), 503–509.

Shamaei, M., Tabarsi, P., Pojhan, S., Ghorbani, L., Baghaei, P., Marjani, M., & Masjedi, M. R. (2011). Tuberculosis-associated secondary pneumothorax: A retrospective study of 53 patients. *Respiratory Care, 56*(3), 298–302.

Shu, C. C., Wang, J. T., Wang, J. Y., Lee, L. N., & Yu, C. J. (2011). In-hospital outcome of patients with culture-confirmed tuberculous pleurisy: Clinical impact of pulmonary involvement. *BMC Infectious Diseases, 11*(1), 46–52.

Siqueira, M. A., Brunini, T. M., Pereira, N. R., Martins, M. A., Moss, M. B., Santos, S. F., . . . Mendes-Ribeiro, A. C. (2011). Increased nitric oxide production in platelets from severe chronic renal failure patients. *Canadian Journal of Physiology and Pharmacology, 89*(2), 97–102.

Soti, V. K., Sarangi, B., Deb, B., Alekya, K., Thomas, S., & Elango, K. (2012). Assessment of the prescribing pattern of antibiotics with corticosteroids in infective acute exacerbation of chronic bronchitis: A case series. *International Journal of Research in Pharmacy & Science, 2*(1), 84–88.

Sudderth, G. M. (2011). Multidisciplinary team management of the patient with tracheostomy. *The Journal for Respiratory Care Practitioners, 24*(11), 20–23.

Summerfield, D. T., Desai, H., Levitov, A., Grooms, D. A., & Marik, P. E. (2012). Inhaled nitric oxide as salvage therapy in massive pulmonary embolism: A case series. *Respiratory Care, 57*(3), 444–448.

Swigris, J. J., Fairclough, D. L., Morrison, M., Make, B., Kozora, E., Brown, K. K., & Wamboldt, F. S. (2011). Benefits of pulmonary rehabilitation in idiopathic pulmonary fibrosis. *Respiratory Care, 56*(6), 783–789.

Tae-Bum, K., Yeon, M. O., Yoon-Seok, C., You, S. C., An-Soo, J., Sang-Heon, C., . . . Hee-Bom, M. (2012). The reality of an intermediate type between asthma and COPD in practice. *Respiratory Care, 57*(8), 1248–1253.

Tashkin, D. P. (2012). Is it asthma, COPD, or something in between, and does it matter? *Respiratory Care, 57*(8), 1354–1356.

Thiem, U., Heppner, H., & Pientka, L. (2011). Elderly patients with community-acquired pneumonia optimal treatment strategies. *Drugs & Aging, 28*(7), 519–537.

Torheim, H., & Gjengedal, E. (2010). How to cope with the mask? Experiences of mask treatment in patients with acute chronic obstructive pulmonary disease-exacerbations. *Scandinavian Journal of Caring Sciences, 24*(3), 499–506.

Toworakul, C., Kasitanon, N., Sukitawut, W., Wichinun, R., & Louthrenoo, W. (2011). Usefulness of pleural effusion antinuclear antibodies in the diagnosis of lupus pleuritis. *Lupus, 20*(10), 1042–1046.

Trethewy, C. E., Burrows, J. M., Clausen, D., & Doherty, S. R. (2012). Effectiveness of cricoid pressure in preventing gastric aspiration during rapid sequence intubation in the emergency department: Study protocol for a randomized controlled trial. *Trials, 13*, 17.

Türkay, C., Özol, D., Kasapoğlu, B., Kirbas, I., Yıldırım, Z., & Yiğlitoğlu, R. (2012). Influence of obstructive sleep apnea on fatty liver disease: Role of chronic intermittent hypoxia. *Respiratory Care, 57*(2), 244–249.

Ulku, R., Avci, A., Onat, S., Nasir, A., & Ozcelik, C. (2009). Spontaneous pneumothorax in systemic sclerosis. *Internet Journal of Thoracic & Cardiovascular Surgery, 14*(1), 1–4.

Vallamkondu, V., & Visvanathan, V. (2011). Clinical review of adult tracheostomy. *Journal of Perioperative Practice, 21*(5), 172–176.

Vasu, T. S., Cavallazzi, R., Hirani, A., Sharma, D., Weibel, S. B., & Kane, G. C. (2009). Clinical and radiologic distinctions between secondary bronchiolitis obliterans organizing pneumonia and cryptogenic organizing pneumonia. *Respiratory Care, 54*(8), 1028–1032.

Vulović, T., & Dordević, G. (2008). Tension pneumothorax in intensive care units. *Military-Medical and Pharmaceutical Review, 65*(3), 245–248.

Wang, H., Xu, Q., Xiao, Y., Zhang, J., & Sperry, A. (2011). Cardiac response and N-terminal-pro-brain natriuretic peptide kinetics during exercise in patients with COPD. *Respiratory Care, 56*(6), 796–799.

Warren, E. (2012). When to use steroids in COPD. *Practice Nurse, 42*(13), 12–16.

Watcher, R. (2012). *Understanding patient safety* (2nd ed.). Los Altos, CA: Lange.

White, A. C., Kher, S., & O'Connor, H. H. (2010). When to change a tracheostomy tube. *Respiratory Care, 55*(8), 1069–1075.

Wilkerson, R. G., & Stone, M. B. (2010). Sensitivity of bedside ultrasound and supine anteroposterior chest radiographs for the identification of pneumothorax after blunt trauma. *Academic Emergency Medicine, 17*(1), 11–17.

Xue-Jun, L., Qi, L., Liang-Yi, S., & Qiao-Ying, Y. (2011). Bacteriological differences between COPD exacerbation and community-acquired pneumonia. *Respiratory Care, 56*(11), 1818–1824.

Yamada, S., Tabata, C., Tabata, R., Fukuoka, K., & Nakano, T. (2011). Clinical significance of pleural effusion mesothelin in malignant pleural mesothelioma. *Clinical Chemistry and Laboratory Medicine, 49*(10), 1721–1726.

Yazkan, R., & Han, S. (2010). Pathophysiology, clinical evaluation and treatment options of spontaneous pneumothorax. *Tüberküloz Ve Toraks, 58*(3), 334–343.

Youssef, T. F., Ahmed, M. R., & Saber, A. (2011). Percutaneous dilatational versus conventional surgical tracheostomy in intensive care patients. *North American Journal of Medical Sciences, 3*(11), 508–512.

Zierold, D., & Chauviere, M. (2012). Hydrogen fluoride inhalation injury because of a fire suppression system. *Military Medicine, 177*(1), 108–112.

Section 6

Endocrine

SECTION 6: ENDOCRINE QUESTIONS

1. **What conditions or medications can trigger the renin–angiotensin mechanism?**
   A. Aldosterone, diuretics
   B. Diuretics, decreased renal blood flow
   C. Diuretics, adrenergic blockers
   D. Increased renal blood flow, diuretics

2. **What is the correct order of response of the renin–angiotensin mechanism when there is a decrease in blood flow to the kidneys?**
   A. Renin, aldosterone, angiotensin I, angiotensin I converting enzyme, angiotensin II
   B. Increased ADH, renin, angiotensin I, angiotensin II
   C. Renin, angiotensinogen, angiotensin I, angiotensin I converting enzyme, angiotensin II, aldosterone
   D. Renin, ACTH, angiotensin

3. **Which of the following statements is true about cortisol?**
   A. Cortisol increases glucose uptake in muscle and adipose tissue
   B. Cortisol increases protein stores
   C. Cortisol decreases tissue response of other hormones, such as glucagon and catecholamines
   D. Cortisol exerts negative feedback on the hypothalamus and the anterior hypothalamus

4. **Use of systemic steroids may cause**
   A. Decreased ability to perspire
   B. Hyperactivity
   C. Increased ability to tolerate cold and heat
   D. Polydipsia

5. **One of your coworkers has been trying to lose weight for the past six months. She lost 10 pounds initially, but now appears to be gaining weight, has become irritable at work, is occasionally depressed, and states she cannot sleep. She also states she thinks management is "out to get her" because she is having difficulty arriving to work on time. This individual may be suffering from**
   A. Chronic hypoglycemia
   B. Overuse of steroids
   C. Hypothyroidism
   D. Hyperthyroidism

6. **Cortisol, glucagon, catecholamines, and growth hormone (GH) as a group are classified as**
   A. Neuroprotective hormones
   B. Serotonin inhibitors
   C. Insulin-antagonistic hormones
   D. Gluconeogenic hormones

7. **Gluconeogenesis may be impaired by**
   A. Increased food intake
   B. Excessive alcohol intake
   C. Use of medications that impair the action of sulfonylureas
   D. An insulin dose less than body requirements

8. **Which of the following medications is used in the treatment of SIADH?**
   A. High-dose steroids
   B. Sandostatin
   C. Demeclocycline
   D. Pitressin

9. **What is the most common cause of hyperparathyroidism?**
   A. Chronic anabolic steroid use
   B. Chronic obstructive pulmonary disease
   C. Chronic renal failure
   D. Tumors of the parathyroid gland

10. **What is the purpose of testing HgbA1c in patients with diabetes mellitus?**
    A. It is of little help in managing diabetes mellitus
    B. It measures blood sugars over a 6-month period
    C. It measures the effectiveness of diabetes mellitus therapy
    D. It measures red blood cell activity in diabetes mellitus

11. **What are the most common presenting symptoms of myxedema coma?**
    A. Facial swelling, ptosis, altered mental status, alopecia
    B. Ptosis, goiter, tachycardia, hypertension
    C. Altered mental status, hypertension, bradycardia
    D. Hypothermia, altered mental status, tachycardia

12. **There are no intensive care unit beds for your patient with myxedema coma, so initial treatment will be done in the PCU until a bed is available. What treatments do you anticipate for this patient?**
    A. Tapazole, fluids and electrolyte replacement
    B. Levothyroxine, fluids and electrolyte replacement, correction of cause of myxedema
    C. Fluids and electrolyte replacement, levothyroxine, methimazole
    D. Levothyroxine, beta-blockers, fluids and electrolyte replacement

13. **The anterior pituitary gland controls which of the following glands?**
    A. Parathyroid, adrenal medulla, gonads
    B. Thyroid, adrenal cortex, gonads

C. Parathyroid, thyroid, gonads
D. Thyroid, adrenal medulla, gonads

14. Which of the following conditions inhibits the release of thyroxine?
A. Hypocalcemia
B. Hyperthermia
C. Hypernatremia
D. Hypokalemia

15. What is the function of ADH (antidiuretic hormone)?
A. Aldosterone production
B. Sodium balance
C. Water balance
D. Potassium balance

16. Your patient has a tumor on her anterior pituitary gland. As a progressive care nurse, you know stimulation of the anterior pituitary gland is from the hypothalamus by way of the
A. Sympathetic nervous system
B. Feedback mechanism
C. Vascular system
D. Parasympathetic nervous system

17. Calcitonin is released by the
A. Thyroid gland
B. Adrenal medulla
C. Hypothalamus
D. Anterior pituitary gland

18. Your patient's serum calcium level is high. An increase in serum calcium, glucagon, or magnesium will stimulate the release of
A. Parathyroid hormone
B. Calcitonin
C. Endogenous epinephrine
D. Aldosterone

19. Mr. M. has been diagnosed with SIADH. What is the most common presentation of a patient with SIADH (syndrome of inappropriate antidiuretic hormone)?
A. Excessive, dilute urine output
B. Seizures
C. Hypotension
D. Tetany

20. Which of the following statements is true regarding glucagon?
A. Glucagon promotes glycolysis
B. Glucagon enables glucose to move into the cells
C. Glucagon helps the body store glycogen
D. Glucagon is released from the alpha cells in the pancreas

21. An increase in catecholamines and amino acids with a decrease in serum glucose stimulates the release of

A. Calcitonin
B. Insulin
C. Aldosterone
D. Glucagon

22. A high serum magnesium or phosphate level, low serum calcium, with catecholamine release, results in secretion of

A. Aldosterone
B. Parathyroid hormone
C. Glyceride
D. Phosphates

23. An important nursing consideration in the patient with HHNS is

A. To prevent alkalosis
B. The administration of corticosteroids
C. To prevent hyperglycemia
D. To monitor electrolytes

24. The most common cause of hypothyroidism is

A. Graves' disease
B. Acromegaly
C. Hashimoto's disease
D. Decreased cortisol levels

25. Which of the following conditions must be present for calcium to be optimally utilized by the body?

A. Increased oral calcium intake
B. Increased phosphorus
C. A euthyroid state
D. Adequate vitamin D levels

26. Your patient is having aldosterone levels monitored daily. Which of the following is a primary effect of aldosterone?

A. Aldosterone promotes sodium loss
B. Aldosterone increases renal potassium excretion
C. Aldosterone decreases potassium excretion
D. Aldosterone increases water loss

27. Aldosterone is secreted by the

A. Zona reticularis of the adrenal cortex
B. Zona glomerulus of the adrenal cortex
C. Posterior pituitary gland
D. Adrenal medulla

28. Aldosterone secretion is regulated by

A. The anterior hypothalamus
B. Potassium ions in intracellular fluid

C. Angiotensin II
D. Hypercalcemia

29. Your patient's aldosterone levels are low. As his nurse, you know a factor that suppresses aldosterone production is
A. Hypocalcemia
B. Hyperkalemia
C. Stress
D. Atrial natriuretic hormone

30. Functions of the thyroid gland, adrenal gland, and male and female reproductive glands are regulated by the
A. Thyroid gland
B. Pineal gland of the brain
C. Pineal–pituitary axis
D. Hypothalamic–pituitary axis

31. Where is the pituitary gland located?
A. Superior to the hypothalamus gland near the optic chiasm
B. Inferior to the hypothalamus and sits in the sella turcica of the skull
C. Between the thalamus and hypothalamus in the midbrain
D. Superior to the pons and brainstem

32. Cortisol is a glucocorticoid. A major effect of cortisol in the body is to
A. Increase the loss of sodium from small intestines
B. Lower blood pressure in times of stress
C. Raise the level of free amino acids in the serum
D. Stimulate urine loss

33. How does hyperglycemic, hyperosmolar, nonketotic syndrome (HHNS) differ from diabetic ketoacidosis (DKA)?
A. HHNS has the same onset, higher blood sugars, more dehydration than DKA
B. HHNS has slower onset, lower blood sugars, less dehydration than DKA
C. HHNS has a slower onset, much higher blood sugar, more profound dehydration than DKA
D. HHNS has the same onset, lower blood sugar, no dehydration than DKA

34. Your patient has been diagnosed with HHNS. What lab results would you anticipate for this patient?
A. Glucose 550, positive ketones, serum osmolality 280 mOsm/L
B. Glucose 1258, negative ketones, serum osmolality 375 mOsm/L
C. Glucose 700, negative ketones, serum osmolality 270 mOsm/L
D. Glucose 600, positive ketones, serum osmolality 240 mOsm/L

35. Congenital hypothyroidism is manifested by
A. A decreased TSH and a decreased T4
B. A euthyroid state
C. An elevated TSH and a decreased T4
D. A decreased TSH and an elevated T4

36. **Which of the following conditions contributes to the development of acute hypoglycemia?**
    A. Insulinoma
    B. Glucose consumption exceeds glucose production
    C. Oral anithyperglycemic agents
    D. Alcoholism

37. **Recurrent episodes of acute hypoglycemia have led to a male patient's admission to your unit. What therapies may be used to treat acute hypoglycemia (blood sugar less than 50 mg/dl)?**
    A. Small, frequent meals, increased carbohydrate consumption
    B. Intravenous D50 administration, oral glucose, and treat the cause
    C. Increased carbohydrate diet, intravenous glucose
    D. Treat the cause, increased carbohydrate consumption

38. **A 30 year old male was admitted to the PCU with a diagnosis of diabetic ketoacidosis. As his nurse you know his insulin drip will be titrated by sliding scale and his anion gap. What does the anion gap measure?**
    A. An estimate of cations and anions
    B. An estimate of unmeasured anions
    C. An estimate of potassium in the blood
    D. An estimate of the correction of the acid-base balance

39. **Your patient with diabetic ketoacidosis has an HCO_3 level of 10 mEq/L. In addition to an insulin drip, you should anticipate which of the following orders?**
    A. Increase the insulin drip to hasten the resolution of the metabolic acidosis
    B. Sodium bicarbonate bolus and repeat every 4–6 hours
    C. Sodium bicarbonate drip with frequent HCO_3 levels
    D. Decrease the insulin drip as the acidosis is resolving

40. **Your patient is suffering from myxedema coma. He is receiving intravenous thyroid replacement therapy when he suddenly develops hypotension, hypoglycemia, nausea, and vomiting. What has happened to this patient?**
    A. An allergic response to the thyroid medication
    B. He needs an increased dose of thyroid medication
    C. He needs a lower dose of thyroid medication
    D. He is experiencing an Addisonian crisis

41. **Which glands regulate thyroid function?**
    A. Posterior pituitary and hypothalamus
    B. Anterior pituitary and thalamus
    C. Anterior pituitary and hypothalamus
    D. Posterior pituitary and thalamus

42. **What is the treatment of choice once a diagnosis of pheochromocytoma is made?**
    A. Diet changes
    B. Antihypertensive medications
    C. Surgical removal of the tumor
    D. Diuretics

43. Which drug is known to cause nephrogenic diabetes insipidus?

A. Demeclocycline
B. Amiloride
C. Celecoxib
D. Indomethicin

44. Part of your patient education for the family of a patient with pheochromocytoma should include dietary restrictions. Which of the following foods should the patient avoid?

A. Cream cheese
B. Red meat
C. Chocolate
D. Aged cheddar cheese

45. Your patient's calcium level is 11.9 mg/dl. This value may be the result of which of the following conditions?

A. Hypoparathyroidism
B. Hyperparathyroidism
C. Excessive calcium intake
D. Recent fracture of a long bone

46. Treatment for a thyrotoxic crisis includes

A. No need for treatment, the crisis will resolve spontaneously
B. Symptomatic care and wait for symptoms to subside
C. Synthroid administration and supportive care
D. Administration of PTH and symptomatic care

47. What is an important teaching point for a patient with hypothyroidism?

A. Take the medication at the same time every day, no need to fast
B. Take thyroid medication at the same time every day, 30 minutes before breakfast
C. Take the thyroid medicine each evening before bed
D. Take daily with food

48. Your patient's TSH (thyroid-stimulating hormone) level is 0.001. What condition does this value indicate?

A. Hypoactive anterior pituitary function
B. Hyperactive anterior pituitary function
C. Hypothyroidism
D. Hyperthyroidism

49. A fellow nurse asks you to explain the differences between the Somoygi effect and the Dawn phenomenon. What are the major differences between the Somoygi effect and the Dawn phenomenon?

A. They are essentially the same process
B. The Dawn phenomenon is nocturnal hypoglycemia, and the Somoygi effect is greatly increased blood sugars in the early morning
C. The Somoygi effect is nocturnal hypoglycemia with rebound hyperglycemia, and the Dawn phenomenon is increased morning glucose without nocturnal hypoglycemia
D. The Dawn phenomenon is morning hypoglycemia, and the Somoygi effect is nocturnal hyperglycemia

50. **Your patient was found unconscious in his backyard by his brother. His blood sugar is 1545, he has negative serum ketones, and his serum osmolality is 340. What fluids do you anticipate administering for medical treatment of this condition?**
    A. D_5 ½NS intravenous fluids 300 ml/hour and an insulin drip with sliding scale coverage
    B. Normal saline at 100 ml/hour, subcutaneous insulin with sliding scale coverage every 4 hours, and monitor potassium
    C. Intravenous fluids with normal saline in high volumes, insulin drip with sliding scale coverage, and monitor electrolyte levels
    D. Normal saline intravenously, bicarbonate drip, and monitor electrolytes

51. **Where is renin stored in the body?**
    A. Renal tubule
    B. Loop of Henle
    C. Juxtoglomerular cells of the nephron
    D. Adrenal cortex

52. **A 28 year old female is being treated for new onset of diabetic ketoacidosis. You have referred her to a diabetic educator and are now teaching her about diabetes mellitus and HgbA1c. Which of the following HgbA1c test results should be the goal for good control of her diabetes mellitus?**
    A. 7–8%
    B. 4–5%
    C. 6–7%
    D. 8–9%

53. **Temperature regulation is controlled by the hypothalamus with the release of which of the following hormones?**
    A. Dopamine
    B. Norepinephrine
    C. Cortisol
    D. Epinephrine

54. **Which of the following diabetic patients is most likely to develop DKA?**
    A. Type 1 well-controlled on 70/30 insulin
    B. Type 1 who is noncompliant with cellulitis of his left leg
    C. Type 2 with an HgbA1c of 6.5 and minor surgery
    D. Type 2 with asthma

55. **Which of the following conditions can cause a thyroid storm in a patient with hyperthyroidism?**
    A. An overdose of PTU (propylthyrouricil)
    B. Increased iodine intake
    C. Trauma or infection
    D. Decreased iodine intake

56. **Your patient is having a thyrotoxic crisis. Which medication is given to reduce symptoms?**
    A. Propranolol
    B. Levophed

C. Adenosine
D. Digoxin

57. **What symptoms are to be expected when a patient is having a thyrotoxic crisis?**
A. Hyperthermia, bradycardia
B. Hypotension, bradycardia
C. Flushing, hypoventilation
D. Hypertension, hyperthermia

58. **Trousseau's sign is seen with which of the conditions listed below?**
A. Increased serum calcium
B. Decreased serum calcium
C. Decreased serum phosphorus
D. Hypothyroidism

59. **Which of the following signs may be elicited in a patient with hypocalcemia?**
A. Short QT interval
B. Hyperparathyroidism
C. Chvostek's sign
D. Cullen's sign

60. **Which of the following hormones is responsible for the symptoms of hypothyroidism?**
A. Low levels of T4 (thyroxine)
B. Low levels of T3 (thriothyroxine)
C. Decreased thyrocalcitonin
D. Increased thyrocalcitonin

61. **Where in the body are the catecholamines produced?**
A. Liver
B. Kidneys
C. Adrenal cortex
D. Adrenal medulla

62. **What is the origin of microvascular disease associated with diabetes mellitus?**
A. Vasoconstriction from hyperglycemia
B. Changes in the capillary basement membrane causing hypoxia on the cellular level
C. Increased atherosclerotic plaques on the intima
D. Repeated hypoglycemic events

63. **What are the three major problems associated with macrovascular disease in a patient with diabetes mellitus?**
A. Diabetic peripheral neuropathy, peripheral vascular disease, cerebral vascular accident
B. Peripheral neuropathy, coronary artery disease, cerebral vascular accident
C. Coronary artery disease, cerebral vascular accident, peripheral vascular disease
D. Retinopathy, coronary artery disease, cerebral vascular accident

64. **What is the role of glucophage in the body?**
A. Glucophage acts on the liver to decrease blood sugar
B. Glucophage acts on the liver to increase blood sugar

C. Glucophage acts on the pancreas to decrease blood sugar
D. Glucophage acts on the pancreas to increase blood sugar

65. Where is the pancreas located in the abdomen?
A. Right lower quadrant of the abdomen
B. Left upper quadrant of the abdomen
C. Right upper quadrant of the abdomen
D. Left lower quadrant of the abdomen

66. Where are the parathyroid glands located?
A. Anterior to the thyroid gland
B. Posterior to the thyroid gland
C. They sit atop the thyroid gland
D. Below the thyroid gland

67. Where is the thyroid gland located?
A. Just below the hyoid bone
B. In the throat on either side of the trachea
C. Above the larynx
D. It sits on top of the thymus gland

68. What physical symptoms do you expect a patient to exhibit if diagnosed with Cushing syndrome?
A. Moon facies, edema, weight loss
B. Moon facies, acne, weight loss
C. Moon facies, purple striae on trunk, buffalo hump
D. Moon facies, easy bruising, weight loss

69. Which of the following hormones are produced by the anterior pituitary gland?
A. Vasopressin and oxytocin
B. FSH, LH, TSH, ACTH
C. ADH, TSH, FSH
D. GRF, TSH, Substance P

70. Your patient has been preliminarily diagnosed with Cushing syndrome. What diagnostic tests do you anticipate the physician ordering for this patient?
A. Computerized tomography of the brain, chest, and abdomen; 24-hour urine cortisol levels; ACTH serum concentrations
B. Computerized tomography of the brain, chest, and abdomen; thyroid levels; basic metabolic panel
C. Serum and urine cortisol levels, thyroid panels, beta-natriuretic peptide levels
D. Urine ACTH concentrations, thyroid panel, C-reactive protein level

71. Your patient has DKA. She has a blood glucose level of 460 mg/dl and also has a potassium level of 6.2. You have started an insulin drip. You know that the insulin drip will
A. Move potassium back into the intracellular space
B. Not change potassium levels
C. Draw more potassium from the intracellular space
D. Draw more potassium from the extracellular space

72. **What are some of the signs and symptoms associated with DKA (diabetic ketoacidosis)?**
    A. Polyuria, polydipsia, polyphagia, dilute urine
    B. Polyuria, polydipsia, polyphagia, fruity breath, dehydration, marked fatigue
    C. Hyperactivity, confusion, nausea, vomiting
    D. Kussmaul's respirations, dilute urine

73. **How is insulin secretion regulated?**
    A. Hormonal, exocrine gland secretion, and glucose controls
    B. Hormonal, insulin and neuronal controls
    C. Chemical, glucagon and insulin controls
    D. Chemical, hormonal and neuronal controls

74. **Which of the following are risk factors for the development of diabetes mellitus?**
    A. Obesity (BMI of 42), blood pressure 160/95, HDL 28, brother with diabetes mellitus
    B. Obesity (BMI of 27), blood pressure 120/70, HDL 42, no family history of diabetes mellitus
    C. Obesity (BMI of 26), Caucasian ancestry, blood pressure 190/100, family history of diabetes mellitus
    D. Obesity (BMI of 40), blood pressure 100/50, HDL 50, no family history of diabetes mellitus

75. **Why are hyperglycemia and hyperlipidemia seen concurrently in patients with diabetes mellitus?**
    A. VLDL (very-low-density lipoprotein) production increases in response to increased insulin production
    B. Insulin resistance promotes VLDL (very-low-density lipoprotein) production
    C. Lipid breakdown is hindered by hyperinsulinemia
    D. Glucose increases cause the liver to increase lipid production

76. **What is the most common complaint with Addison's disease?**
    A. Increased appetite, weight loss, insomnia
    B. Weight gain, anorexia, constipation
    C. Weakness, fatigue, weight loss
    D. Salt craving, weight loss, constipation

77. **Which of the following should be included in patient education for the patient with Addison's disease?**
    A. Lifelong condition, follow-up labs, hydrocortisone injection
    B. Follow-up labs, Medic-Alert bracelet, no-added-salt diet
    C. Lifelong condition, no-added-salt diet, push oral fluids
    D. Liberal sodium diet, self-limiting disease

78. **What are the 5 S's for the management of a patient with Addison's disease in an adrenal crisis?**
    A. Steroids, saline, sulfa antibiotics, supplemental oxygen, struma
    B. Steroids, salt, sugar, support, search for cause
    C. Steroids, sugar, stress test, serologic tests, salt
    D. Steroids, search for cause, serial labs, salt, stress test

79. **Your patient on oral amiodarone has been admitted with myxedema. What symptoms do you expect to see in this patient?**
   A. Periorbital edema and facial puffiness
   B. Tibial and pedal edema
   C. Anasarca
   D. No edema

80. **Which of the following are signs of myxedema coma?**
   A. Fever, elevated T4 and T3
   B. Decreased level of consciousness, hypotension
   C. Decreased T4 and T3, hyperthermia
   D. Hypothermia, decreased thyroid-stimulating hormone

81. **What is the pathophysiology of pheochromocytoma?**
   A. Tumor of the renal gland secreting excessive angiotensinogen
   B. Tumor of the adrenal glands secreting excessive catecholamines
   C. Tumor of the pituitary gland secreting excessive ADH
   D. Tumor of the adrenal glands secreting excessive angiotensin I

82. **Which of the following can lead to hyperparathyroidism?**
   A. Low vitamin D levels, phenytoin, phenobarbital, laxatives
   B. Phenytoin, calcium supplements, renal failure
   C. Low phosphate levels, excessive vitamin D, laxatives
   D. Low vitamin D levels, excessive vitamin K, phenytoin

SECTION 6: ENDOCRINE ANSWERS

1. **Correct answer: B**
   Anything that causes a perceived drop in renal blood flow triggers the renin–angiotensin mechanism. Renin release can also be triggered by sodium and volume depletion such as seen with diuretic use.

2. **Correct answer: C**
   The correct order of response of the renin–angiotensin mechanism when there is a decrease in blood flow to the kidneys is renin, angiotensinogen, angiotensin I, angiotensin I converting enzyme, angiotensin II, and aldosterone. The kidneys perceive a drop in blood flow, leading to the release of renin from the juxtoglomerular cells of the nephron. This stimulates the release of angiotensinogen, which stimulates the release of angiotensin I. If the blood pressure is not corrected, the lungs release angiotensin I converting enzyme, which in turn causes the secretion of angiotensin II. Angiotensin II causes the release of aldosterone from the adrenal glands, causing the retention of sodium and water, as well as increased blood pressure.

3. **Correct answer: D**
   Cortisol exerts negative feedback on the hypothalamus and the anterior hypothalamus. Cortisol has an insulin antagonistic effect and decreases glucose uptake in muscle and adipose tissue.

4. **Correct answer: D**
   Use of systemic steroids may cause polydipsia. The patient will have a decreased ability to tolerate cold and heat, will suffer from excess perspiration, and will likely be fatigued and weak.

5. **Correct answer: B**
   The symptoms of weight gain, irritability at work (emotional lability), occasional depression, and statements that she cannot sleep, coupled with paranoia (she also states she thinks management is "out to get her") are classic signs of overuse of steroids. Because she is having difficulty arriving to work on time, she may be suffering from lack of coping ability and impairment of ability to perform ADLs. These are also indicators of overuse of steroids.

6. **Correct answer: C**
   Cortisol, glucagon, catecholamines, and growth hormone (GH) as a group are classified as insulin-antagonistic hormones.

7. **Correct answer: B**
   Gluconeogenesis may be impaired by excessive alcohol intake.

8. **Correct answer: C**
   Demeclocycline is used in the treatment of SIADH. Its use in treatment of SIADH is because of its side effect; demeclocycline induces nephrogenic diabetes insipidus. The patient becomes dehydrated due to the inability to concentrate urine.

9. **Correct answer: C**
   Chronic renal failure is the most common cause of hyperparathyroidism.

10. **Correct answer: C**
HgbA1c measures the effectiveness of diabetes mellitus therapy. Hemoglobin and glucose have an affinity for each other and join together to form a glycolated hemoglobin. The HgbA1c rises and falls in direct correlation with blood sugars. The American College of Endocrinologists recommends a HgbA1c of less than 6.5%, whereas the American Diabetes Association recommends a HgbA1c less than 7%. Patients with a HgbA1c less than 6% are considered nondiabetic.

11. **Correct answer: A**
There are numerous symptoms of myxedema coma, which include facial swelling, altered mental status, alopecia, hypotension, bradycardia, hypothermia, ptosis, periorbital edema and macroglossia. The symptoms that are not seen with myxedema are tachycardia, hypertension, and goiter. These symptoms are seen with hyperthyroidism.

12. **Correct answer: B**
Intravenous administration of levothyroxine and replacement of fluids and electrolytes are initial therapies for myxedema coma. The patient must also be supported to prevent potential cardiopulmonary collapse, sometimes requiring mechanical ventilation.

13. **Correct answer: B**
The anterior pituitary, or adenohypophysis, controls the function of the thyroid gland with TSH (thyroid-stimulating hormone). The anterior pituitary also controls the adrenal cortex with ADH (antidiuretic hormone) and the gonads with LH (luteinizing hormone) or ICSH (interstitial cell-stimulating hormone).

14. **Correct answer: B**
Hyperthermia inhibits the release of thyroxine.

15. **Correct answer: C**
ADH (antidiuretic hormone) deals with the functions of thirst and water balance. It is produced by the posterior pituitary gland. When the plasma becomes concentrated, or there is a reduced blood volume, the posterior pituitary gland releases ADH, causing water retention and concentration of urine. ADH is regulated by a feedback mechanism in the pituitary gland.

16. **Correct answer: C**
Stimulation of the anterior pituitary gland is from the hypothalamus by way of the vascular system.

17. **Correct answer: A**
Calcitonin is released by the thyroid gland.

18. **Correct answer: B**
An increase in serum calcium, glucagon, or magnesium stimulates the release of calcitonin. Calcitonin reduces serum calcium levels, targets bone and kidney cells to inhibit bone cell lysis, and decreases calcium reabsorption by the kidney.

19. **Correct answer: B**
Seizures are one of the most common presenting symptoms of SIADH. SIADH causes hemodilution and a relative decrease in serum sodium levels. Once the sodium falls below 120, the patient is at great risk for seizures. Excessive urine output and hypotension are symptoms of diabetes insipidus.

20. **Correct answer: D**
Glucagon is released from the alpha cells in the pancreas. Glucagon inhibits glycolysis, increases lipolysis, and increases blood glucose by stimulating glycogenolysis and gluconeogenesis.

21. **Correct answer: D**
An increase in catecholamines and amino acids with a decrease in serum glucose stimulates the release of glucagon. If one becomes low on serum glucose from exercise, for example, glucagon is released to help produce an increase in blood glucose.

22. **Correct answer: B**
A high serum magnesium or phosphate level, low serum calcium, with catecholamine release results in secretion of parathyroid hormone. Bone breakdown is accelerated, releasing calcium into the blood. Calcium reabsorption is increased in the intestine, and kidney tubule reabsorption is decreased. Phosphate loss is increased in the urine, which decreases serum phosphate. Parahormone increases reabsorption of magnesium by renal tubules. Renal calculi may develop.

23. **Correct answer: D**
An important nursing consideration in the patient with HHNS monitor electrolytes and treat dysrhythmias. The severe hypokalemia is the result of no intracellular-to-extracellular shift occurring because the patient is not usually acidotic. When the patient is hypokalemic, hypocalcemia and hypomagnesemia also occur. Cardiac tissue may be compromised due to electrolyte imbalances and life-threatening dysrhythmias may occur.

24. **Correct answer: C**
Hashimoto's disease, or chronic lymphocytic thyroiditis, is the most common cause of hypothyroidism. Hashimoto's disease is an autoimmune disorder. In Hashimoto's disease, the immune system makes antibodies against the thyroid and interferes with production of thyroid hormone.

25. **Correct answer: D**
Calcium cannot be utilized by the body without adequate vitamin D levels. Fifteen minutes of daylight on the skin without use of sun block allows the body to create its own vitamin D. An increased phosphorus level would bind the calcium, making it unavailable.

26. **Correct answer: B**
The primary effects of aldosterone are to increase reabsorption of water and sodium, which results in an increased extracellular fluid volume. Renal excretion of potassium is increased.

27. **Correct answer: B**
Aldosterone is secreted by the zona glomerulus of the adrenal cortex.

28. **Correct answer: C**
Aldosterone secretion is regulated by angiotensin II. When renal blood flow is decreased, angiotensin is released, and it stimulates aldosterone secretion. An increase in potassium ions in extracellular fluid also stimulates the release of aldosterone. Adrenocorticotropic hormone stimulates aldosterone production for short periods of time.

29. **Correct answer: D**
A factor that suppresses aldosterone production is atrial natriuretic hormone. Hypercalcemia and hypokalemia also suppress aldosterone production.

30. **Correct Answer: D**
Functions of the thyroid gland, adrenal gland, and male and female reproductive glands are regulated by the hypothalamic–pituitary axis. The hypothalamic–pituitary axis releases a number of hormones that inhibit or release several other hormones that affect body functions.

31. **Correct answer: B**
The pituitary gland is inferior to the hypothalamus and sits in the sella turcica of the sphenoid bone.

32. **Correct answer: C**
Cortisol raises the free amino acids in the serum by inhibiting collagen formation and protein synthesis. Cortisol stimulates gastric acid secretion, inhibits loss of sodium from the small intestines, acts as an antidiuretic hormone, and works with epinephrine and norepinephrine to increase blood pressure.

33. **Correct answer: C**
HHNS develops slowly in type 2 diabetes, most often in elderly patients or those with undiagnosed diabetes mellitus. The blood sugars are generally more than 600 mg/dl and can go over 1500 mg/dl. The other differentiation between HHNS and DKA is the lack of ketones with HHNS.

34. **Correct answer: B**
Blood sugars over 600 mg/dl with negative serum ketones and a serum osmolality greater than 310 are typical of hyperglycemic, hyperosmolar, nonketotic syndrome (HHNS). The pH is usually greater than 7.3, and the BUN (blood urea nitrogen) may be elevated. Osmolality is the best predictor of survivability than the blood sugar levels.

35. **Correct answer: C**
Congenital hypothyroidism is manifested by an elevated TSH and a decreased T4. This disease is usually autosomal recessive, but some cases are autosomal dominant. Congenital hypothyroidism occurs when the thyroid gland fails to develop or function properly. The thyroid gland may be absent, hypoplastic, or displaced. In a few cases, the gland is enlarged, but the production of thyroid hormones is deficient or absent.

36. **Correct answer: B**
Acute hypoglycemia occurs if glucose consumption exceeds glucose production. Lack of food, or if the liver is unable to provide glucogenesis, causes a drop in blood glucose can drop to less than 50 mg/dl.

37. **Correct answer: B**
D50, oral glucose, and treating the cause are the most effective ways to treat acute hypoglycemia. Increased carbohydrate consumption would be prohibited. The optimal diet would consist of small, frequent meals and reduced carbohydrates.

38. **Correct answer: B**
The anion gap measures anions not generally measured in routine labs. It is an estimate of the degree of lactic acidosis. The formula for figuring the anion gap is

Na (HCO_3 + Cl). The normal level is 10–20 mEq/L. With diabetic ketoacidosis the anion gap is greater than 30 mEq/L.

39. **Correct answer: C**
A sodium bicarbonate drip should be anticipated to replace the HCO_3. This helps to resolve the metabolic acidosis. Boluses would be given only if the pH was very low. The insulin drip will not directly correct the HCO_3.

40. **Correct answer: D**
Your patient is having an Addisonian crisis. Subclinical adrenal insufficiency may coexist with myxedema. The treatment of choice is intravenous hydrocortisone therapy.

41. **Correct answer: C**
The anterior pituitary and hypothalamus glands regulate thyroid function. The anterior pituitary gland secretes TSH (thyroid-stimulating hormone) and the hypothalamus regulates the anterior pituitary gland with thyrotropin-releasing hormone (TRH).

42. **Correct answer: C**
The best option for pheochromocytoma is surgical removal of the tumor. It is important to remove the tumors, as they can rupture and lead to the patient's death. Alpha-adrenergic blockers or beta-adrenergic blockers may be used to treat hypertension until surgery can be performed.

43. **Correct answer: A**
Demeclocycline is the only tetracycline known to cause nephrogenic diabetes insipidus. In few cases, amiloride and prostoglandin inhibitors such as celecoxib and indomethicin have been noted to be effective treatments for nephrogenic diabetes insipidus.

44. **Correct answer: D**
Hypertension with pheochromocytoma can be triggered by foods such as cheese, alcohol, yogurt, and caffeine. It is important to give the patient a list of foods to avoid. Crises often occur after life events where these foods might be consumed.

45. **Correct answer: B**
A calcium level of 11.9 mg/dl indicates hyperparathyroidism. Hyperparathyroidism can be either primary or secondary in nature. Primary hyperparathyroidism is the excess secretion of PTH (parathyroid hormone) and may be related to a breakdown of the feedback system to the glands or overgrowth of the glands. Secondary hyperparathyroidism is generally related to a chronic disorder such as chronic renal failure or a malabsorption state.

46. **Correct answer: D**
Treatment of thyrotoxic crisis includes PTH to decrease thyroid-stimulating hormone and thyroid hormones, plus treatment based on presenting symptoms.

47. **Correct answer: B**
Thyroid medications should be taken on an empty stomach 30 minutes before breakfast, at the same time every day. Other teaching points include regular follow-up labs of TSH and T4, and watching for symptoms of myxedema and hyperthyroidism. Taking thyroid medication in the evening can lead to insomnia.

48. **Correct answer: D**
A TSH (thyroid-stimulating hormone) level of 0.001 indicates hyperthyroidism or thyrotoxicosis. Causes can include goiter, Graves' disease, thyroid carcinoma, and TSH secreting pituitary adenoma. Hyperthyroidism without toxicosis is most often related to excessive intake of thyroid hormones.

49. **Correct answer: C**
The Somoygi effect is nocturnal hypoglycemia with rebound hyperglycemia. It is more common in Type 1 diabetics, especially children. The Dawn phenomenon is morning hyperglycemia without nocturnal hypoglycemia, and it is caused by growth hormone secretion in the early morning hours.

50. **Correct answer: C**
The patient has HHNS. Normal saline should be given in large volumes until depletion is corrected and then D_5NS once blood glucose is in the 250–300 mg/dl range. An insulin drip with a sliding scale and hourly glucose monitoring would probably be ordered. Frequent electrolyte monitoring would also be performed. If the patient was given D_5 ½NS too early in the treatment, it could lead to cerebral edema.

51. **Correct answer: C**
Renin is stored in a crystalline form in the juxtoglomerular cells of the kidneys. When the kidneys perceive a decreased blood flow, the sympathetic response triggers the release of renin, which converts angiotensinogen to angiotensin I, a mild vasoconstrictor. If the problem is not resolved, the lungs release angiotensin I converting enzyme to create angiotensin II, a powerful vasoconstrictor. Angiotensin II triggers the release of aldosterone from the adrenal glands, which causes sodium and water retention, thereby increasing the blood pressure.

52. **Correct answer: C**
A HgbA1c of 6–7% will mean this patient's glucose was 100–150 mg/dl over a 3-month period. Four to 5% is normal, and 7–8% and 8–9% or more are indicative of poorly controlled diabetes mellitus.

53. **Correct answer: B**
Norepinephrine is released by the hypothalamus in response to chemical and temperature receptors in the skin, face, and along the spinal column. Norepinephrine triggers a cascade of actions within the body to retain or create heat in the core. The efficiency of this cascade is impaired by weight, disease process, and respiratory function. Peripheral vasoconstriction shunts blood flow to internal organs to control heat loss through the abdomen. Norepinephrine also causes pulmonary vasoconstriction, which inhibits normal blood flow through the lungs, inhibiting blood oxygenation. The best treatment for hypothermia or cold stress is appropriate and timely prevention.

54. **Correct answer: B**
The patient most likely to develop DKA is the one who is noncompliant with cellulitis. DKA is more common in insulin-dependent diabetics, especially those with an illness or infection such as cellulitis. However, 20–30% of DKA patients have no identified precipitating factors. A well-controlled diabetic is at low risk for DKA. Type 2 diabetics are more likely to develop HHNS.

55. **Correct answer: C**
Injury or infection, as well as manipulation, of the thyroid gland can trigger a thyroid storm and thyrotoxicosis.

56. **Correct answer: A**
Propranolol (Inderal) is used for a patient having a thyrotoxic crisis. Propranolol is a beta-blocker and decreases the effects of the sympathetic stimulation of thyrotoxic crisis. It controls heart rate, hypertension, and oxygen consumption.

57. **Correct answer: D**
Thyrotoxic crisis symptoms include: hypertension, hyperthermia, flushing, tachycardia (especially atrial tachyarrhythmias), high output heart failure, nausea and vomiting, psychosis, and delirium. Treatment includes supportive care and medications to block catecholamine effects.

58. **Correct answer: B**
Trousseau's sign is known as carpal-pedal spasm and is seen with decreased calcium levels. Hypocalcemia can occur with end stage renal disease (increased phosphorus) and decreased vitamin D levels. It is also seen in patients who receive 3 or more units of red blood cells that are treated with calcium citrate.

59. **Correct answer: C**
Chvostek's sign is seen with hypocalcemia. It is elicited by tapping the cheek over the zygomatic arch and causes facial twitching. The QT interval would be prolonged with hypocalcemia. Cullen's sign is ecchymosis around the umbilicus and is often seen in pancreatitis.

60. **Correct answer: A**
A low level of thyroxine is responsible for the symptoms of hypothyroidism. The decreased T4 leads to hypothyroid symptoms of cold, dry skin, hair loss, periorbital edema, and possible thyroid enlargement.

61. **Correct answer: D**
The adrenal medulla produces 75–85% of the catecholamine epinephrine and 25% of norepinephrine from phenylalanine.

62. **Correct answer: B**
The origins of microvascular disease associated with diabetes mellitus are due to changes in the capillary basement membrane, causing hypoxia on the cellular level. Prolonged hyperglycemia thickens the capillary basement membrane. This thickening leads decreased blood flow, hypoxia, and a lack of nutrients at the cellular level. The eye and kidney are the organs most susceptible to this process.

63. **Correct answer: C**
Coronary artery disease, cerebral vascular accident, and peripheral vascular disease are the three major problems associated with macrovascular disease seen in type 2 diabetes mellitus. Mortality or morbidity in these patients is due to macrovascular changes. Diabetes leads to early atherosclerosis and atherosclerotic heart disease. The other problems listed (retinopathy, peripheral neuropathy, and diabetic nephropathy) are microvascular diseases.

64. **Correct answer: A**
The role of glucophage in the body is as an antihyperglycemic agent, which improves glucose tolerance in patients with type 2 diabetes. Glucophage (Metformin) decreases liver glucose production and also acts to decrease intestinal absorption of glucose.

65. **Correct answer: B**
The pancreas is located in the left upper quadrant of the abdomen and sits behind the stomach near the spleen and duodenum. This is a basic question, but one that has caught many an unwary nurse.

66. **Correct answer: B**
The parathyroid glands are located posterior to the thyroid gland and may consist of four to six small glands. The parathyroid glands produce PTH (parathyroid hormone), which regulates serum calcium, magnesium, and phosphorus levels. PTH also stimulates the kidney to produce bioavailable vitamin D.

67. **Correct answer: B**
The thyroid gland is located below the larynx on either side of the trachea.

68. **Correct answer: C**
Numerous physical changes occur with Cushing syndrome or Cushing disease: thinning hair, acne, moon facies, increased body hair, buffalo hump on the upper back, purple striae on the trunk, truncal obesity with thin extremities, and easy bruising.

69. **Correct answer: B**
The anterior pituitary gland produces numerous hormones, which include TSH, LH, FSH, ACTH, and melanocyte-stimulating hormone. Substance P is a hormone released by the hypothalamus. Vasopressin and oxytocin are released by the posterior pituitary gland.

70. **Correct answer: A**
Cushing syndrome is usually seen with Cushing disease. Anticipated diagnostic tests include computerized tomography of the brain, chest, and abdomen, 24-hour urine cortisol levels, and ACTH serum concentrations. It is important to rule out tumors of the pituitary gland, chest (small cell cancer of the lung), adrenal tumors, and pheochromocytomas. These tumors cause excessive ACTH production leading to physical changes seen with Cushing syndrome, such as moon facies, buffalo hump, truncal obesity, and purple striae on the abdomen.

71. **Correct answer: A**
An insulin drip moves potassium back into the intracellular space, then potassium is pulled from the intracellular space due to metabolic acidosis. The insulin drip helps correct the metabolic acidosis, allowing the potassium to return to normal levels.

72. **Correct answer: B**
Signs and symptoms of DKA include polyuria, polydipsia, and polyphagia, known as the "3 P's." The fruity breath is from ketone production when fatty acids are broken down. Dehydration is due to the osmotic diuresis. Fatigue is due to potassium shifting from inside the cell to the intravascular space.

73. **Correct answer: D**
Insulin secretion is controlled by chemicals such as glucose and amino acids. Hormones such as GI hormones and prostaglandin will also control insulin secretion.

74. **Correct answer: A**
Risk factors for the development of diabetes mellitus include: blood pressure greater than 140/90 or higher than accepted for age, first-degree relative with diabetes mellitus, non-White ancestry, obesity (BMI greater than 30), and HDL (high-density lipoproteins) less than 35.

75. **Correct answer: B**
Insulin resistance predisposes the patient to elevated blood glucose and increased insulin production. VLDL (very-low-density lipoproteins) production increases with hyperinsulinemia.

76. **Correct answer: C**
The most common symptoms of Addison's disease are weakness, fatigue, and weight loss. One unique symptom is salt cravings. Weight gain and constipation are more commonly seen with hypothyroidism. Addison's disease is caused by deficient ACTH (adrenocorticotropic hormone) due to a problem with the adrenal cortex.

77. **Correct answer: A**
There are many important teaching points for patient Addison's disease. It is important for the patient to understand this is a lifelong illness that has to be monitored regularly. They will need to know how to inject themselves with hydrocortisone for emergency situations. A Medic-Alert bracelet is necessary. A liberal sodium diet, up to 3 grams a day, is recommended. Include family in the education.

78. **Correct answer: B**
The 5 S's in the management of a patient in adrenal crisis include intravenous steroids, salt, sugar, support, and search for a cause. The patient may not need sulfa antibiotics, supplemental oxygen, or a stress test. Struma is synonymous for goiter.

79. **Correct answer: A**
Patients with myxedema often have periorbital edema and facial puffiness.

80. **Correct answer: D**
Myxedema coma is a life-threatening emergency. The patient has severe hypothyroidism that leads to hypothermia, hypotension, low blood sugar, and lactic acidosis. It is often seen in elderly patients with concomitant vascular disease.

81. **Correct answer: B**
Pheochromocytomas are tumors of the adrenal glands that cause excessive secretion of the catecholamines such as norepinephrine, epinephrine, and dopamine. Symptoms include sudden increase of blood pressure, headache, chest pain, tachycardia, profuse sweating, and palpitations.

82. **Correct answer: A**
Aside from chronic renal failure, low vitamin D levels, phenytoin, phenobarbital, and laxatives can lead to hyperparathyroidism. The patient can present with pathologic fractures.

ENDOCRINE REFERENCES

Abbott, K. C., Bernet, V. J., Agodoa, L. Y., & Yuan, C. M. (2003). Diabetic ketoacidosis and hyperglycemic hyperosmolar syndrome after renal transplantation in the United States. *BMC Endocrine Disorders, 3,* 1–14.

Ahmed, S., Van Gelder, I. C., Wiesfeld, A. C., Van Veldhuisen, D. J., & Links, T. P. (2011). Determinants and outcome of amiodarone-associated thyroid dysfunction. *Clinical Endocrinology, 75*(3), 388–394.

Ahrens, T., Prentice, D., & Kleinpell, R. M. (2011). *Progressive care nursing certification: Preparation, review and practice exams.* St. Louis, MO: McGraw-Hill.

American Association of Critical-Care Nurses [AACN]. (2006). *AACN core curriculum for critical care nursing.* St. Louis, MO: Saunders.

Ballard, E. (2009). Adult onset type 1 diabetes mellitus versus type 2 diabetes mellitus: A case study. *Internet Journal of Advanced Nursing Practice, 10*(1), 1–19.

Brimioulle, S., Orellana-Jimenez, C., Aminian, A., & Vincent, J. L. (2008). Hyponatremia in neurological patients: Cerebral salt wasting versus inappropriate antidiuretic hormone secretion. *Intensive Care Medicine,* 34(1), 125–131.

Brorsen, A. (2012). *CEN examination review.* Burlington, MA: Jones & Bartlett Learning.

Brorsen, A., & Rogelet, K. (2009). *PCCN certification review.* Sudbury, MA: Jones and Bartlett.

Brownlie, B. E., & Turner, J. G. (2011). Lithium-associated thyrotoxicosis. *Clinical Endocrinology, 75*(3), 402–403.

Carmona-Calero, E. M., Castañeyra-Ruiz, L., Gonzalez-Marrero, I., Gonzalez-Toledo, J. M., Paz-Carmona, H. D., . . . Castañeyra-Perdomo, A. (2012). Vasopressin, angiotensin II and tyrosine-hydroxylase expression in the hypothalamus of the syndrome of inappropriate ADH: A case report. *Open Pathology Journal,* 6, 1–7.

Caspersen, C. J., Thomas, G. D., Boseman, L. A., Beckles, G .L. A., & Albright, A. L. (2012). Aging, diabetes, and the public health system in the United States. *American Journal of Public Health, 102*(8), 1482–1497.

Chulay, M., & Burns, S. (2010). *Essentials of progressive care nursing* (2nd ed.). St. Louis, MO: McGraw-Hill.

Conradie, M., Koegelenberg, C., Ascott-Evans, B. H., & Hough, F. S. (2012). Pulmonary hypertension and thyrotoxicosis. *Journal of Endocrinology, Metabolism, & Diabetes of South Africa, 17*(2), 101–104.

Cullen, K. W., & Buzek, B. B. (2009). Knowledge about type 2 diabetes risk and prevention of African American and Hispanic adults and adolescents with family history of type 2 diabetes. *Diabetes Educator, 35*(5), 836–839.

Curley, M. A. Q. (2007). *Synergy: The unique relationship between nurses and patients.* St. Louis, MO: Saunders.

Daly, M. D., Liam, D. P. P., & MacLachlan, M. (2011). The role of awakening cortisol and psychological distress in diurnal variations in affect: A day reconstruction study. *Emotion,* 11(3), 524–532.

Donohoe-Dennison, R. (2007). *Pass CCRN* (3rd ed.). St. Louis, MO: Mosby.

Drews, H. L., Castiglione, A. L., Brentin, S. N., Ersig, C. R., Dukatz, T. K., Harrison, B. E., . . . Rosenblatt, S. I. (2012). Perioperative hypoglycemia in patients with diabetes: Incidence after low normal fasting preoperative blood glucose versus after hyperglycemia treated with insulin. *AANA Journal, 80*(Suppl. 4), S17–S24.

Eldin, W. S., Ragheb, A., Klassen, J., & Shoker, A. (2008). Evidence for increased risk of prediabetes in the uremic patient. *Nephron, 108*(1), c47–c55.

"Effects of diabetes on women's reproductive health." (2012). *Nursing Standard, 26*(38), 35–40.

Gassanov, N., Semmo, N., Semmo, M., Nia, A., Fuhr, U., & Er, F. (2011). Arginine vasopressin (AVP) and treatment with arginine vasopressin receptor antagonists (vaptans) in congestive heart failure, liver cirrhosis and syndrome of inappropriate antidiuretic hormone secretion (SIADH). *European Journal of Clinical Pharmacology, 67*(4), 333–346.

Hardin, S., & Kaplow, R. (2005). *Synergy for clinical excellence: The AACN synergy model for patient care*. St. Louis, MO: Saunders.

Hibel, L. C., Mercado, E., & Trumbell, J. M. (2012). Parenting stressors and morning cortisol in a sample of working mothers. *Journal of Family Psychology, 26*(5), 738–746.

Hildebrandt, T., Yehuda, R., & Olff, M. (2012). Effects of traumatic stress molecular and hormonal mechanism. *European Journal of Psychotraumatology, 3*, Special section 1–123.

Holt, P. (2012). Pre and post-operative needs of patients with diabetes. *Nursing Standard, 26*(50), 50–56.

Ionită, A., Copotoiu, M., Hutan, A., & Copotoiu, R. (2011). Assessment of the level of burnout in several medical fields by studying the diurnal profile of salivary cortisol. *Acta Medica Marisiensis, 57*(6), 645–648.

Jaber, J. A., Haque, S., Noor, H., Ibrahim, B., & Al Suwaidi, J. (2010). Thyrotoxicosis and coronary artery spasm: Case report and review of the literature. *Angiology, 61*(8), 807–812.

Jones & Bartlett Learning. (2011). *2012 nurse's drug handbook* (11th ed.). Sudbury, MA: Jones & Bartlett Learning.

Kinoshita, H., Yasuda, M., Kaneko, S., Usui, R., Inoshita, S., Furumoto, Y., . . . Yakushiji, F. (2010). Thyroid hormones, their carrier proteins, and thyroid antibodies in the pleural effusion of two patients with Graves' disease-induced thyrotoxicosis. *Endocrine Research, 35*(4), 183–187.

Korytnaya, E., Rao, N. G., & Mayrin, J. V. (2011). An unusual case of hypercalcemia associated with Graves' disease and vitamin D deficiency. *Clinical Medicine Insights: Endocrinology & Diabetes*, 4, 25–28.

Kung, A. W. (2007). Neuromuscular complications of thyrotoxicosis. *Clinical Endocrinology*, 67(5), 645–650.

Lynn-McHale Wiegand, D. J. (Ed.). (2011). *AACN procedure manual for critical care* (6th ed.). St. Louis, MO: Saunders.

Magon, N., & Chauhan, M. (2012). Pregnancy in type 1 diabetes mellitus: How special are special issues? *North American Journal of Medical Sciences, 4*(6), 250–256.

Mäntyselkä, P., Korniloff, K., Saaristo, T., Koponen, H., Eriksson, J., Puolijoki, H., . . . Vanhala, M. (2011). Association of depressive symptoms with impaired glucose regulation, screen-detected, and previously known type 2 diabetes: Findings from the Finnish. *Diabetes Care, 34*(1), 71–76.

Mellor, D. (2012). A review of the current nutritional guidelines for diabetes. *Practice Nursing, 23*(5), 234–240.

Mishra, N. K., Son, R. Y., & Arnzen, J. J. (2012). Towards automatic diabetes case detection and ABCs protocol compliance assessment. *Clinical Medicine & Research, 10*(3), 106–121.

Mongardon, N., Bruneel, F., Henry-Lagarrigue, M., Legriel, S., Revault d'Allonnes, L., Guezennec, P., . . . Bedos, J. P. (2007). Shock during heparin-induced thrombocytopenia: Look for adrenal insufficiency! *Intensive Care Medicine, 33*(3), 547–548.

O'Shaughnessey, C., & Shubrook, J. H. (2012). Hypoglycemia. *Primary Care Reports, 18*(5), 49–63.

O'Shaughnessey, C., & Shubrook, J. H. (2012, May 21). Hypoglycemia in adults. *Emergency Medicine Reports*, 133–146.

Park, A. R. (2010). A review on hyperthyroidism: Thyrotoxicosis under surveillance. *Pakistan Journal of Biological Sciences, 13*(22), 1066–1076.

Rosner, M. H. (2011). Hyponatremia: An update on the management of SIADH. *Renal & Urology News, 10*(10), 26–30.

Sakurai, K., Fukazawa, H., Arihara, Z., & Yoshida, K. (2010). Sunitinib-induced thyrotoxicosis followed by persistent hypothyroidism with shrinkage of thyroid volume. *The Tohoku Journal of Experimental Medicine, 222*(1), 39–44.

Sarkissian, C., Gámez, A., & Scriver, C. (2009). What we know that could influence future treatment of phenylketonuria. *Journal of Inherited Metabolic Disease, 32*(1), 3–9.

Schopman, J. E., Geddes, J., & Frier, B. M. (2011). Frequency of symptomatic and asymptomatic hypoglycaemia in Type 1 diabetes: Effect of impaired awareness of hypoglycaemia. *Diabetic Medicine, 28*(3), 352–355.

Shimshi, M., & Davies, T. F. (2010). Hypothyroidism. In R. E. Rakel & E. T. Bope (Eds.), *Conn's current therapy 2010* (pp. 672–676). Philadelphia, PA: Saunders Elsevier.

Shin, I. Y., Joo, H. M., Chung, Y. G., Kim, M. S., Park, J. W., & Ahn, R. S. (2011). Abnormal diurnal pattern of cortisol secretion in patients after aneurysmal subarachnoid hemorrhage. *The International Journal on the Biology of Stress, 14*(2), 156–165.

Takata, K., Amino, N., Kubota, S., Sasaki, I., Nishihara, E., Kudo, T., . . . Miyauchi, A. (2010). Benefit of short-term iodide supplementation to antithyroid drug treatment of thyrotoxicosis due to Graves' disease. *Clinical Endocrinology, 72*(6), 845–850.

Tandon, N., Ali, M. K., & Narayan, K. M. (2012). Pharmacologic prevention of microvascular and macrovascular complications in diabetes mellitus: Implications of the results of recent clinical trials in type 2 diabetes. *American Journal of Cardiovascular Drugs: Drugs, Devices, and Other Interventions, 12*(1), 7–22.

Tantisattamo, E., & Ng, R. C. (2011). Dual paraneoplastic syndromes: Small cell lung carcinoma-related oncogenic osteomalacia, and syndrome of inappropriate antidiuretic hormone secretion: Report of a case and review of the literature. *Hawaii Medical Journal, 70*(7), 139–143.

Tsai, S. H., Lin, Y. Y., Hsu, C. W., Cheng, C. S., & Chu, D. M. (2011, November). Hypoglycemia revisited in the acute care setting. *Yonsei Medical Journal, 52*(6), 898–908.

Vincent, R. P., Etogo-Asse, F. E., Dew, T., Bernal, W., Alaghband-Zadeh, J., & le Roux, C. W. (2009). Serum total cortisol and free cortisol index give different information regarding the hypothalamus-pituitary-adrenal axis reserve in patients with liver impairment. *Annals of Clinical Biochemistry, 46*(Pt. 6), 505–507.

Watcher, R. (2012). *Understanding patient safety* (2nd ed.). Los Altos, CA: Lange.

Yam, F. K., & Eraly, S. A. (2012). Syndrome of inappropriate antidiuretic hormone associated with moxifloxacin. *American Journal of Health-System Pharmacy, 69*(3), 217–220.

Section 7

Hematology/Immunology

SECTION 7: HEMATOLOGY/IMMUNOLOGY QUESTIONS

1.A function of a red blood cell is

A. Cell humoral mediation
B. To function as a macrophage
C. To initiate hemostasis
D. Carbonic acid dissociation

2. An adverse effect of an antihistamine would include

A. Anticholenergic effects
B. Itching and anxiety
C. Central nervous system depression
D. Sodium channel blockade

3. After an antigenic substance has been eliminated, what type of cell plays an active role in suppression of an immune response?

A. A segmented neutrophil
B. Eosinophils
C. Band neutrophils
D. T8 lymphocytes

4. A blood differential test measures the percentage of each type of white blood cell found in the blood. Which type of cell makes up the largest percent of WBCs normally found in the blood?

A. Band neutrophils
B. Segmented neutrophils
C. Lymphocytes
D. Monocytes

5. Your patient's differential results show a decreased percentage of neutrophils. This result may be due to

A. Trauma
B. Chemotherapy
C. Gout
D. Eclampsia

6. If differential results show an increase in neutrophils, this increase may be the result of

A. Gout
B. Neoplastic anemia
C. Pneumonia
D. Aplastic anemia

7. **The differential drawn with your patient's A.M. labs shows a lymphocyte count of 22%. This result may be indicative of**
   A. Infectious mononucleosis
   B. Infectious hepatitis
   C. Sepsis
   D. Lymphocytic leukemia

8. **If a patient's differential shows an increase in the percentage of lymphocytes, this result may be due to**
   A. Multiple myloma
   B. Radiation therapy
   C. Leukemia
   D. Sepsis

9. **Which condition listed below would result in an increased percentage of monocytes?**
   A. Pneumonia
   B. Overwhelming bacterial infection
   C. Bone marrow damage
   D. A parasitic infection

10. **Your patient is suffering from an infection and this is the first time the patient has been exposed to the bacteria responsible for the infection. Which of the following types of cells would be the first to respond to the antigen?**
    A. T8 lymphocytes
    B. Eosinophils
    C. T4 lymphocytes
    D. Segmented neutrophils

11. **Your patient is a 35 year old female with Hodgkin's disease. She has developed respiratory distress secondary to her chemotherapy treatment. She was placed on a nasal cannula and labs were drawn. The results of this patient's CBC with differential are as follows:**
    WBCs 1,450/mm^3
    Segmented neutrophils 23%
    Banded neutrophils 11%
    Lymphocytes 29%
    Platelets 17,000/mm^3
    aPTT 105 seconds
    Based on the available lab data, which of the following complications is likely to occur with this patient?
    A. Pulmonary embolus and infection
    B. Systemic infection
    C. Heart failure
    D. Infection and bleeding

12. **Which of the cells listed below secrete lymphokines?**
    A. Segmented neutrophils
    B. T lymphocytes

C. Eosinophils
D. B lymphocytes

13. Which of the following antibodies mediates allergic reactions?
A. IgG
B. IgE
C. IgM
D. IgD

14. Your patient is suffering from pneumococcal pneumonia. What antibiotics would you expect to be prescribed for this patient?
A. Aminoglycosides
B. Vancomycin
C. Cephalosporins
D. Amphotericin B

15. The initial response to promote coagulation of an injured blood vessel is
A. Platelet aggregation
B. Fibrin formation
C. Thrombin formation
D. Vasoconstriction

16. The electrolyte necessary for normal coagulation that acts as an enzyme cofactor via the intrinsic, extrinsic, and common pathways is
A. Potassium
B. Sodium
C. Calcium
D. Magnesium

17. Which of the following actions affects the thrombotic effect of plasmin?
A. Calcium ionization
B. Fibrin breakdown
C. Prevention of platelet aggregation
D. Magnesium

18. A clotting factor most likely synthesized in the spleen is
A. Factor II
B. Factor IIa
C. Factor VIII
D. Calcium

19. Actions of histamine include
A. Vasodilation
B. Vasoconstriction
C. Production of smooth muscle contractions
D. Increased capillary permeability

20. Actions of leukotriene include
A. Production of smooth muscle contractions
B. Vasodilation

C. Development of fever
D. Activation of lymphocytes

21. **An action of serotonin would be**
A. Pulmonary vasoconstriction
B. Smooth muscle relaxation
C. Promotion of platelet aggregation
D. Decreasing capillary permeability

22. **Which of the following statements is true about the immunoglobulin IgA?**
A. IgA kills bacteria in the bloodstream
B. IgA attaches to mast cells and basophils, then causes them to release their contents
C. IgA coats bacteria and viruses to enhance phagocytosis
D. IgA activates the complement system

23. **Which of the following statements is true about prothrombin?**
A. Fibrinogen becomes prothrombin
B. Prothrombin is synthesized in the spleen
C. Prothrombin is vitamin K dependent
D. Prothrombin is the precursor to fibrin

24. **Days or weeks after a transfusion, a patient may develop a delayed hemolytic reaction. Symptoms of this condition would include**
A. Hypoxemia
B. Chills
C. Crackles
D. Mild jaundice

25. **To help prevent dilutional coagulopathy during transfusions, it is advised to administer**
A. Only packed cells
B. Fresh frozen plasma
C. Cryoprecipitate
D. Only whole blood

26. **A treatment used for disseminated intravascular coagulation (DIC) that decreases the amount of fibrin-split products is**
A. Antithrombin III
B. Desmopressin
C. Fresh frozen plasma
D. Amicar

27. **Which of the following statements is true about the use of colloids?**
A. Colloids should be used in initial burn resuscitations
B. Colloids are large-molecule protein or starch solutions
C. Colloids provide greater hydrostatic pressure to help push fluids into the interstitial spaces
D. Colloids should be used concurrently with whole blood products

28. Use of the colloid Hetastarch may affect your patient in which of the following ways?

A. Hetastarch may elevate serum amylase levels
B. Hetastarch may decrease serum potassium levels
C. Hetastarch will increase capillary permeability
D. Hetastarch will cause acute tubular necrosis

29. You are caring for a 45 year old woman with mononucleosis. What symptoms do you expect this patient to exhibit?

A. Fever, chills, sore throat, cough
B. Sore throat, lymphadenopathy, maculopapular rash
C. Hepatosplenomegaly, nasal congestion, maculopapular rash
D. Lymphadenopathy, fever, cough

30. What teaching should be done for the patient with infectious mononucleosis when discharging them from the progressive care unit?

A. There are no special precautions
B. Avoid contact sports and activities that increase intra-abdominal pressure
C. Antibiotics will cure the mononucleosis
D. Expect to feel better in 7 to 10 days

31. What treatment do you anticipate for a patient with infectious mononucleosis?

A. Supportive therapy for most patients
B. Intravenous antibiotics and contact isolation
C. Acyclovir 400 mg orally every 8 hours for 10 days
D. High-dose intravenous steroids

32. What is the causative agent in infectious mononucleosis?

A. *Streptococcus pyogenes*
B. *Streptococcus mutans*
C. Epstein–Barr virus
D. Herpes simplex I

33. The major immunoglobulin of serum and interstitial fluid is

A. IgG
B. IgA
C. IgE
D. IgM

34. A decrease in the available number of erythrocytes caused by bone marrow production failure is known as

A. Chronic anemia
B. Hemolytic anemia
C. Aplastic anemia
D. Pernicious anemia

35. Your patient was admitted to the PCU for low H and H secondary to epistaxis, as well as bleeding into the diaphragm. She bleeds from the gums, even with only

the lightest stimulus. Petechiae are noted on her chest and arms. Her platelet count is <100,000. Her probable diagnosis is

A. Idiopathic thrombocytopenia purpura
B. Pernicious anemia
C. Aplastic anemia
D. Hemolytic anemia

36. **High blood viscosity and low oxygen tension are the cause of which of the following types of anemia?**
A. Pernicious anemia
B. Aplastic anemia
C. Sickle cell anemia
D. Hemolytic anemia

37. **Your patient has been prescribed Epogen. As a progressive care nurse, you know adverse effects of Epogen include**
A. Decreased thrombosis
B. Increased iron
C. Hypertension
D. Decreased BUN

38. **Cellular humoral immunity is mediated by which of the following types of cells?**
A. Eosinophils
B. B lymphocytes
C. T Lymphocytes
D. Killer cells

39. **All the clotting factors in blood are synthesized in the liver except**
A. VIII and XII
B. VII and IX
C. IX and III
D. IIa and IXa

40. **The synthesis of hemoglobin is regulated by**
A. A myeloid stem cell
B. Erythropoietin
C. Thromboplastin
D. Thrombopoietin

41. **The physician has ordered an MCH test for your patient. This test evaluates**
A. The average concentration of RBCs in a single sample
B. The average amount (by weight) of hemoglobin in each RBC
C. The average size and volume of a single RBC
D. The average concentration of hemoglobin per single RBC

42. **Which of the following statements regarding ABO incompatibilities is true?**
A. ABO incompatibility is more frequent in mothers with type O blood
B. ABO incompatibility is more severe in mothers with type AB blood

C. ABO incompatibility is more severe than Rh incompatibility
D. ABO incompatibility is more frequent in mothers with type B blood

43. Your patient has been diagnosed with DIC. Which of the following drugs is useful in the treatment of DIC to inhibit fibrinolysis?
A. Heparin
B. Cryoprecipitate
C. Prednisone
D. Amicar

44. Your patient has a history of hemolytic anemia. She was admitted today for chest pain, fever, and heart failure. These symptoms indicate the patient is probably suffering from
A. A hemolytic crisis
B. Pulmonary edema
C. DIC
D. A myocardial infarction

45. Immune-mediated HITT usually begins about _______ after the initiation of heparin therapy.
A. 24 hours
B. 72 hours
C. Three days
D. 5–7 days

46. A partial thromboplastin time (PTT) is used to assess
A. Intrinsic and common portions of the coagulation cascade
B. The number of fibrin degradation products present
C. The number of platelets
D. The number of hemoglobin molecules

47. The extrinsic system of the coagulation cascade is initiated by
A. Exposure to cell membrane tissue factor
B. Vascular endothelial injury
C. Irritation of the intimal lining of blood vessels
D. Hypocalcemia

48. Which of the following tests is used to assess the extrinsic and common pathways of the coagulation cascade?
A. Split fibrin product
B. Prothrombin time
C. Partial thromboplastin time
D. Activated clotting time

49. A transfusion reaction that usually occurs within 5–30 minutes of the start of the transfusion is known as
A. An allergic reaction
B. A febrile reaction

C. An acute intravascular hemolytic reaction
D. An acute extravascular hemolytic reaction

50. Pernicious anemia results from a lack of
A. Vitamin B_6
B. Vitamin A
C. Vitamin B_{12}
D. Vitamin E

51. A pharmacologic antagonist to vitamin K is
A. Neostigmine
B. Digoxin
C. Amiodarone
D. Phenobarbital

52. Your patient is being treated for respiratory difficulty. He has been increasingly restless and now has petechiae on the trunk, arms, and legs. His abdomen is slightly distended, and he demonstrates increased respiratory effort. He is now obtunded. During your assessment, you note pink-tinged urine in the Foley bag, generalized ecchymosis, and oozing from the IV line insertion point. You suspect this patient may be suffering from
A. DIC
B. Pulmonary emboli
C. A fat embolism
D. Meningitis

53. Cyclosporine has significant adverse effects that include
A. Hepatotoxicity
B. Hypertension
C. Acute pancreatitis
D. Hypokalemia

54. An antirejection drug classified as an antimetabolite is
A. Cyclosporine
B. Terralimus
C. Prednisolone
D. Imuran

55. Factor VIII deficiency is also known as
A. Hemophilia B
B. Sickle-cell anemia
C. Von Willebrand's disease
D. Aplastic anemia

56. The blood component that contains factor VIII is
A. FFP
B. PRBCs

C. Salt-poor albumin
D. Cryoprecipitate

57. A fluid that causes decreased platelet aggregation and possible allergic reactions is
A. Hetastarch
B. Dextran
C. Lactated Ringer's
D. D_5/Isolyte M

58. Your patient is to receive two units of packed cells over the next 4 hours. When patients receive multiple transfusions, they are susceptible to increased
A. Bilirubin and amylase levels
B. BUN and creatinine levels
C. Serum potassium levels
D. Sodium and magnesium retention

59. A medication that may cause hemolytic anemia is
A. Phenobarbital
B. Furosemide
C. Quinidine
D. Captopril

60. Your patient was admitted with a factor VIII deficiency. In addition to specific factor VIII, the blood component that carries factor VIII, factor XIII, and fibrinogen is
A. FFP
B. PRBC
C. Salt-poor albumin
D. Cryoprecipitate

61. Possible causes of thrombocytopenia could include
A. Alcoholism
B. Portal hypertension
C. Latex sensitivity
D. A low-protein diet

62. Nursing interventions should include which of the following to minimize risk to a patient with HIT?
A. Avoid the use of heparin flushes
B. Assess the need for manual blood pressure measurements
C. Monitor platelet counts
D. Observe for petechiae

63. Type II HIT patients are at great risk for developing
A. Generalized bleeding
B. Pericarditis

C. Thrombosis
D. Limb amputation

64. **Your patient was evenomated by a rattlesnake on the right lower leg this morning while crawling under a neighbor's porch. The entire right lower leg is ecchymotic. The best course of treatment would be to provide**
A. Clotting factors and anti-venin
B. Clotting factors and heparin
C. IV at 100 ml/hour and anti-venin
D. IV at 100 ml/hour and heparin

65. **A snake bite results in activation of which of the following responses to physiologic insult to the body?**
A. Fibrinolytic system
B. Antithrombin system
C. Intrinsic cascade
D. Extrinsic cascade

66. **Your patient was thrown from the back of a truck onto a road and suffered abdominal abrasions and lacerations with a splenic rupture and a fractured right humerus. While in surgery, he received 6 units of PRBCs. As his nurse you know that this patient should also receive**
A. FFP
B. Platelets
C. Whole blood
D. Heparin

67. **Your patient has a history of acute lymphoblastic leukemia. During your assessment you note she is confused, hypotonic, and starts having generalized seizures. You would anticipate receiving orders for which of the following tests?**
A. A spinal tap
B. CT scan
C. MRI
D. PET scan

68. **Blood component replacement therapy for DIC may include all but which of the following?**
A. FFP
B. Cryoprecipitate
C. Amicar
D. Platelets

69. **Your patient is 26 years old and presented with chest pain and respiratory distress. He weighs approximately 150 pounds. During your assessment you note he is short of breath and has a dry cough. On the patient's chest you find irregularly shaped lumps near the left infraclavicular border. Based on these findings, which of the following questions should you ask the patient?**
A. "Have you suddenly gained weight in the last 2 months?"
B. "Have you noticed skin patches that are itchy and with a green cast?"

C. "Have you noticed any stomach pain or swelling?"
D. "Has your appetite increased over the last few months?"

70. Your patient has been diagnosed with anemia. She will be receiving Epogen. Adverse effects of Epogen include
A. Iron depletion
B. Hypokalemia
C. Decreased creatinine
D. Decreased ability to clot

71. Clopidogrel may interfere with the metabolism of which of the following drugs?
A. Phenobarbital
B. Phenytoin
C. Cimetidine
D. Estrogen

72. How does low-molecular-weight heparin (LMWH) differ from unfractionated heparin?
A. It is more difficult to administer
B. There are more side effects with LMWH
C. LMWH is more stable
D. Unfractionated heparin is easier to administer

73. Hemoglobin is primarily phagocytized in the
A. Liver
B. Gallbladder
C. Spleen
D. Pancreas

74. Your patient has been diagnosed with an oat cell carcinoma. Oat cell carcinomas are primarily found in the
A. Central airways
B. Genital area
C. Bronchial wall
D. Pancreas

75. Why is DIC usually fatal if untreated?
A. Exsanguination
B. Intracranial hemorrhage
C. Myocardial infarction
D. Cerebral thrombosis

76. Your patient had a previous transplant 2 years ago. She is now experiencing severe back pain. Back pain or abdominal pain with itching can be indicators of acute rejection in which of the following organs?
A. Pancreas
B. Lung
C. Liver
D. Kidney

77. **The ACT (activated coagulation time) is more sensitive to _______ and _______ than whole blood clotting time.**
A. Oxygenation, hemofiltration
B. Factor VIII, heparin
C. Warfarin, leukemia
D. Liver disease, calcium

78. **What is the most common cause of a fatal transfusion reaction?**
A. Immune-compromised recipient
B. Volume overload
C. Mismatched blood
D. Severe hyperkalemia

79. **Rejection of a transplanted organ usually occurs as a result of**
A. Cellular immunity
B. Humoral immunity
C. Delayed hypersensitivity reaction
D. Complement cascade

80. **Organ rejection that occurs 3–5 days after transplant that is antibody mediated, with fever and oliguria, is known as**
A. A chronic rejection
B. An acute rejection
C. An accelerated acute rejection
D. A hyperacute rejection

81. **Your patient had a renal transplant about 1 year ago. She is now being seen for severe flu-like symptoms. What sign or symptom would lead you to suspect that this patient is having an acute rejection episode?**
A. Hypotension
B. Pelvic pain
C. Increased urine output
D. Decreased urine osmolality

82. **The most prevalent type of anemia is known as**
A. Chronic anemia
B. Acute anemia
C. Pernicious anemia
D. Iron-deficiency anemia

83. **Acute posthemorrhagic anemia develops after**
A. Bone marrow is damaged
B. The spleen is damaged
C. Iron levels decrease by more than 15%
D. A rapid loss of erythrocytes

84. **Which of the following types of cells would be considered nongranular leukocytes?**
A. Eosinophils
B. Neutrophils

C. Monocytes
D. Basophils

85. Your patient has immune thrombocytopenic purpura that has worsened and become refractory to treatments, including plasmapheresis and injections of gamma globulin. Glucocorticoid therapy has also not been successful. The patient will be undergoing a splenectomy. One of the preoperative treatments to expect is
A. Interferon
B. Anti-Rh immunoglobulin
C. *Haemophilus influenzae* type B vaccination
D. Colchicine

86. Your patient's mother carries the sickle cell trait. Which statement about sickle cell anemia is true?
A. Sickle cell anemia always results in death by age 40
B. Sickle cell anemia causes a loss of protein intrinsic factor
C. High blood viscosity and low oxygen tension may cause a sickle cell crisis
D. Sickle cell disease is limited to the African American and Caucasian populations

87. The Kleihauer–Betke test identifies
A. Sickle cell trait in utero
B. Common blood group antigens
C. Bone marrow lymphocyte precursors
D. Fetal hemoglobin in maternal blood

88. Your patient is 21 years old and plans to breastfeed her newborn. A mother's breastmilk contains the immunoglobulin known as
A. IgG
B. IgX
C. IgY
D. IgB

89. If an 18 year old mother received an incompatible transfusion of Rh-positive platelets following a placental rupture, it would be appropriate to administer
A. Neostigmine
B. FFP
C. RhoGAM
D. CuroSurf

90. Your patient is 32 years old and was admitted for a liver transplant. A thorough history was obtained by the transplant coordinator prior to admission to the PCU. Patients can become presensitized and are more likely to experience organ rejection if they have a history of
A. Multiple pregnancies
B. Small or reduced lumens in the bile ducts
C. Destruction of small airways
D. Cytomegalovirus (CMV) infections

91. Your patient was stung by a bee and had an anaphylactic reaction. She has received epinephrine both via Epi-Pen and intravenously because she had severe airway obstruction due to swelling. Epinephrine is given for anaphylactic reactions because

A. It prevents localized edema
B. It promotes temporary changes in ST segments
C. It prevents third space fluid loss
D. It promotes bronchodilation and inhibits additional mediator release

92. A 25 year old patient has been treated in your unit for an exacerbation of his thalassemia. Patient and family teaching for a patient with thalassemia would include

A. Keeping the limbs flat to avoid a stasis ulcer
B. Avoiding oral stimulants (e.g., caffeine)
C. Eating fewer, larger, high-protein meals
D. Using warm water to cleanse the skin

93. Your patient is an 18 year old who has not been eating correctly for about 2 weeks because he is stressed out about asking a girl to their college prom. He eats a diet of toaster pastries, pastas, and high-calorie, high-sugar foods and drinks large quantities of Red Bull. He collapsed at home today after becoming dyspneic. His EKG shows sinus tachycardia without ectopy; he is pale, somewhat irritable, and complains of a headache. His initial diagnosis is folic acid deficiency. Tomorrow the patient is scheduled for more tests to determine if there is an underlying disease process. You suspect that he simply has a dietary deficiency and prepare to instruct him about foods that contain high amounts of folic acid. These foods would include

A. Green beans
B. Peanut butter
C. Oranges
D. Fish

94. Your patient is an 18 year old diagnosed with Hodgkin's lymphoma. Which of the following techniques is important to teach her about skin care?

A. Use an alcohol-based cleaner to treat acne
B. Use a moisturizer containing lidocaine
C. Use ice packs directly on the skin to decrease swelling
D. Scrub daily with a pumice-based soap

95. Which of the following statements is true about hepatitis D?

A. Hepatitis D is detectable only when the patient has concurrent HBV infection
B. IgM rises late in the course of infection
C. IgG rises slowly and the increase is limited to the acute phase of infection
D. Hepatitis D is an RNA virus that is able to self-replicate when it is present concurrently with HBV

SECTION 7: HEMATOLOGY/IMMUNOLOGY ANSWERS

1. **Correct answer: D**
A red blood cell has multiple functions, including carbonic acid dissociation to form bicarbonate ions. The RBC provides oxygen transport via hemoglobin and carbon dioxide transport via carboxyhemoglobin. The RBC buffers protons by binding with hemoglobin to form acid hemoglobin.

2. **Correct answer: A**
An adverse effect of an antihistamine would include anticholenergic effects. An antihistamine is indicated for itching and anxiety and is a mild central nervous system depressant.

3. **Correct answer: D**
After an antigenic substance has been eliminated, a T8 lymphocyte plays an active role in suppression of an immune response. T8-lymphocytes become activated by antigen-presenting cells and subsequently proliferate. These cells then differentiate into cytotoxic T-lymphocytes to kill infected and tumor cells within the body.

4. **Correct answer: B**
Segmented neutrophils make up the largest percent of WBCs normally found in the blood. A differential result should be in the range of
Neutrophils: 40% to 60%
Lymphocytes: 20% to 40%
Monocytes: 2% to 8%
Eosinophils: 1% to 4%
Basophils: 0.5% to 1%
Bands (immature neutrophils): 0% to 3%

5. **Correct answer: B**
Your patient's differential results show a decreased percentage of neutrophils. This result may be due to chemotherapy. Other potential causes of decreased neutrophils include aplastic anemia, viral infections, pneumonia, systemic bacterial infections, and radiation exposure.

6. **Correct answer: A**
If differential results show an increase in neutrophils, this increase may be the result of gout. Additional causes of increased neutrophils are rheumatoid arthritis, rheumatic fever, thyroiditis, acute stress, infection, myelocytic leukemia, trauma, and eclampsia.

7. **Correct answer: C**
The differential drawn with your patient's A.M. labs shows a lymphocyte count of 22%. This result may be indicative of sepsis. The normal range for lymphocytes on a differential is 20–40%, so this patient is deficient in lymphocytes. All the other conditions listed (infectious mononucleosis, infectious hepatitis, and lymphocytic leukemia) would cause an increase in lymphocytes.

8. **Correct answer: A**
If a patient's differential shows an increase in the percentage of lymphocytes, this result may be due to multiple myloma, viral infections such as infectious mononucleosis, measles, and mumps, and infectious hepatitis. Additional causes of

increased lymphocytes could be lymphocytic leukemia, radiation treatment (or exposure) and chronic bacterial infections.

9. **Correct answer: D**
   A parasitic infection would increase the percentage of monocytes as reflected on a differential. Additional possible reasons the monocytes would be elevated are tuberculosis, infectious mononucleosis, or chronic inflammatory diseases.

10. **Correct answer: D**
    If your patient is suffering from an infection and this is the first time the patient has been exposed to the bacteria responsible for the infection, segmented neutrophils would be the first to respond to the antigen.

11. **Correct answer: D**
    This patient is likely to develop an infection and bleeding.

12. **Correct answer: B**
    T lymphocytes secrete lymphokines. As part of the inflammatory response, lymphokines encourage cell growth, promote cell activation, and destroy target cells.

13. **Correct answer: B**
    Allergic reactions are mediated by IgE.

14. **Correct answer: C**
    Cephalosporins are generally used to treat pneumococcal pneumonia. Cephalosporins have a beta-lactam ring structure that interferes with synthesis of the bacterial cell wall, so the cell breaks down and dies.

15. **Correct answer: D**
    The initial response to promote coagulation of an injured blood vessel is vasoconstriction.

16. **Correct answer: C**
    The electrolyte necessary for the normal coagulation process via the intrinsic, extrinsic, and common pathways is calcium.

17. **Correct answer: B**
    Fibrin breakdown affects the thrombotic effect of plasmin.

18. **Correct answer: C**
    A clotting factor most likely synthesized by macrophages in the spleen is factor VII, which also may work in conjunction with macrophages.

19. **Correct answer: A**
    Actions of histamine include vasodilation, increased capillary permeability, inhibition of T cells, initiation of bronchospasms, increased secretion of mucus, and increased heart rate and contractility.

20. **Correct answer: A**
    Actions of leukotriene include production of smooth muscle contractions, vasoconstriction and increased capillary permeability.

21. **Correct answer: A**
    Actions of serotonin include pulmonary vasoconstriction, smooth muscle contractions (bronchospasms), vasodilation (systemic), and increased capillary permeability.

22. **Correct answer: D**
IgA activates the complement system, protects epithelial surfaces and protects against entry into the respiratory, genitourinary, and gastrointestinal tracts.

23. **Correct answer: C**
Prothrombin is vitamin K dependent, is synthesized in the liver, and is the precursor to thrombin (IIa).

24. **Correct answer: D**
Days or weeks after a transfusion, a patient may develop a delayed hemolytic reaction. Symptoms of this condition would include mild jaundice, purpura, anemia, and fever. It is incumbent on the nurse to monitor strict I&O, especially urine output and hematocrit and hemoglobin results.

25. **Correct answer: B**
Dilutional coagulopathy results when excess units of packed cells are administered. Bleeding may occur at the puncture site and the PT and PTT will be prolonged. It is good practice to administer 2 units of fresh frozen plasma for every 10 units of packed cells.

26. **Correct answer: D**
A treatment used for disseminated intravascular coagulation (DIC) that decreases the amount of fibrin split products is Amicar. The fibrinolytic system is blocked so stable clots do not become degraded. The Amicar decreases the amount of fibrin split products (which are anticoagulants).

27. **Correct answer: B**
Colloids are large-molecule protein or starch solutions. Dextran and Hetastarch may decrease platelet aggregation.

28. **Correct answer: A**
Hetastarch may elevate serum amylase levels, but the levels will return to normal within a week after administration. Hetastarch will not increase serum potassium levels or increase capillary permeability. Hetastarch must be used with caution in patients in anaphylactic or septic shock because capillary permeability is already increased. Dextran may cause acute tubular necrosis.

29. **Correct answer: B**
Infectious mononucleosis presents with severe sore throat, lymphadenopathy, maculopapular rash, and, at times, hepatosplenomegaly. The patient may also experience mild to moderate abdominal discomfort and fatigue. In severe cases, the spleen may rupture. It is important to teach the patient the importance of rest and to follow up with their primary care provider to prevent relapse. It can take several weeks to months to recover from infectious mononucleosis.

30. **Correct answer: B**
It is important to tell a patient with infectious mononucleosis to avoid strenuous activities that increase intra-abdominal pressure, such as heavy lifting, overexertion, minor trauma, and contact sports. These activities may lead to splenic rupture. The patient must be taught to return to the ED or primary care provider if severe abdominal pain develops.

31. **Correct answer: A**
For most patients with infectious mononucleosis, supportive therapy is all that is necessary. NSAIDs may be prescribed for pain or fever, along with increased oral fluids and rest. Steroids are sometimes necessary to manage more severe cases. Acyclovir is not indicated and has no value for these patients even though the Epstein–Barr virus is the causative agent.

32. **Correct answer: C**
The Epstein–Barr virus is the causative agent in infectious mononucleosis. It is spread by contact with body fluids, most often saliva. This disease is predominantly seen in teens and 30 year olds, but people of any age may become infected. *Streptococcus pyogenes* causes strep throat. *Streptococcus mutans* causes tooth decay. Herpes simplex I cause cold sores and is one form of genital herpes.

33. **Correct answer: A**
The major immunoglobulin of serum and interstitial fluid is immunoglobulin G (IgG). This immunoglobulin provides immunity against viral and bacterial pathogens.

34. **Correct answer: C**
A decrease in the available number of erythrocytes caused by bone marrow production failure is known as aplastic anemia. About 50% of all the cases of aplastic anemia are caused by toxins. The other 50% have an unknown cause. Some of the known causes are radiation (x-rays, radioactive isotopes, radium), benzene, streptomycin, carbon tetrachloride, DDT, chloramphenicol, and sulfonamides. Many types of pesticides other than DDT are thought to contribute to aplastic anemia.

35. **Correct answer: A**
Idiopathic thrombocytopenia purpura (ITP) is the result of a low platelet count. Sometimes platelets are destroyed early and systematically. The cause is thought to be an autoimmune response. Hemorrhages may occur in the brain, which may lead to stroke and an increased intracranial pressure.

36. **Correct answer: C**
Sickle-cell anemia occurs primarily in the African American population. These people are homozygous for HgS and have more HgS than HgA. This causes some of the cells to form a "sickle" shape—curved with rough edges. A crisis can occur when the low oxygen tension (postulated) causes a proliferation of these cells. The sharp edges of these cells travel through the microcirculation and damage capillaries. A simple thing like cold weather can precipitate massive sickling. Other identified factors include dehydration, vomiting, diarrhea, high altitude, excessive exercise, and stress. When these cells break apart, they occlude the microcirculation and lower oxygen tension, which initiates more sickling. This is a very painful time for the patient, and oxygen, pain management, and fluids are very important.

37. **Correct answer: C**
Epogen and Procrit are recombinant erythropoietin, and they are used to correct anemia that can occur with chronic renal failure and an adverse effect would be hypertension. Additional adverse effects include clotting at the site of vascular access, depletion of iron, and increased potassium, creatinine, and BUN.

38. Correct answer: B
Cellular humoral immunity is mediated by B lymphocytes. The B lymphocytes originate in bone marrow and mature there. The B lymphocytes form antibodies (immunoglobulins) that regulate a response to a specific antigen that has bound itself to the B cell's receptor sites. The B cell then forms a specific antibody for that particular antigen. Five different types of immunoglobulins are available: IgG, IgA, IgM, IgE, and IgD. After the antibodies are synthesized, the specific antibody can attach to its antigen and set off the reaction to allow for phagocytosis. The cells retain a "memory" for the specific antigen, and if another exposure occurs, the response will be quicker and stronger.

39. Correct answer: A
All factors except VIII and XII are synthesized in the liver, so that is why liver injuries can bleed so much and are so dangerous. At this time it is postulated that some of these factors may actually be synthesized in the spleen as well, but that information is unlikely to be tested.

40. Correct answer: B
Erythropoietin is a hormone responsible for the synthesis of hemoglobin. Erythropoietin levels increase in response to anemia and low oxygen states and decrease in response to hypertransfusion. Levels are also increased in infants with Down syndrome and intrauterine growth restriction. Erythropoietin may also be elevated in infants born to mothers with pregnancy-induced hypertension or diabetes.

41. Correct answer: B
A mean corpuscular hemoglobin (MCH) test measures the average amount (by weight) of hemoglobin in each RBC. A mean corpuscular hemoglobin concentration (MCHC) test measures the average concentration of hemoglobin per single RBC. A mean corpuscular volume (MCV) test measures the average size and volume of a single RBC.

42. Correct answer: A
ABO incompatibility is most often seen in mothers with type O blood, which has an absence of antigens. If the mother is exposed to A and B antigens from the fetus, an ABO incompatibility will exist. The mother can also be exposed to A and B antigens carried in food, bacteria, and pollen. This can make the first pregnancy perilous. ABO incompatibility is less severe than Rh incompatibility and occurs more frequently. ABO incompatibility protects against fetal Rh disease because of rapid destruction of A and B cells. This rapid destruction prevents Rh antigen exposure and resultant maternal antibody production.

43. Correct answer: D
Aminocaproic acid (Amicar) interferes with plasmin and inhibits fibrinolysis. Synthetic antithrombin III inhibits thrombin and can be very useful in DIC.

44. Correct answer: A
Your patient has a history of hemolytic anemia. She was admitted today for chest pain, fever, and heart failure. These symptoms indicate the patient is probably suffering from a hemolytic crisis. Patients who have hemolytic anemia may be fine until they are exposed to a major stressor like infection, trauma, or surgery. A psychological stressor,

such as divorce, may also initiate a crisis. The patient may be overwhelmed, so hemolysis accelerates and may cause tissue hypoxia, ischemia, and progress to necrosis and infarction. Treatment is supportive and targeted to presenting symptoms.

45. **Correct answer: D**
Immune-mediated HITT usually begins about 5 to 7 days after the initiation of heparin therapy. If a severe reaction develops, the patient will have chest pain due to cardiac ischemia, neurologic impairment and LOC changes, and paresthesias because of cerebral ischemia. The patient may develop pulmonary emboli, dyspnea, extremity pain and pallor due to thrombosis, and possible arterial thrombosis. It usually takes 5–7 days to manifest, but it can take much less.

46. **Correct answer: A**
A partial thromboplastin time (PTT) is used to assess intrinsic and common portions of the coagulation cascade. The results may be affected by an absence of clotting factors, anticoagulants, low levels of clotting factors, inhibitors, and an increased use of clotting factors.

47. **Correct answer: A**
The extrinsic system of the coagulation cascade is initiated by exposure of cell membrane tissue factor from tissue injury. The intrinsic system is initiated by vascular endothelial injury.

48. **Correct answer: B**
The prothrombin time (PT) is used to assess the extrinsic and common pathways of the coagulation cascade. The test used to assess the intrinsic and common pathways of the coagulation cascade is the partial thromboplastin time (PTT).

49. **Correct answer: C**
A transfusion reaction that usually occurs within 5–30 minutes of the start of the transfusion is known as an acute intravascular hemolytic reaction. The patient may experience chills, fever, tachycardia, hypotension, hematuria, back pain, and may exhibit additional signs of shock. The extravascular hemolytic reaction may manifest as fever, low H and H even after transfusion, and elevated bilirubin.

50. **Correct answer: C**
Pernicious anemia results from a lack of vitamin B_{12}. This disease results from lack of protein intrinsic factor in the stomach that helps the body absorb vitamin B_{12}. This stress on the heart from resultant hypoxia can cause heart murmurs, tachycardias, arrhythmias, hypertrophy, and heart failure. A lack of vitamin B_{12} raises the homocysteine level. High levels of homocysteine add to the buildup of fatty deposits. A lack of vitamin B_{12} can damage nerve cells and cause problems such as paresthesias in hands and feet and problems with ambulation and balance. Memory loss, visual disturbances, and confusion may develop. The condition was named "pernicious" because it was often fatal before the cause was discovered to be a lack of vitamin B_{12}.

51. **Correct answer: D**
Pharmacologic antagonists to vitamin K are phenobarbital and hydantoin (anticonvulsants) and heparin and warfarin (anticoagulants). These drugs induce hepatic enzymes and increase vitamin K degradation. Vitamin K transport across the placenta is inhibited, and vitamin K-dependent clotting factors are depressed.

52. **Correct answer: A**
This patient probably has DIC. Disseminated intravascular coagulation is an overstimulation of the clotting cascade. Both the intrinsic and extrinsic pathways are activated at the same time, which causes an acceleration of the clotting process. When the clots lyse, the fibrin split products are anticoagulants. Eventually, all the clotting factors are used up, and no further clots can form. Neonates are at increased risk for DIC secondary to inappropriate levels of anticoagulants and fibrinolytics, along with decreased levels of antithrombin and protein. One of the treatments for DIC is antithrombin III, which sometimes attenuates organ failure and reverse coagulopathy.

53. **Correct answer: B**
Cyclosporine has significant adverse effects that include nephrotoxicity, hypertension, hyperkalemia, leg cramps, headache, seizures, and development of neoplasms.

54. **Correct answer: D**
An antirejection drug classified as antimetabolite is Imuran. Antimetabolites interfere with RNA and DNA synthesis and inhibit T and B lymphocyte proliferation.

55. **Correct answer: C**
Factor VIII deficiency is also known as Von Willebrand's disease. Hemophilia A and B are factor IX deficiencies.

56. **Correct answer: D**
The blood component that contains factor VIII is cryoprecipitate. Cryoprecipitate means it is quick-frozen. It contains large amounts of factor VIII. Cryoprecipitate does have disadvantages. It is expensive and there are newer recombinant factor VIII products available. There also is the risk of transmission of hepatitis A, hepatitis C, hepatitis G, and HIV.

57. **Correct answer: B**
A fluid that causes decreased platelet aggregation and possible allergic reactions is Dextran. Sometimes Dextran causes acute tubular necrosis because it is made of polymers of high-molecular-weight polysaccharides.

58. **Correct answer: C**
When patients receive multiple transfusions, they are susceptible to increased serum potassium levels. When blood is transfused, sometimes the cells lyse and the intracellular potassium is released. This can also occur as the cells strike the floating ball in the infusion chamber. It is sound practice to monitor electrolytes after every two units of blood given. Remember to monitor the patient for dysrhythmias.

59. **Correct answer: C**
A medication that may cause hemolytic anemia is quinidine. In addition, quinidine, procainamide, and acetaminophen may cause hemolytic anemia. Phenobarbital may actually cause aplastic anemia, and furosemide may cause a generalized anemia. Captopril causes pancytopenia.

60. **Correct answer: D**
Cryoprecipitate, as mentioned previously, does carry factors VIII, XIII, and fibrinogen. There is a risk of disease transmission and transfusion reactions.

61. **Correct answer: B**
Possible causes of thrombocytopenia could include portal hypertension. Other potential causes include sepsis, viral infection, burns, and radiation therapy. Medications such as thiazides, furosemide, penicillins, sulfonomides, ranitidine, and heparin may cause thrombocytopenia. Chemotherapy is another cause.

62. **Correct answer: A**
HIT is heparin-induced thrombocytopenia, so it is best to eliminate the use of heparin.

63. **Correct answer: B**
Type II HIT patients are at great risk for developing pericarditis. Type II HIT is sometimes called "white clot syndrome." Thrombi are primarily venous in origin and can lead to DVT, pulmonary emboli, thrombotic stroke, limb ischemia, and myocardial infarction.

64. **Correct answer: A**
Treatment should include clotting factors and anti-venin. Rattlesnakes evenomate with an enzyme called hyaluronidase, which breaks down the hyaluronic acid barriers on cells. The cells lyse and exudative products enter the blood stream. Treatment is very similar to a patient with DIC because fibrin split products (anticoagulants) are released. The patient may have to receive multiple vials of anti-venin.

65. **Correct answer: D**
Damage to the tissues and vessels as a result of a snakebite initiates the extrinsic cascade. Thromboplastin and factor VII are released and are activated in the presence of calcium.

66. **Correct answer: B**
This patient should also receive platelet infusions. PRBCs contain no platelets and platelets must be given to aid in hemostasis.

67. **Correct answer: A**
This patient's presentation of confusion, hypotonia, and seizures is indicative of spinal cord involvement. A spinal tap would provide proof of the presence of blast cells in the spinal fluid. Rapid, aggressive chemotherapy treatment is indicated.

68. **Correct answer: C**
Blood component (factor) replacement therapy for DIC does not include amicar. Amicar is used to inhibit fibrinolysis, not replace clotting factors. It is used in the treatment of DIC, but it may change a simple bleeding issue into DIC. It must be used in combination with heparin. DIC is usually treated with FFP, cryoprecipitate, and platelets. Cryoprecipitate contains more than 5–10 times more fibrinogen than FFP. A good rule of thumb is to give 10 units of cryoprecipitate for every 3 units of FFP. If the patient is actively bleeding, platelets are commonly used.

69. **Correct answer: C**
An irregularly shaped lump near the infraclavicular border and respiratory distress with dry cough is suspicious for lymphoma. The nurse should ask if there has been any abdominal pain or distension, which might be indicative of hepatosplenomegaly. Rapid tumor growth is associated with Burkitt's non-Hodgkin lymphoma. Additional questions will assist in determining which type of lymphoma may be present.
A sudden weight loss, fever, and nausea/vomiting with decreased appetite have been

associated with lymphomas. The nurse's findings and history assessment should be reported to the physician immediately. As this patient is also suffering respiratory distress, the physician may perform a biopsy to determine type of lymphoma and additional tests to determine spread of disease.

70. **Correct answer: A**
Epogen and Procrit are recombinant erythropoietin and they are used to correct anemia. Adverse effects include clotting at the site of vascular access, depletion of iron, and may cause increases of potassium, creatinine, and BUN.

71. **Correct answer: B**
Clopidogrel (Plavix) interferes with phenytoin, tamoxifen and tolbutamide, fluvastin, toresemide, and warfarin. It also may affect nonsteroidal anti-inflammatories. Plavix does not seem to affect estrogen, cimetidine, or phenobarbital.

72. **Correct answer: C**
Low-molecular-weight heparin is more stable than unfractionated heparin. LMWH (i.e., Lovenox) is so stable and predictable that PTTs are not required. It is also easy to administer at home.

73. **Correct answer: A**
Hemoglobin is phagocytized primarily in the liver. Hemoglobin is comprised of two parts. The first part is "heme" that causes the reddish color and contains iron and porphyrin. The second part is a protein called "globin." Hemoglobin combines with oxygen to form oxyhemoglobin. Hemoglobin also binds with CO_2 and carries it to alveoli to be expired. When the hemoglobin is phagocytized in the liver, it breaks down into the heme and globin.

74. **Correct answer: C**
Oat cell carcinomas are primarily found in the bronchial wall. Oat cell carcinoma is a small cell carcinoma. On CXR, a central mass will be seen. This type of carcinoma easily spreads to the brain, bone, liver, and adrenal glands. Prognosis is very poor.

75. **Correct answer: A**
DIC is usually fatal if untreated because the patient exsanguinates.

76. **Correct answer: C**
Back pain or abdominal pain with itching can be indicators of acute rejection of the liver. Additional indicators would include elevated liver enzymes, elevated bilirubin, jaundice, and elevated ammonia levels (a late sign). The itching is a result of bilirubin deposits in the skin.

77. **Correct answer: B**
The ACT (activated coagulation time) is more sensitive to factor VIII and heparin than whole blood clotting time. The test is easy to do and is reliable. The ACT measures the ability of the blood to clot. Fresh, whole blood is added to a test tube that contains an activator. The activator can be glass particles, kayolin, or diatomaceous earth. The result will be the time it takes for a clot to form.

78. **Correct answer: C**
The most common cause of a fatal transfusion reaction is mismatched blood. Mismatched blood causes a hemolytic reaction, resulting in systemic cellular lysis.

The overwhelming destruction of cells cannot be corrected rapidly enough by the bone marrow.

79. **Correct answer: A**
Rejection of a transplanted organ usually occurs as a result of cellular immunity. The function of T cells is cellular immunity. These cells recognize the transplanted organ cells as foreign, resulting in a mounted attack leading to rejection. Immunosuppressive drugs suppress this normal response.

80. **Correct answer: C**
Organ rejection that occurs 3–5 days after transplant that is antibody mediated, with fever and oliguria, is known as an accelerated acute rejection. This is the standardized definition of this type of rejection.

81. **Correct answer: B**
The transplanted kidney is placed in the pelvic area. Pelvic pain is an ominous sign. Patients who have undergone kidney transplants should be educated to notify their physicians immediately if suffering from pelvic pain, as it is a symptom of rejection.

82. **Correct answer: D**
Iron-deficiency anemia is the most frequently occurring anemia seen around the world. It can be caused by either consumption of an iron-poor diet or an excessive loss of iron. Trauma is a primary cause of acute loss, with the anemia then resulting from bleeding. Blood donations, menses, GI bleeding, malabsorption syndromes, pica, and excessive diarrhea are all potential causes of this type of anemia. If you could view the erythrocytes under a microscope, they look kind of "puny". They are pale from lack of hemoglobin and tend to be smaller than normal red blood cells.

83. **Correct answer: D**
Acute post- hemorrhagic anemia may be the result of hemorrhage, cancerous lesion, an ulcerative lesion that erodes an arterial wall, trauma to a major vessel, or rupture of an aneurysm. After hemorrhage, plasma is lost and vasoconstriction takes place. The concentration of erythrocytes is increased because the volume is low—in other words, the same number of cells are in less fluid, so the count is artificially high. It can take approximately 6 weeks for hemoglobin levels to return to normal.

84. **Correct answer: C**
A monocyte would be considered a non-granular leukocyte. Both monocytes and lymphocytes are classified as agranulocytes. Monocytes are the largest leukocytes, but account for only a small portion of the total cell count for WBCs. When the monocytes mature, they become tissue macrophages and work as phagocytes. When a phagocyte lives in the liver, it is called a Kupffer cell. When it is in the lungs, it is called an alveolar macrophage. When it is found in connective tissues, it is a histiocyte.
Macrophages contain lysosomal enzymes and chemicals that can destroy bacteria. If a macrophage is activated by an antigen, it will secrete monokines, which control communication between all the cells involved in the immune response.

85. **Correct answer: C**
Preoperative treatment would include a *Haemophilus influenzae* type B vaccination. Interferon is not applicable. Anti-Rh immunoglobulin and colchicine are treatments for ITP that will have probably been tried prior to the decision to perform a

splenectomy. The patient should also be vaccinated for pneumococcal and meningococcal organisms to lower the risk of postoperative infection.

86. **Correct answer: C**
High blood viscosity and low oxygen tension may cause a sickle cell crisis.

87. **Correct answer: D**
The Kleihauer–Betke test identifies fetal hemoglobin in maternal blood. The results of this test allow for calculations to determine the amount of fetal–maternal hemorrhage and the amount of immune globulin (RhoGAM) necessary to prevent sensitization. If a patient has a positive test, follow-up testing at a postpartum check-up should be done to rule out the possibility of a false-positive result. For example, a false-positive result in the mother could be caused by sickle cell trait, which causes persistent elevation of fetal hemoglobin.

88. **Correct answer: A**
A mother's breastmilk contains multiple immunoglobulins including IgG, IgA, IgM, IgD and IgE. IgA provides anitbodies specific to environmental antigens. IgA specifically provides protection to the infant's gastrointestinal system by protecting against viruses and bacteria-associated food. IgE plays a key role in histamine release and allergic response.

89. **Correct answer: C**
If an 18 year old mother received an incompatible transfusion of Rh-positive platelets following a placental rupture, it would be appropriate to administer RhoGAM.

90. **Correct answer: A**
Patients can be presensitized and are more likely to develop organ rejection if they have a history of multiple pregnancies. It is becoming more common in some areas for teenagers to have had multiple pregnancies by age 15. Other possible causes of organ rejection include transfusions, previous organ transplants, and blood type incompatibilities. Answers B, C and D are the results of organ rejection, not causes.

91. **Correct answer: D**
Epinephrine is given for anaphylactic reactions because it promotes bronchodilation and inhibits additional mediator release. Epinephrine counteracts the bronchoconstrictive and vasodilator actions of histamine by stimulating alpha, beta1, and beta2 receptors. Epinephrine is also useful in treating hay fever and urticaria.

92. **Correct answer: B**
In thalassemia, the erythrocytes—known as "target cells"— are very thin and fragile. Use of oral stimulants could lead to vasoconstriction. The serum bilirubin is elevated in this disease, so you should caution the patient against scratching. Cool water and lotion may be used for skin care. The integrity of the skin is weakened, so careful positioning is paramount. The patient may require ongoing transfusions. Multiple transfusions may actually lead to the presence of too much iron, which might then have to be removed through chelation.

93. **Correct answer: B**
Peanut butter contains large amounts of folic acid. Other foods that are high in folic acid include red beans, broccoli, asparagus, liver, and beef.

94. **Correct answer: B**
Your patient is 18 years old and may have body image issues related to her Hodgkin's lymphoma and treatment. Patients with Hodgkin's lymphoma often have severe itching and bruising. The itching is caused by an increase of eosinophils in the blood stream. If liver impairment and hepatomegaly are present, patients may have difficulty clotting and present with bruising and petechiae. Skin care should focus on maintaining skin integrity and soothing itching. A moisturizer containing lidocaine may sooth itching and prevent skin compromise. Alcohol-based cleaners and soaps with pumice will dry the skin and be too abrasive. Ice may be used to sooth itching, but the patient should use a barrier when it is applied to prevent damage to the dermal layer.

95. **Correct answer: A**
Hepatitis D (HDV) can replicate only when hepatitis B (HBV) is present. When HDV is present, either as a co-infection or as a super-infection, liver disease and progression are more rapid and severe. IgM levels rise early in infection and may remain chronically high. IgG levels rise more slowly during infection, but will continue to be elevated for the remainder of the patient's life.

HEMATOLOGY/IMMUNOLOGY REFERENCES

Addis, G. (2010). Sickle cell disease, part 1: Understanding the condition. *British Journal of School Nursing, 5*(5), 231–234.

Ahmad, Z. (2009). A study of the knowledge and attitudes of emergency physicians and plastic surgeons in the management of snakebites. *European Journal of Plastic Surgery, 32*(3), 141–145.

Ahrens, T., Prentice, D., & Kleinpell, R. M. (2011). *Progressive care nursing certification: Preparation, review and practice exams*. St. Louis, MO: McGraw-Hill.

Akin, M., Balkan, C., Karapinar, D. Y., & Kavakli, K. (2012). The influence of the ABO blood type on the distribution of von Willebrand factor in healthy children with no bleeding symptoms. *Clinical and Applied Thrombosis/Hemostasis, 18*(3), 316–319.

Amarapurkar, P. D., & Amarapurkar, D. N. (2011). Management of coagulopathy in patients with decompensated liver cirrhosis. *International Journal of Hepatology,* 1–5.

American Association of Critical-Care Nurses. (2006). *AACN core curriculum for critical care nursing*. St. Louis, MO: Saunders.

Amir, A., Gilad, O., Yacobovich, J., Scheuerman, O., Tamary, H., & Garty, B. Z. (2010). Post-varicella thrombocytopenic purpura. *Acta Paediatrica, 99*(9), 1385–1388.

Baer, D. M. (2010). Tips from the clinical experts. What does the CBC include? *Medical Laboratory Observer, 42*(2), 34.

Barnett, R., & Kendrick, B. (2010). HELLP syndrome – a case study. *New Zealand Journal of Medical Laboratory Science, 64*(1), 14–17.

Biswajit, H., Pratim, P. P., Kumar, S. T., Shilpi, S., Krishna, G. B., & Aditi, A. (2012). Aplastic anemia: A common hematological abnormality among peripheral pancytopenia. *North American Journal of Medical Sciences, 4*(9), 384–388.

Blood management: Reducing blood use reduces risk and lowers cost. (2012). *OR Manager, 28*(1), 1, 8–10, 12.

Bocşan, C., & Cristea, V. (2011). The anti-inflammatory effect of H1 antihistamines in allergic rhinitis. *Therapeutics, Pharmacology & Clinical Toxicology, 15*(1), 13–17.

Bostock, B. (2011). Anaemias of chronic disease and sickle cell anaemia. *Practice Nurse, 41*(20), 21–24.

Brorsen, A. (2012). *CEN examination review.* Burlington, MA: Jones & Bartlett.

Brorsen, A., & Rogelet, K. (2009). *PCCN certification review.* Sudbury, MA: Jones and Bartlett.

Bross, M. H., Soch, K., & Smith-Knuppel, T. (2010). Anemia in older persons. *American Family Physician, 82*(5), 480–487.

Brown, M. (2012). Managing the acutely ill adult with sickle cell disease. *British Journal of Nursing, 21*(2), 90–96.

Camp-Sorrell, D., & Moore, S. (2008). Clinical challenges. Hemolytic uremic syndrome. *Oncology Nursing Forum, 35*(4), 593–596.

Casey, G., & Kai, T. (2011). Blood transfusion: The high-risk life-saving therapy. *Nursing New Zealand, 17*(4), 20–25.

Choudhury, N., Aimone, A., Hyder, S. M., & Zlotkin, S. H. (2012). Relative efficacy of micronutrient powders versus iron-folic acid tablets in controlling anemia in women in the second trimester of pregnancy. *Food and Nutrition Bulletin, 33*(2), 142–149.

Chulay, M., & Burns, S. (2010). *Essentials of progressive care nursing* (2nd ed.). St. Louis, MO: McGraw-Hill.

Church, M. K., Maurer, M., Simons, F. E. R., Bindslev-Jensen, C., van Cauwenberge, P., Bousquet, J., . . . Zuberbier, T. (2010). Risk of first-generation H1–antihistamines: A GA2LEN position paper. *Allergy, 65*(4), 459–466.

Connes, P., Machado, R., Hue, O., & Reid, H. (2011). Exercise limitation, exercise testing and exercise recommendations in sickle cell anemia. *Clinical Hemorheology and Microcirculation, 49*(1–4), 151–163.

Coyer, S. M., & Lash, A. A. (2008). Pathophysiology of anemia and nursing care implications. *MEDSURG Nursing, 17*(2), 77–83, 91.

Cuker, A., Arepally, G., Crowther, M. A., Rice, L., Datko, F., Hook, K., . . . Cines, D. B. (2010). The HIT Expert Probability (HEP) Score: a novel pre-test probability model for heparin-induced thrombocytopenia based on broad expert opinion. *Journal of Thrombosis & Haemostasis, 8*(12), 2642–2650.

Curley, M. A. Q. (2007). *Synergy: The unique relationship between nurses and patients.* St. Louis, MO: Saunders.

Donohoe-Dennison, R. (2007). *Pass CCRN* (3rd ed.). St. Louis, MO: Mosby.

Dressler, D. K. (2012). Coagulopathy in the intensive care unit. *Critical Care Nurse, 32*(5), 48–60.

Dubyk, M. D., Card, R. T., Whiting, S. J., Boyle, C. A., Zlotkin, S. H., & Paterson, P. G. (2012). Iron deficiency anemia prevalence at first stroke or transient ischemic attack. *The Canadian Journal of Neurological Sciences, 39*(2), 189–195.

Dymond, M. M. (2009). Case study: The link between severe traumatic brain injury and coagulopathy. *NENA Outlook, 32*(2), 27–29.

Evans, G. (2012). Time to put the gloves on: C. diff patient deaths hit a historic high. *Hospital Infection Control & Prevention, 39*(4), 37–42.

Floresca, D., Dupree, L., Basile, S., & Tan, P. (2012). Evaluation of appropriate serologic testing for suspected heparin-induced thrombocytopenia. *American Journal of Health-System Pharmacy, 69*(18), 1581–1587.

Fransson, M., Rydningen, H., & Henriksson, A. E. (2012). Coagulopathy in patients with ruptured abdominal aortic aneurysm. *Clinical and Applied Thrombosis/Hemostasis, 18*(1), 96–99.

Frazier, T. (2012). Disseminated intravascular coagulation and implications for medical-surgical nurses. *Med-Surg Matters, 21*(3–4), 8–11.

Ganesan, C., & Maynard, S. E. (2011). Acute kidney injury in pregnancy: The thrombotic microangiopathies. *Journal of Nephrology, 24*(5), 554–563.

Gatt, A., Riddell, A., Calvaruso, V., Tuddenham, E. G., Makris, M., & Burroughs, A. K. (2010). Enhanced thrombin generation in patients with cirrhosis-induced coagulopathy. *Journal of Thrombosis & Haemostasis, 8*(9), 1994–2000.

Gómez-Almaguer, D. (2012). Monoclonal antibodies in the treatment of immune thrombocytopenic purpura (ITP). *Hematology, 17*(S1), S25–27.

Gu, X., Yang, X., Lu, Z., & Wang, J. (2011). Alteration in cellular immunity after chronic hepatitis B deteriorated into severe hepatitis and its significance. *Hepatitis Monthly, 11*(10), 810–815.

Habib, A. G. (2011). Effect of pre-medication on early adverse reactions following antivenom use in snakebite. *Drug Safety, 34*(10), 869–880.

Hardin, S., & Kaplow, R. (2005). *Synergy for clinical excellence: The AACN synergy model for patient care.* St. Louis, MO: Saunders.

Ibis, S., Hazar, S., & Gokdemir, K. (2012). Acute effects of the cellular immune system on aerobic and anaerobic exercises. *HealthMed, 6*(4), 1248–1257.

Isbister, G. K., Scorgie, F. E., O'Leary, M. A., Seldon, M., Brown, S. G. A., & Lincz, L. F. (2010). Factor deficiencies in venom-induced consumption coagulopathy resulting from Australian elapid envenomation: Australian Snakebite Project (ASP-10). *Journal of Thrombosis & Haemostasis, 8*(11), 2504–2513.

Jantsch, J., Chikkaballi, D., & Hensel, M. (2011). Cellular aspects of immunity to intracellular Salmonella enterica. *Immunological Reviews, 240*(1), 185–195.

Jones & Bartlett Learning. (2011). *2012 nurse's drug handbook.* (11th ed.). Sudbury, MA: Jones & Bartlett Learning.

Jung, F., Clevert, D., Connes, P., Machado, R., Hue, O., & Reid, H. (2011). Exercise limitation, exercise testing and exercise recommendations in sickle cell anemia. *Clinical Hemorheology & Microcirculation, 49*(1–4), 151–163.

Kaygusuz, I., Firatli-Tuglular, T., Toptas, T., Ugurel, V., & Demir, M. (2011). Low levels of protein Z are associated with HELLP syndrome and its severity. *Clinical and Applied Thrombosis/Hemostasis, 17*(2), 214–219.

Keating, G. M. (2012). Romiplostim: A review of its use in immune thrombocytopenia. *Drugs, 72*(3), 415–435.

Kikuchi, M., Inagaki, T., Miyagawa, K., Ueda, R., Shinagawa, N., & Hanaki, H. (2006). Risk factors of disseminated intravascular coagulation in septic systemic inflammatory response syndrome in nursing home residents. *Geriatrics & Gerontology International, 6*(2), 109–115.

Kirkham, K., & Nero, A. C. (2011). Adult sickle cell anemia. *Primary Care Reports, 17*(12), 121–135.

Kolde, H. J., Dostatni, R., & Mauracher, S. (2011). Rapid and simple IgG specific test for the exclusion of heparin induced thrombocytopenia (HIT). *Clinical Chemistry & Laboratory Medicine, 49*(12), 2065–2068.

Koliscak, L., & Maynor, L. (2012). Pharmacologic prophylaxis against venous thromboembolism in hospitalized patients with cirrhosis and associated coagulopathies. *American Journal of Health-System Pharmacy, 69*(8), 658–663.

Kyriazi, V. I. (2011). A holistic approach of erythropoiesis and iron in anemia. *Health Science Journal, 5*(3), 176–181.

Laurent, C. (2012). Screening for sickle cell disease and thalassaemia in primary care. *Primary Health Care, 22*(7), 22–24.

Leightner, J. M., Jilma, B., Spiel, A. O., Sterz, F., Laggner, A. N., & Janata, K. M. (2010). Massive pulmonary embolism leading to cardiac arrest is associated with consumptive coagulopathy presenting as disseminated intravascular coagulation. *Journal of Thrombosis & Haemostasis, 8*(7), 1477–1482.

Levi, M., Toh, C. H., Thachil, J., & Watson, H. G. (2009). Guidelines for the diagnosis and management of disseminated intravascular coagulation. British Committee for Standards in Haematology. *British Journal of Haematology, 145*(1), 24–33.

Linder, J., & Zahniser, D. J. (2012). Digital imaging in hematology. . . New approaches to the CBC and WBC differential. *Medical Laboratory Observer, 44*(5), 14–18.

Lochmanova, A., & Lochman, I. (2011). Immunity to cytomegalovirus. *Journal of Antivirals & Antiretrovirals, 3*(3), 40–44.

Loirat, C., & Frémeaux-Bacchi, V. (2011). Atypical hemolytic uremic syndrome. *Orphanet Journal of Rare Diseases, 6*, 60.

Luzuriaga, K., & Sullivan, J. L. (2010). Infectious mononucleosis. *The New England Journal of Medicine, 362*(21), 1993–2000.

Lynn-McHale Wiegand, D. J. (Ed.). (2011). *AACN procedure manual for critical care* (6th ed.). St. Louis, MO: Saunders.

Machado, R. F., Hildesheim, M., Mendelsohn, L., Remaley, A. T., Kato, G. J., & Gladwin, M. T. (2011). NT-pro brain natriuretic peptide levels and the risk of death in the cooperative study of sickle cell disease. *British Journal of Haematology, 154*(4), 512–520.

Mahmoud, A. A., & Ismail, M. A. (2012). Anemia, iron status and calcium-phosphorus levels in rheumatoid arthritis patients. *Nature & Science, 10*(7), 110–114.

Mansour, A., Anginot, A., Mancini, S. J., Schiff, C., Carle, G. F., Wakkach, A., & Blin-Wakkach, C. (2011). Osteoclast activity modulates B-cell development in the bone marrow. *Cell Research, 21*(7), 1102–1115.

Martinez-Vea, A., Marcas, L., Bardaji, A., Romeu, M., Gutierrez, C., Garcia, C., . . . Giralt, M. (2012). Role of oxidative stress in cardiovascular effects of anemia treatment with erythropoietin in predialysis patients with chronic kidney disease. *Clinical Nephrology, 77*(3), 171–181.

Mathias, S. D., Gao, S. K., Miller, K. L., Cella, D., Snyder, C., Turner, R., . . . Nichol, J. L. (2008). Impact of chronic Immune Thrombocytopenic Purpura (ITP) on health-related quality of life: A conceptual model starting with the patient perspective. *Health and Quality of Life Outcomes, 6*, 13.

Matsukawa, Y., Iwamoto, M., Kato, K., Mizuno, S., Gon, Y., Hemmi, A., . . . Sawada, S. (2010). Long term changes in platelet counts after H. pylori eradication in non-ITP patients. *Platelets, 21*(8), 628–631.

Matzdorff, A. C., Arnold, G., Salama, A., Ostermann, H., Eberle, S., & Hummler, S. (2011). Advances in ITP -- Therapy and Quality of Life -- A Patient Survey. *PLoS ONE, 6*(11), 1–6.

Medina, V. A., Croci, M., Carabajal, E., Bergoc, R. M., & Rivera, E. S. (2010). Histamine protects bone marrow against cellular damage induced by ionising radiation. *International Journal of Radiation Biology, 86*(4), 283–290.

Milman, N. (2011). Anemia: Still a major health problem in many parts of the world! *Annals of Hematology, 90*(4), 369–377.

Mosad, E., Elsayh, K. I., & Eltayeb, A. A. (2011). Tissue factor pathway inhibitor and P-selectin as markers of sepsis-induced non-overt disseminated intravascular coagulopathy. *Clinical and Applied Thrombosis/Hemostasis, 17*(1), 80–87.

Mousa, S. A., Al Momen, A., Al Sayegh, F., Al Jaouni, S., Nasrullah, Z., Al Saeed, H., . . . Qari, M. (2010). Management of painful vaso-occlusive crisis of sickle-cell anemia: consensus opinion. *Clinical and Applied Thrombosis/Hemostasis, 16*(4), 365–376.

Murakami, H., Gando, S., Hayakawa, M., Sawamura, A., Sugano, M., Kubota, N., . . . Jesmin, S. (2012). Disseminated intravascular coagulation (DIC) at an early phase of trauma continuously proceeds to DIC at a late phase of trauma. *Clinical and Applied Thrombosis/Hemostasis, 18*(4), 364–369.

Musumadi, L., Westerdale, N., & Appleby, H. (2012). An overview of the effects of sickle cell disease in adolescents. *Nursing Standard, 26*(26), 35–40.

Myers, L. (2010). Postpartum plasma exchange in a woman with suspected Thrombotic Thrombocytopenic Purpura (TTP) vs. Hemolysis, Elevated Liver Enzymes, and Low Platelet Syndrome (HELLP): A case study. *Nephrology Nursing Journal, 37*(4), 399–402.

Na, Y. K., Hye, J. C., Heun, Y. K., Kwang, M. Y., Hyun, K. A., Thornton, S., . . . Kwak-Kim, J. (2011). Thyroid autoimmunity and its association with cellular and humoral immunity in women with reproductive failures. *American Journal of Reproductive Immunology, 65*(1), 78–87.

Nelson, J. (2011). Sickle cell disease in the workplace. *Occupational Health, 63*(8), 26–29.

Newton, J. L., Reese, J. A., Watson, S. I., Vesely, S. K., Bolton-Maggs, P. H. B., George, J. N., & Terrell, D. R. (2011). Fatigue in adult patients with primary immune thrombocytopenia. *European Journal of Haematology, 86*(5), 420–429.

Ninkovich, G. M., Miller, S. K., & Alpert, P. T. (2010). Sickle-cell anemia and pulmonary hypertension. *Journal of the American Academy of Nurse Practitioners, 22*(4), 198–204.

O'Connor, T. E., Skinner, L. J., Kiely, P., & Fenton, J. E. (2011). Return to contact sports following infectious mononucleosis: The role of serial ultrasonography. *Ear, Nose, & Throat Journal, 90*(8), E21–E24.

Ogbe, P. J., Idoko, O. A., Ezimah, A. C. U., Digban, K. A., & Oguntayo, B. O. (2012). Evaluation of iron status in anemia of chronic disease among patients with HIV infection. *Clinical Laboratory Science, 25*(1), 7–12.

Olson, D., & Huntington, M. K. (2009). Co-infection with cytomegalovirus and Epstein–Barr virus in mononucleosis: Case report and review of literature. *South Dakota Medicine, 62*(9), 349, 351–353.

Parle-Pechera, S., Powers, L., St. Anna, L., & Guirguis-Blake, J. (2012). Intranasal steroids vs antihistamines: Which is better for seasonal allergies and conjunctivitis? *Journal of Family Practice, 61*(7), 429–448.

Paul, J., & Dasgupta, S. (2012). Early prediction of acute kidney injury by clinical features of snakebite patients at the time of hospital admission. *North American Journal of Medical Sciences, 4*(5), 216–220.

Plana, M., Garcia, F., Darwich, L., Romeu, J., López, A., Cabrera, C., . . . Bofill, M. (2011). The reconstitution of the thymus in immunosuppressed individuals restores CD4–specific cellular and humoral immune responses. *Red de Investigación en Sida (RIS), Immunology, 133*(3), 318–328.

Pluta, A., Gutkowski, K., & Hartleb, M. (2010). Coagulopathy in liver diseases. *Advances in Medical Sciences, 55*(1), 16–21.

Ponte, J. F., Ponath, P., Gulati, R., Slavonic, M., Paglia, M., O'Shea, A., . . . Rosenzweig, M. (2010). Enhancement of humoral and cellular immunity with an anti-glucocorticoid-induced tumour necrosis factor receptor monoclonal antibody. *Immunology, 130*(2), 231–242.

Qari, M. H., Dier, U., & Mousa, S. A. (2012). Biomarkers of inflammation, growth factor, and coagulation activation in patients with sickle cell disease. *Clinical and Applied Thrombosis/Hemostasis, 18*(2), 195–200.

Radaideh, S. M., Frenkel, E. P., Dowell, J. E., Sarode, R., & Shen, Y. M. (2012). Incidence of isolated heparin-induced thrombocytopenia and risk of thrombosis by IgG-specific anti-PF4/heparin ELISA. *Clinical and Applied Thrombosis/Hemostasis, 18*(2), 215–217.

Rahman, S., Cichon, M., Hoppensteadt, D., Cunanan, J., Jeske, W., Thethi, I., & Fareed, J. (2011). Upregulation of microparticles in DIC and its impact on inflammatory processes. *Clinical and Applied Thrombosis/Hemostasis, 17*(6), E202–E204.

Renouf, L. S., Sheps, S., Hubley, A., Pick, N., Johansen, D., & Tyndall, M. W. (2012). The role of diet in predicting iron deficiency anemia in HIV-positive women. *Canadian Journal of Dietetic Practice & Research, 73*(3), 128–133.

Rollins, K. E., Trim, N. L., Luddington, R. J., Colah, S., Klein, A., Besser, M. W., & Nair, S. K. (2012). Coagulopathy associated with massive cell salvage transfusion following aortic surgery. *Perfusion, 27*(1), 30–33.

Sabol, V. K., Resnick, B., Galik, E., Gruber-Baldini, A., Morton, P. G., & Hicks, G. E. (2010). Anemia and its impact on function in nursing home residents: What do we know? *Journal of the American Academy of Nurse Practitioners, 22*(1), 3–16.

Sakabe, K., Fukui, M., Ushigome, E., Hamaguchi, M., Tanaka, T., Atsuta, H., . . . Nakamura, N. (2012). Second measurement of morning systolic blood pressure is more closely associated with albuminuria. *Clinical Nephrology, 78*(2), 129–134.

Sari, I., Birlik, M., Akar, S., Onen, F., Kargi, A., & Akkoc, N. (2009). Atypical infectious mononucleosis in a patient receiving tumor necrosis factor alpha inhibitory treatment. *Rheumatology International, 29*(7), 825–826.

Sarpatwari, A., Provan, D., Erqou, S., Sobnack, R., David Tai, F. W., & Newland, A. C. (2010). Autologous 111 in-labelled platelet sequestration studies in patients with primary immune thrombocytopenia (ITP) prior to splenectomy: A report from the United Kingdom ITP Registry. *British Journal of Haematology, 151*(5), 477–487.

Sater, M. S., Mahdi, N., Al-Absi, I. K., Al-Subaie, A. M., Al-Ola, K., Mohammed, F. A., & Almawi, W. Y. (2011). Anti-annexin V IgG and IgM antibodies in sickle cell disease patients with vaso-occlusive crisis. *Annals of Hematology, 90*(9), 1031–1036.

Sathappan, S. S., Ginat, D., & Di Cesare, P. E. (2006). Multidisciplinary management of orthopedic patients with sickle cell disease. *Orthopedics, 29*(12), 1094–1103.

Serjeant, G. R. (2010). One hundred years of sickle cell disease. *British Journal of Haematology, 151*(5), 425–429.

Shahid, S. M., Nawab, S. N., Shaikh, R., & Mahboob, T. (2012). Glycemic control, dyslipidemia and endothelial dysfunction in coexisted diabetes, hypertension and nephropathy. *Pakistan Journal of Pharmaceutical Sciences, 25*(1), 123–129.

Smythe, M. A., Mehta, T. P., Koerber, J. M., Forsyth, L. L., Sykes, E., Corbets, L. R., . . . Parikh, R. (2012). Development and implementation of a comprehensive heparin-induced thrombocytopenia recognition and management protocol. *American Journal of Health-System Pharmacy, 69*(3), 241–248.

Snyder, S. R., Kivlehan, S. M., & Collopy, K. T. (2011). Prehospital management of the anemia patient. *EMS World, 40*(9), 65–72.

Tavare, A. N., Wrench, D., & Cooper, N. (2012). Acute splenic sequestration crisis in an adult with sickle cell anaemia. *British Journal of Hospital Medicine, 73*(3), 168–169.

Taylor, J. G., Darbari, D. S., Maric, I., McIver, Z., & Arthur, D. C. (2011). Therapy-related acute myelogenous leukemia in a hydroxyurea-treated patient with sickle cell anemia. *Annals of Internal Medicine, 155*(10), 722–724.

Thoms, K. M., Kuschal, C., Oetjen, E., Mori, T., Kobayashi, N., Laspe, P., . . . Emmert, S. (2011). Cyclosporin A, but not everolimus, inhibits DNA repair mediated by calcineurin: Implications for tumorigenesis under immunosuppression. *Experimental Dermatology, 20*(3), 232–236.

Thorsen, K., Ringdal, K. G., Strand, K., Søreide, E., Hagemo, J., & Søreide, K. (2011). Clinical and cellular effects of hypothermia, acidosis and coagulopathy in major injury. *British Journal of Surgery, 98*(7), 894–907.

Tripathi, A., Jerrell, J. M., & Stallworth, J. R. (2011). Cost-effectiveness of adenotonsillectomy in reducing obstructive sleep apnea, cerebrovascular ischemia, vaso-occlusive pain, and ACS episodes in pediatric sickle cell disease. *Annals of Hematology, 90*(2), 145–150.

Tutanc, M., Arica, V., Yılmaz, N., Nacar, A., Zararsiz, I., Basarslan, F., . . . Nacar, E. (2012). Effects of erdosteine on cyclosporin-A-induced nephrotoxicity. *Human & Experimental Toxicology, 31*(6), 565–573.

Understanding blood results: Urea and electrolytes. (2012). *Practice Nurse, 42*(5), 20–24.

Warkentin, T. E. (2011). HIT paradigms and paradoxes. *Journal of Thrombosis & Haemostasis, 9*(7), 105–117.

Watcher, R. (2012). *Understanding Patient Safety* (2nd ed.). Los Altos, CA: Lange.

Watson, S. (2009). Global issues facing the ITP community. *Pharmaceuticals Policy & Law, 11*(4), 269–274.

Wilbur, K., Lynd, L. D., & Sadatsafavi, M. (2011). Low-molecular-weight heparin versus unfractionated heparin for prophylaxis of venous thromboembolism in medicine patients: A pharmacoeconomic analysis. *Clinical and Applied Thrombosis/Hemostasis, 17*(5), 454–465.

Yohannes, A. M., & Ershler, W. B. (2011). Anemia in COPD: A systematic review of the prevalence, quality of life, and mortality. *Respiratory Care, 56*(5), 644–652.

Yontz, C. J., & Waller, K. V. (2011). Homozygous sickle cell anemia and secondary complications: A case study. *Clinical Laboratory Science, 24*(2), 78–84.

Yu, J. M., Shord, S. S., & Cuellar, S. (2011). Transfusions increase with nationally driven reimbursement changes of erythropoiesis stimulating agents for chemotherapy-induced anemia. *Journal of Oncology Pharmacy Practice, 17*(4), 360–365.

Yucesoy, G., Cakiroglu, Y., Bodur, H., Ozkan, S., & Tan, T. (2011). An analysis of HELLP syndrome cases: Does platelet count predict adverse maternal and fetal outcomes in women with HELLP syndrome? *Archives of Gynecology and Obstetrics, 283*(5), 941–945.

Section 8

Neurology

SECTION 8: NEUROLOGY QUESTIONS

1. **A 69 year old man is complaining a left chest pain that radiates to his back. He thinks he somehow burned himself. When you remove his shirt there are erythematous blisters from the spine to the sternum. The blisters are most likely which of the following disorders?**
   A. Herpes zoster infection (shingles)
   B. Sjögren's syndrome
   C. Stevens–Johnson syndrome
   D. A second-degree burn
2. **Your patient has been diagnosed with sine shingles. What lab test(s) do you anticipate the physician will order?**
   A. CBC, CMP, sedimentation rate
   B. Varicella-zoster virus culture
   C. CBC, CMP, varicella titer
   D. Blood culture, wound swab
3. **Under which of the following circumstances is a lumbar puncture contraindicated?**
   A. Signs of increased cranial pressure of unknown origin
   B. Signs of an intracranial hemorrhage
   C. Signs of Guillain–Barré syndrome
   D. Obtaining a specimen for laboratory study
4. **If your patient scores 15 on the Adult Glasgow Coma Scale**
   A. The patient has a poor chance of survival physically and neurologically
   B. The patient has a fair chance of survival neurologically intact
   C. The patient is likely to survive neurologically intact
   D. The patient will have no discernible brain function
5. **Patients who have right hemispheric involvement will often**
   A. Use great caution when making decisions
   B. Tend to underestimate their abilities
   C. Move slowly
   D. Display poor judgment
6. **In a patient with a complete transection of the spinal cord at the C2-3 level, you expect which of the following findings?**
   A. Full sensation of the face, intermittent breathing, shoulder shrug
   B. Some sensation on the occiput, face, and ears, no diaphragm movement
   C. Complete loss of sensory and motor function below the level of the injury
   D. No movement of the diaphragm, shoulder shrug

7. **What is the highest level of cervical spinal cord injury at which a patient can survive without ventilator assistance?**
   A. C3-4
   B. C7-8
   C. C5-6
   D. C1-2

8. **Where does the dermatome for the fifth thoracic spinal nerve cross the anterior portion of a patient's body?**
   A. At the level of the axilla
   B. At the level of the xyphoid process
   C. At the level of the clavicular line
   D. At the nipple line

9. **Your head-injured patient has developed nystagmus. Nystagmus may be defined as**
   A. Eyes deviated to the side of the injury
   B. A convergent gaze
   C. Rhythmic tremor or shaking of the eyes
   D. Divergent gaze

10. **Spinal reflexes indicate**
    A. Functional upper motor neurons
    B. Nonfunctional lower motor neurons
    C. Nonfunctional upper motor neurons
    D. Functional lower motor neurons

11. **A sympathetic response to a stimuli results in**
    A. Heightened awareness, increased blood pressure, bronchial dilation, and increased glucogenosis
    B. Dilated pupils, bronchial relaxation, increased gastric motility, and normal urine output
    C. Vasodilatation, increased blood pressure, decreased gastric secretions, and pupils at 3 mm
    D. Relaxation, decreased blood pressure, bronchial dilation

12. **Normal intracranial pressure is in the range of**
    A. 0–5 mmHg
    B. 4–5 mmHg
    C. 16–20 mmHg
    D. 20–40 mmHg

13. **Which of the following mechanisms decreases intracranial pressure?**
    A. CO_2 retention
    B. PaO_2 less than 50 mmHg
    C. Increased cerebrospinal fluid absorption
    D. Increased metabolic activity

14. **What is autonomic hyperreflexia?**
    A. Malfunction of the autonomic nervous system seen with head injury
    B. Malfunction of the autonomic nervous system seen with spinal cord injury
    C. Malfunction of the autonomic nervous system seen with pituitary tumor removal
    D. Malfunction of the autonomic nervous system seen with epidural bleeds

15. **Your patient has a gunshot wound to his T11-12 spine. Upon assessment you find motor paralysis on the same side as the gunshot wound but loss of pain and temperature sensation on the opposite side. This phenomenon is known as**
    A. Grey–Turner syndrome
    B. Cushing syndrome
    C. Syndrome X
    D. Brown Sequard syndrome

16. **What is the most common etiology of meningococcal meningitis?**
    A. *Streptococcus pneumonia*
    B. *Neisseria meningitidis*
    C. *Staphylococcus aureus*
    D. *Haemophilius influenza*

17. **What is the hallmark symptom of meningococcal meningitis?**
    A. Headache
    B. Petechiae
    C. Malaise
    D. Vomiting

18. **What is the proper technique for eliciting a Babinski response?**
    A. Stroke the sole of the foot from side to side
    B. Stroke the sole of the foot along the lateral sole from the heel up toward the toes and across the ball of the foot
    C. Strike the heel and the ball of the foot
    D. Strike the Achilles tendon with a reflex hammer

19. **What effect is seen with a normal response to the Doll's eyes maneuver?**
    A. Disconjugate gaze with head turn
    B. Conjugate gaze in the opposite direction as the head is turned
    C. Conjugate gaze in the same direction as the head is turned
    D. Nystagmus with head turning

20. **Cerebrospinal fluid is formed in which of the following locations in the brain?**
    A. Lateral ventricles
    B. Choroid plexus
    C. Subarachnoid space
    D. Arachnoid villi

21. **Patients who have left hemispheric involvement will often**
    A. Overestimate their abilities
    B. Move slowly

C. Display impulsive behavior
D. Use poor judgment

22. **A 55 year old man with meningitis is having a lumbar puncture. As his progressive care nurse, you know the cerebrospinal fluid (CSF) should be**
A. Hazy with a glucose level of 85
B. Clear with RBCs present
C. Clear and colorless with less than 45 mg/dl of protein
D. Clear and colorless with a white blood cell count greater than 150 cells/mm^3

23. **What does the acronym RIND represent?**
A. Recurrent ischemic neurologic default
B. Reversible intracerebral neurologic deficit
C. Recurrent intracerebral neurologic default
D. Reversible ischemic neurologic deficit

24. **You are educating your patient and his family about stroke. Part of your talk involves modifiable risk factors for stroke. Which of the following are modifiable risk factors for stroke?**
A. Alcohol use, obesity, family history
B. Alcohol use, smoking, obesity
C. Alcohol use, family history, smoking
D. Alcohol use, family history, hypertension

25. **What are the two major types of stroke?**
A. Ischemic and lacunar
B. Ischemic and hemorrhagic
C. Hemorrhagic and transient ischemic attack
D. Hemorrhagic and reversible ischemic neurologic deficit

26. **You are caring for a 72 year old man with a left-sided cerebrovascular accident. Which symptoms do you expect to see?**
A. Hearing deficits, left vision problems, left facial droop
B. Speech deficits, loss of right visual field, right facial droop
C. Loss of right visual field, receptive aphasia, left facial droop
D. Speech deficits, left visual field loss, left facial droop

27. **Which area in the cerebrum controls verbal expression?**
A. Wernicke's area
B. Broca's area
C. Limbic area
D. Pontine area

28. **A 35 year old woman has Guillain–Barré syndrome. What is the most important diagnostic parameter for this patient?**
A. Blood pressure
B. Negative inspiratory force (NIF)
C. Pain level
D. Cerebrospinal fluid study results

29. Which of the following descriptions would be the most appropriate for the patient with Guillain–Barré syndrome?

A. Impaired motor weakness, impaired respiratory function, acute pain
B. Impaired respiratory function, impaired nutrition, acute pain
C. Impaired motor weakness, impaired bowel function, acute pain
D. Impaired respiratory function, impaired bowel function, acute pain

30. Death from status epilepticus is usually caused by which of the following mechanisms?

A. Airway blockage leads to severe cerebral hypoxia
B. A hypermetabolic state within the brain
C. Falls from seizure causing head trauma
D. Aspiration pneumonia

31. Mrs. C. is a patient with new onset grand mal seizures. While moving her to the gurney, you witness a seizure. What is the first action you should take to protect this patient?

A. Hold the patient down to prevent injury
B. Roll the patient to her right side and protect the airway
C. Insert an oral airway and call for help
D. Hit the Code Blue button

32. Your patient had a grand mal seizure lasting 70 seconds. As soon as the seizure passed, he was fully awake and asking for food. Given the patient's reaction to his seizure, you should

A. Tell the patient you know he faked the seizure
B. Feed the patient
C. Notify the attending physician and anticipate a psychological evaluation
D. Give Dilantin 1 g IV slowly

33. Aggrenox is commonly used to treat

A. Myocardial infarction
B. Cerebrovascular accident
C. Pulmonary embolism
D. Deep vein thrombosis

34. Your patient has been diagnosed with multiple sclerosis (MS). She was admitted to the PCU after an acute exacerbation during which she experienced left-side weakness. You know that multiple sclerosis is classified as which of the following types of disease?

A. Motor disorder of the spinal cord
B. Demyelinating disorder of the brain and spinal cord
C. Motor disorder of the brain and spinal cord
D. Demyelinating disease of the spinal cord

35. A depressed patient states, "I don't want to die like my mother did with MS." She is exhibiting behavior consistent with which Kubler-Ross stage of grief?

A. Denial
B. Bargaining

C. Anger
D. Acceptance

36. **What are the four types of Guillain–Barré syndrome?**
A. Ascending, progressive, relapsing–remitting, pure motor
B. Ascending, descending, Miller–Fisher variant, pure motor
C. Ascending, descending, relapsing, pure sensory
D. Ascending, relapsing–remitting, pure motor, pure sensory

37. **Common symptoms of an exacerbation of multiple sclerosis can include which of the following?**
A. Hyperesthesia, fatigue, and hyporeflexia
B. Paresthesias, urinary incontinence, and constipation
C. Diplopia, ataxia, and emotional lability
D. Ataxia, dementia, and temporal neuralgia

38. **What is the postulated etiology of multiple sclerosis?**
A. Heredity
B. Autoimmune disorder
C. Chemical exposure
D. Heavy metal poisoning

39. **Myasthenia gravis is diagnosed using which of the following tests?**
A. Weber test
B. Rinne test
C. Tensilon test
D. Clonus test

40. **Which of the following statements about Bell's palsy is true?**
A. The patient will have to take long-term steroid treatments
B. The patient will have to wear sunglasses when outside
C. The patient will develop a secondary petechial rash
D. The patient will no longer require the use of thermal packs to the face

41. **A 62 year old woman has had several months of declining fine motor skills. Her family brought her to the hospital because of a sudden onset of dementia and incontinence. Following a CT scan she was diagnosed with normal pressure hydrocephalus. What is the most common cause of normal pressure hydrocephalus?**
A. Cerebrovascular accident
B. Deep vein thrombosis
C. An idiopathic cause
D. Recreational drug use

42. **Your patient has suffered a stroke. He has been evaluated using the NIH stroke scale and received a score of 26. This score indicates that this patient has suffered**
A. A minor stroke
B. A severe stroke
C. A moderate stroke
D. A moderate/severe stroke

43. One of the primary purposes of using the NIH scale is to determine whether or not the degree of disability will merit

A. Extended rehabilitation
B. A DNR order
C. Additional speech therapy
D. Use of tPA

44. Which of the following is not considered a testable aspect of brain function when using the NIH stroke scale?

A. Language
B. Ethnicity
C. Sensation
D. Vision

45. Your patient is being evaluated for meningitis. The patient is placed supine, with hips and knees flexed. When the physician attempts to extend the leg past 135 degrees, the patient complains of pain. This response is known as

A. Cullen's sign
B. Moses' sign
C. Trevell's sign
D. Kernig's sign

46. What patient parameters does the Glasgow Coma Scale measure?

A. Verbal response, orientation, and activity
B. Eye opening, motor response, and verbal response
C. Eye opening, orientation, and motor response
D. Verbal response, orientation, and eye opening

47. What results do you anticipate from a lumbar puncture in a patient with suspected Guillain–Barré syndrome?

A. The cerebrospinal fluid (CSF) is normal
B. The glucose level is down but the CSF is otherwise normal
C. There is a high red blood cell count in the CSF
D. The CSF protein level is elevated but the cell count is normal

48. A 24 year old female is brought to the PCU directly from her physician's office by paramedics. The primary physician did not obtain a temperature on this patient. She has a fever of 105.7° F. The hospitalist called a neurologist to evaluate the patient. He performs a lumbar puncture for evaluation of this patient's cerebrospinal fluid. Which of the following results would you expect to see if this patient has bacterial meningitis?

A. Xanthochromia, elevated CSF glucose, decreased protein
B. Decreased CSF specific gravity, increased protein levels, normal cell count
C. Elevated specific gravity, cloudy CSF, decreased glucose, elevated WBCs
D. Increased protein levels, elevated cell count and CSF glucose

49. Your patient has an old injury to C5. He has a blood pressure of 215/129 and his pulse is 175. What is the cause of his symptoms?

A. Autonomic dysreflexia
B. Hypertension

C. Spinal shock
D. Neurogenic shock

50. Cerebral aneurysms are most often found in the
A. Internal carotid arteries
B. Bifurcations of the anterior-posterior Circle of Willis
C. Temporal artery
D. Vertebral arteries

51. The most common first symptom of a rupturing cerebral aneurysm is
A. Fever
B. Nuchal rigidity
C. Nausea and vomiting
D. An explosive headache, often "worst headache of my life."

52. Nursing management of a patient with a cerebral aneurysm includes
A. Ambulation, monitoring of vital and neurologic signs
B. Glasgow Coma Scale assessments and monitoring for cerebral vascular spasm
C. Maintaining normal intracranial pressure
D. Maintaining systolic blood pressure less than 120 mmHg

53. What is the formula for cerebral perfusion pressure (CPP)?
A. CPP = SBP + MAP and ICP
B. CPP = MAP – ICP
C. CPP = ICP – MAP
D. CPP = MAP – CVP and ICP

54. The goal for cerebral perfusion pressure (CPP) is a pressure of
A. 50–80 mmHg
B. 20–40 mmHg
C. 10–20 mmHg
D. 40–60 mmHg

55. Spinal shock is defined as a(n)
A. Areflexia at or below the spinal cord injury
B. Hyperreflexia and spasticity after spinal cord injury
C. Areflexia that rises above the site of injury
D. Spasticity below injury site

56. Neurogenic shock differs from spinal shock in which of the following ways?
A. It is a less severe form of shock with spinal cord injury that causes a brief decrease in blood pressure
B. It is a more severe form of shock that causes cardiovascular collapse in patients with a spinal cord injury above T6
C. It is a more severe shock that increases paralysis and death
D. It is a more severe form of shock that occurs within hours after a spinal cord injury and causes increased sympathetic outflow

57. Arteriovenous malformations (AVMs) are
A. Commonly found misshapen blood vessels
B. More common in women than in men

C. A complex tangle of misshapen blood vessels susceptible to hemorrhage
D. Never seen in children

58. The hallmark symptom of encephalopathy from any cause is
A. An altered mental state
B. Liver failure
C. Renal failure
D. Infection

59. Treatment of encephalopathy includes
A. Antibiotics
B. High-dose steroids
C. Treating the underlying cause
D. Electrolyte replacement

60. Diagnostic tests for a patient with encephalopathy could include
A. BMP, CRP, and CXR
B. Blood tests, CSF evaluation, and EEG
C. EEG and Dilantin levels
D. Lumbar puncture and cervical ultrasound

61. What is the effect of Cushing syndrome in a patient with increased intracranial pressure?
A. Increased systolic blood pressure, widening pulse pressure, bradycardia
B. Elevated blood pressure, narrow pulse pressure, tachycardia
C. Bradycardia, low blood pressure, narrow pulse pressure
D. Tachycardia, increased systolic blood pressure, widening pulse pressure

62. Which of the following mechanisms decreases intracranial pressure?
A. CO_2 retention
B. PaO_2 less than 50 mm Hg
C. Increased cerebrospinal fluid absorption
D. Increased metabolic activity

63. Mrs. P., a patient with a closed head injury, has a Foley catheter. In 1 hour, her urine output increased from 30 ml/hour to 1000 ml of very pale, clear urine. As her nurse, you know the increase in urine output is probably due to
A. A volume shift from the third space
B. Syndrome of inappropriate antidiuretic hormone
C. Diabetes insipidus
D. Diuresis from steroids

64. As a progressive care nurse, you know the treatment of diabetes insipidus includes which of the following interventions?
A. Fluid restriction
B. Intravenous replacement to cover the increased urine output
C. Diuretics
D. Demeclocycline

65. What is one cause of autonomic hyperreflexia?
A. Diarrhea
B. Suctioning

C. Constipation
D. Warm breeze

66. A positive Babinski or plantar reflex indicates
A. A reflex elicited with a reflex hammer to the Achilles tendon
B. Normal neurologic functioning
C. Upper motor neuron lesion of the pyramidal tract
D. Lower motor neuron lesion of the pyramidal tract

67. A 21 year old woman was injured in a motor vehicle accident and she is demonstrating decerebrate posturing. As her nurse, you know decerebrate posturing displays as
A. One arm flexed, one flaccid, legs flaccid
B. Both arms fully extended and internally rotated, legs flaccid
C. Both arms fully extended and internally rotated, legs fully extended with toes pointed
D. Flaccid arms and legs extended

68. Your patient suddenly develops right pupil dilation. What significance does this change indicate?
A. Basilar skull fracture
B. Uncal herniation
C. Brainstem herniation
D. Cerebrovascular accident

69. Your patient was an unrestrained driver in a motor vehicle crash where he struck and fractured the windshield. He has a left frontal lobe injury. Which of the following symptoms would you expect in this patient?
A. Hearing and balance impairment
B. Sensory and memory problems
C. Personality changes, poor short-term memory
D. Loss of motor function, hearing problems

70. What differentiates a transient ischemic attack (TIA) from a reversible ischemic neurologic deficit (RIND)?
A. TIA lasts less than 24 hours, a RIND lasts more than 24 hours
B. TIA lasts less than 6 hours, a RIND lasts more than 48 hours
C. TIA lasts more than 24 hours, a RIND lasts less than 24 hours
D. TIA lasts less than 24 hours, a RIND lasts less than 6 hours

71. What volume of cerebrospinal fluid is produced each day?
A. 1000–1200 ml
B. 600–700 ml
C. 400–800 ml
D. 800–900 ml

72. Your patient has had a major left-sided stroke. What is the most common cause of stroke in the United States?
A. Uncontrolled diabetes mellitus
B. Cocaine abuse

C. Uncontrolled hypertension
D. Tobacco addiction

73. Why does diabetes mellitus increase the risk of stroke?
A. DM increases the risk of hypertension
B. DM decreases neuroreceptor response in cerebral circulation
C. DM accelerates atherosclerosis of the large arteries
D. DM increases the risk of clot formation

74. Your patient with uncontrolled hypertension is most likely to have which of the following types of stroke?
A. Ischemic
B. Lacunar
C. Transient ischemic attack
D. Reversible neurologic deficit

75. Which hemisphere, cerebral or cerebellar, is more likely to be affected by stroke?
A. Right cerebellar hemisphere
B. Right cerebral hemisphere
C. Left cerebral hemisphere
D. Left cerebellar hemisphere

76. Your priority in caring for a patient with a cerebrovascular accident is
A. Prevention of decubitus ulcers
B. Prevention of aspiration of food or fluid
C. Prevention of contractures
D. Prevention of depression

77. An 80 year old African American man has had a left temporal cerebrovascular accident due to uncontrolled hypertension. As his nurse, you know that this patient is likely to have which of the following deficits?
A. Motor deficits
B. Expressive aphasia
C. Receptive aphasia
D. Balance deficits

78. Suspected cases of meningitis should be placed in which of the following types of isolation?
A. Universal precautions are all that is needed
B. Contact precautions
C. Reverse isolation
D. Droplet precautions

79. Which results would you expect in the evaluation of the cerebrospinal fluid in a patient with Guillain–Barré syndrome?
A. Increased white blood cells
B. Increased protein levels
C. Increased glucose levels
D. Anaerobic bacteria

80. Which of the following descriptions would be the most appropriate for the patient with Guillain–Barré syndrome?

A. Impaired motor weakness, impaired respiratory function, acute pain
B. Impaired respiratory function, impaired nutrition, acute pain
C. Impaired motor weakness, impaired bowel function, acute pain
D. Impaired respiratory function, impaired bowel function, acute pain

81. Your patient with Guillain–Barré syndrome is experiencing a great deal of pain. Why is this occurring?

A. Parasympathetic function
B. Sympathetic inactivity
C. Autonomic dysfunction
D. Sympathetic function

82. Nursing management of a patient with Guillain–Barré syndrome includes which of the following actions?

A. Monitoring labs and neurologic signs
B. Monitoring respiratory status and neurologic signs
C. Monitoring respiratory status and lab results
D. Monitoring labs results and urinary output

83. A nursing diagnosis for the patient with Guillain–Barré syndrome includes

A. Impaired nutrition
B. Risk for impaired respiratory function
C. Impaired fluid balance
D. Impaired body image

84. Your patient has three large aneurysms in his Circle of Willis. What methods are used to treat these types of aneurysms?

A. Clipping the aneurysms and endovascular coiling
B. Clipping of the aneurysms and tPA administration
C. Medical management of blood pressure and Amicar infusion
D. Amicar infusion and tPA administration

85. Which diagnoses should be considered as the cause of any patient's seizures?

A. Alcohol abuse and hypertension
B. Panic attack and psychological illness
C. Panic attack and transient ischemic attack
D. Cardiac arrhythmias and hypertension

86. Lab studies for multiple sclerosis identification include

A. Cerebrospinal fluid evaluation, sedimentation rate, and fluorescent treponomal antibody absorption
B. Cerebrospinal fluid evaluation, syphilis, and a drug screen
C. Cerebrospinal fluid evaluation, CBC, and HIV
D. Cerebrospinal fluid evaluation, lipids, and sedimentation rate

87. What are the two major types of multiple sclerosis?

A. Progressive and relapsing–resolving
B. Relapsing–remitting and static
C. Progressive and relapsing–relapsing
D. Relapsing–remitting and progressive

88. What is myasthenia gravis?

A. A neuromuscular disorder where myelin is destroyed at varying rates
B. A neuromuscular disorder at the neuromuscular junction
C. A neuromuscular disorder seen after viral infections
D. A fatal neuromuscular disorder of upper motor neurons and lower motor neurons causing muscle wasting

89. What are some common symptoms of myasthenia gravis?

A. Ptosis, proximal muscle weakness, and spasticity
B. Dysphonia and atrophy
C. Fatigue, proximal muscle weakness, and respiratory weakness
D. Generalized weakness, hyperreflexia, and dyspnea

90. A 50 year old woman was admitted to PCU for acute coronary syndrome. She also has myasthenia gravis and has pyridostigmine in her purse so she does not miss a dose. The staff does not know she has this medication. Suddenly, the patient's monitor alarms and indicates a severe bradycardia. You suspect an overdose of pyridostigmine. If that is true, the patient's problem is

A. Cholinergic crisis
B. Acetylcholine crisis
C. Myasthenia gravis crisis
D. The bradycardia is related to the acute coronary syndrome, not myasthenia gravis

91. Assessment of a patient indicated an abnormal response when the patient was tested for pronator drift. This response indicates that the patient probably has

A. A forearm fracture
B. Myasthenia gravis
C. Upper motor neuron disease
D. A skull fracture

92. When you attempt to passively flex your patient's neck and touch his chin to his chest, he complains of a stiff neck and pain. This response indicates

A. Meningeal irritation
B. A basilar skull fracture
C. Labyrinthitis
D. A peritonsilar abscess

SECTION 8: NEUROLOGY ANSWERS

1. **Correct answer: A**
   Shingles on the trunk are characterized by lesions that follow a dermatome. Dermatomes are the paths innervated by the spinal nerves. Shingles may be found anywhere on the body, including inside the mouth.

2. **Correct answer: B**
   Labs are often not required for shingles, but if the patient presents with sine shingles (symptoms without rash), the varicella-zoster viral culture may be necessary. Unless a secondary infection is suspected, blood cultures and a CBC would not be done. A varicella titer only shows immunity to varicella, not an acute illness.

3. **Correct answer: A**
   Contraindications for a lumbar puncture (LP) are signs of increased intracranial pressure, infection in the area where the LP would be performed, and anticoagulant therapy. If an LP is done when there is increased intracranial pressure, the sudden change in pressure in the cerebrospinal space can cause herniation of the brainstem and death.

4. **Correct answer: C**
   If your patient scores 15 on the Adult Glasgow Coma Scale, the patient is likely to survive neurologically intact. GCS scoring is as follows:

   Glasgow Coma Scale (Adult)

Best Eye Response	Best Verbal Response	Best Motor Response
No eye opening (1)	No verbal response (1)	No motor response (1)
Eye opening to pain (2)	Incomprehensible sounds (2)	Extension to pain (2)
Eye opening to verbal command (3)	Inappropriate words (3)	Flexion to pain (3)
Eyes open spontaneously (4)	Confused (4)	Withdrawal from pain (4)
	Oriented (5)	Localizing pain (5)
		Obeys commands (6)

5. **Correct answer: D**
   Patients who have right hemispheric involvement will often display poor judgment, euphoria, impulsive behavior, and overestimate their abilities.

6. **Correct answer: B**
   The patient with a high cervical transection of the spinal cord can present with the following: sensation of the occiput, face, and ears; there is no diaphragmatic movement; no voluntary movement below the injury; and there is loss of bowel and bladder function. Patients with this level of injury often die due to pneumonia.

7. **Correct answer: C**
   At C5-6 there is enough diaphragmatic movement to allow for adequate respiratory function. Injuries above C5-6 require some level of mechanical ventilation.

8. **Correct answer: D**
   The fifth thoracic spinal nerve innervates at the nipple line. The dermatome innervates not only the skin but the organs, muscles, and tendons along the same path. It is important to know the dermatomes when dealing with spinal injuries because they help locate the level of the injury.

9. **Correct answer: C**
   Nystagmus, a rhythmic tremor or shaking of the eyes, indicates pressure or damage to cranial nerve VIII (acoustic) in the vestibular portion. Shaking is usually stronger on one side and may occur in any of the cardinal eye directions.

10. **Correct answer: D**
    The knee jerk, also known as the patellar reflex, is an example of a functional lower motor neuron. These reflexes are also known as deep tendon reflexes. The nerve impulse makes an arc from the tendon to the sensory portion of the spinal cord to the motor root and back to the patella, causing extension of the lower leg.

11. **Correct answer: A**
    A sympathetic response to a stimuli results in heightened awareness, increased blood pressure, bronchial dilation, and increased glucogenosis. Other responses include dilated pupils for increased visual acuity, increased heart rate, increased myocardial contractility, increased blood pressure, increased respiratory rate, decreased gastric motility, decreased gastric secretion, decreased urine output, decreased insulin production, and decreased renal blood flow.

12. **Correct answer: B**
    Four to 15 mmHg is the normal range for intracranial pressure.

13. **Correct answer: C**
    Cerebrospinal fluid absorbed at an increased rate decreases intracranial pressure. CO_2 retention, PaO_2 less than 50 mmHg, and increased metabolic activity contribute to increased intracranial pressure.

14. **Correct answer: B**
    Autonomic hyperreflexia is a potentially life-threatening response to a minor stimuli seen after spinal cord injury at T6 or higher. It occurs after the initial spinal shock has resolved. Symptoms can include severe hypertension, dysrhythmias, severe headache, and photophobia.

15. **Correct answer: D**
    Brown Sequard causes ipsilateral (same side) motor paralysis and contralateral (opposite side) loss of pain and temperature sensation. This syndrome occurs because of the way the pyramidal tracts cross in the spinal column.

16. **Correct answer: B**
    Neisseria meningitidis is the causative agent for meningococcal meningitis. *Streptococcus pneumonia* causes pneumococcal meningitis. *Haemophilius influenza* causes Haemophilius meningitis. *Staphylococcus aureus* is not likely to cause meningitis but can cause infection in the brain with ventriculostomy drains or bolts.

17. **Correct answer: B**
Petechiae are the hallmark symptom of meningococcal meningitis. Headache, malaise, and vomiting can be seen with any form of meningitis.

18. **Correct answer: B**
The proper technique is stroking the lateral sole of the foot from the heel up to and across the ball of the foot. It should be done in one motion with a relatively sharp instrument like the end of a reflex hammer.

19. **Correct answer: B**
With a normal Doll's eyes or oculocephalic reflex, the eyes appear to move to the opposite direction from the head turn. For example, if the head is turned quickly to the patient's left, the eyes normally appear to move to the far right side. If the reflex is absent, the eyes appear fixed and do not move. This is a poor neurologic sign. It represents pontine and midbrain damage. It may be used in determining brain death.

20. **Correct answer: B**
Cerebrospinal fluid is formed by the choroid plexus of the third ventricle. The arachnoid villi, projections from the subarachnoid space, reabsorb the cerebrospinal fluid.

21. **Correct answer: B**
Patients who have left hemispheric involvement will often move slowly with caution and underestimate their abilities.

22. **Correct answer: C**
The cerebrospinal fluid should be clear and colorless with a protein count of 16–45 mg/dl, WBCs 0–5 cells/mm^3, and the glucose level should be approximately 80% of the serum glucose level.

23. **Correct answer: D**
RIND is a reversible ischemic neurologic deficit. It is similar to a TIA, but symptoms last more than 24 hours and the patient recovers completely.

24. **Correct answer: B**
Alcohol use, smoking, and obesity are all modifiable risk factors in preventing stroke.

25. **Correct answer: B**
The two major types of stroke are ischemic and hemorrhagic. Hemorrhagic strokes are usually caused by hypertension and may include aneurysm rupture. Ischemic strokes are usually caused by an occlusion of an atherosclerotic cerebral artery secondary to an embolus or occlusion.

26. **Correct answer: B**
A left-side cerebrovascular accident causes right-side deficits because of crossing of the cerebrospinal tracts in the brain and spinal cord. You would expect the patient to have speech deficits, loss of right visual field, and right facial droop.

27. **Correct answer: B**
Broca's area at the lower edge of the frontal lobe is responsible for verbal expression. A deficit in this area is called expressive aphasia. The patient can comprehend what is said but lacks the ability to form the words due to loss of motor skills.

28. **Correct answer: B**
The negative inspiratory force measures the ability of the patient to take a deep breath to minus 28 mmHg. Once the effort is less than 28 mmHg, the patient should be evaluated for intubation to prevent respiratory arrest.

29. **Correct answer: A**
Guillain–Barré patients experience motor weakness, impaired respiratory function, and acute pain. The pain is due to accentuated sympathetic response secondary to loss of parasympathetic counterbalance.

30. **Correct answer: B**
Death from status epilepticus is usually caused by a hypermetabolic state within the brain. Status epilepticus results in decreased oxygen and glucose levels in the brain, leading to the release of glutamate. The increased glutamate causes the influx of calcium into the neurons, destabilizing them electronically, which leads to cell injury and death.

31. **Correct answer: B**
The best action is to turn the patient to her right side and protect her airway. Because the seizure has already started, it would be impossible to safely insert an oral airway. Never try to restrain a patient having a seizure. Hitting the Code Blue button is certainly an option, but it doesn't help the patient immediately. Precipitating events, aura, onset, duration, nursing actions, and postictal state should be included in the nursing notes.

32. **Correct answer: C**
This patient should be given a psychological evaluation. If he had a genuine grand mal seizure, the postictal state is expected to last several hours and the patient would not be able to request food.

33. **Correct answer: B**
Aggrenox is a persantine-based medication given in twice daily dosing for stroke or TIA patients.

34. **Correct answer: B**
Multiple sclerosis is a demyelinating disorder of the white matter of the brain and spinal cord. It can be intermittent, progressive, or relapsing. It follows an acute or a progressive course. It is the major cause of disability in young adults aged 16–40. Multiple sclerosis affects females more than males.

35. **Correct answer: C**
This patient is angry at her diagnosis and afraid she will suffer the same fate as her mother. The five stages of grief identified by Kubler-Ross in 1969 are denial, anger, bargaining, depression, and acceptance. The patient can move through the stages in any order and can revisit a stage at any time. The nurse should try to encourage the patient to express her feelings. The physician should also be notified, and the patient should receive counseling. Antidepressants may be considered.

36. **Correct answer: B**
Ascending, descending, Miller–Fisher variant, and pure motor are the four types of Guillain–Barré syndrome. Ascending is the classic form of weakness and numbness that starts in the legs and moves up the trunk to involve the cranial nerves in some

patients. The weakness is symmetric. Descending affects the cranial nerves first and the weakness progresses caudally. Respiratory failure is a major problem for these patients. Miller-Fisher variant is a very rare form that has a triad of symptoms that includes ophthalmoplegia, areflexia, and pronounced ataxia. The pure motor form of Guillain–Barré is identical to ascending but there is limited sensory involvement and therefore no pain.

37. **Correct answer: C**
Multiple sclerosis produces a wide variety of symptoms depending on the white matter being affected by the exacerbation. These symptoms include both motor and sensory problems. Symptoms include ataxia, Babinski reflex, vision disturbances (for example, diplopia), clumsiness, emotional lability, fatigue, paresthesias, paralysis, hyperactive deep tendon reflexes, loss of proprioception, loss of vibratory sense, impotence in men, and urinary problems in women.

38. **Correct answer: B**
Although the exact etiology of multiple sclerosis is unknown, it is thought to be an autoimmune disorder triggered by environmental exposure or viral illness. There are clusters in Northern European families, and there is a higher incidence in people who work with manganese.

39. **Correct answer: C**
The tensilon test is often used to test for myasthenia gravis because of the ease of administration. The medication has a quick onset and half-life. Ten milligrams are given intravenously. If there is improvement in a weak muscle, it is considered a positive tensilon test. The Weber and Rinne tests are for hearing. Clonus is a reflex used to test spasticity.

40. **Correct answer: B**
The patient with Bell's palsy will need to wear sunglasses when outside and use artificial tears because the blink reflex is absent. Steroids are often used short term for this condition. Thermal packs, especially cold, may exacerbate the condition.

41. **Correct answer: C**
The most common cause of normal pressure hydrocephalus is idiopathic (unknown). For most patients the cause is idiopathic. The mnemonic for normal pressure hydrocephalus (NPH) is "wet, wobbly, and wacky" due to the symptoms of incontinence, instability, and dementia. This condition can be successfully treated with a ventriculoperitoneal (VP) shunt.

42. **Correct answer: B**
The patient received a score of 26 after an evaluation for a stroke. This value indicates a severe stroke. The NIH scale rankings are

0 = no stroke

1–4 = minor stroke

5–15 = moderate stroke

15–20 = moderate/severe stroke

21–42 = severe stroke

43. **Correct answer: D**
One of the primary purposes of using the NIH scale is to determine whether or not the degree of disability will merit use of tPA. The NIHSS also provides objective comparisons of efficacy between treatment and rehabilitation modalities.

44. **Correct answer: B**
Ethnicity is not considered a testable aspect of brain function when using the NIH stroke scale. Components of the NIHSS include testing for language, sensation, vision, consciousness, movement, and speech.

45. **Correct answer: D**
When the patient is placed supine, with hips and knees flexed, and the physician attempts to extend the leg past 135 degrees, the patient complains of pain. This response is known as Kernig's sign and indicates meningeal irritation.

46. **Correct answer: B**
The Glasgow Coma Scale measures eye opening, motor response, and verbal response. It rates each with a total scale from 3 to 15, with 15 being a fully responsive patient. A score of 6–7 is comatose level. The longer that the patient remains in the lower score ranges, the worse the projected outcome.

47. **Correct answer: D**
The cerebrospinal fluid in a patient with Guillain–Barre syndrome generally shows elevated protein but a normal cell count. A patient with meningitis or a subarachnoid hemorrhage would present with a decreased glucose level in the CSF. A high red blood cell count would be indicative of an intracranial hemorrhage such as a ruptured aneurysm.

48. **Correct answer: C**
With meningitis, the specific gravity is elevated, the CSF cloudy due to the infection, and the white blood cell count elevated. The glucose would be decreased in this case. Xanthochromia is a yellow, orange, or brown color of the CSF due to the breakdown of RBCs from a previous hemorrhage and is not seen with meningitis.

49. **Correct answer: A**
This patient has autonomic dysreflexia also known as autonomic hyperreflexia. This is a life-threatening exaggerated sympathetic response to minor stimuli. The stimuli may be a drafty room, a full bladder, or a bowel obstruction. Treating the cause will fix the problem. The symptoms include hypertension, severe headache, tachycardia or bradycardia, and profuse sweating or flushing.

50. **Correct answer: B**
Eighty-five percent of cerebral aneurysms are located at the anterior bifurcations of the Circle of Willis and 15% at the posterior bifurcations.

51. **Correct answer: D**
An explosive headache, often "worst headache of my life," is a common statement from patients suffering from rupturing cerebral aneurysms. It frequently is the last thing patients say before losing consciousness.

52. **Correct answer: B**
Glasgow Coma Scale assessment is imperative and is helpful in monitoring for vascular spasm, a potentially life-threatening problem for a patient with a cerebral aneurysm. Vascular spasm occurs secondary to meningeal irritation from the blood in the subarachnoid space.

53. **Correct answer: B**
Mean arterial pressure minus intracranial pressures equals cerebral perfusion pressure. Cerebral perfusion pressure is a calculated measurement of the pressure gradient that allows blood to flow to the brain. The CPP may also be calculated using the CVP instead of the ICP because it is a measure of vascular resistance.

54. **Correct answer: A**
As cerebral perfusion pressure is a calculated measurement of the pressure gradient that allows blood to flow to the brain, the goal is a CPP of 50–80 mmHg.

55. **Correct answer: A**
Spinal shock is defined as an areflexia at or below the spinal cord injury. Spinal shock can occur hours to weeks after an injury to the spinal cord. The patient develops flaccidity, loss of sensation, and loss of bowel and bladder function. Hyperreflexia and spasticity occurs after spinal shock resolves.

56. **Correct answer: B**
Neurogenic shock is a much more severe form of shock that may occur with spinal cord injuries at or above T6. The autonomic dysfunction causes increased vagal tone, which results in severe bradycardia, decreased cardiac output, peripheral dilatation, and decreased SVR.

57. **Correct answer: C**
AVMs are a complex tangle of misshapen blood vessels susceptible to hemorrhage. AVMs lack the normal blood flow from arterial to venous flow and do not go through a capillary bed. This high-pressure flow makes them more likely to bleed. They are not common, they occur slightly more often in men, and AVMs are the most common cause of stroke in children under 12 years of age.

58. **Correct answer: A**
An altered mental state is the primary symptom of encephalopathy. The definition of encephalopathy is an umbrella term for a collection of symptoms of other illnesses. This can include liver or renal failure, infection, brain tumors, increasing hydrocephalus, and environmental hazard exposure.

59. **Correct answer: C**
Because there are so many potential causes, encephalopathy must be treated at its cause first. Examples of treatment include antibiotics, hemodialysis, and electrolyte replacement.

60. **Correct answer: B**
Blood tests for a patient with encephalopathy can include CMP, CBC, and sedimentation rate, as well as tests for specific illnesses or toxins. Other tests may be done such as a lumbar puncture to rule out neurologic infection. Additional tests include electroencephalogram (EEG) and imaging studies of specific structures—such as hepatic or renal imaging.

61. **Correct answer: A**
The effect of Cushing syndrome in a patient with increased intracranial pressure is increased systolic blood pressure, widening pulse pressure, and bradycardia. Cushing syndrome is also known as the triad of symptoms. These are late indicators of a serious deterioration of neurologic status. This patient is at very high risk for herniation and death.

62. **Correct answer: C**
Cerebrospinal fluid absorbed at an increased rate decreases intracranial pressure. CO_2 retention, PaO_2 less than 50 mmHg, and increased metabolic activity contribute to increased intracranial pressure.

63. **Correct answer: C**
A sudden increase in urine output from 30 to 1000 ml/hour of pale, clear urine indicates diabetes insipidus. Diabetes insipidus (DI) is a serious decrease in antidiuretic hormone (ADH). The most common causes of neurogenic DI are closed head injury and posterior pituitary tumor removal. ADH is produced by the posterior pituitary gland. Closed head injury and cerebral edema lead to pressure on the pituitary gland, thus decreasing ADH. Other common causes of DI are lung cancer (small or oat cell carcinoma), leukemia, and lymphoma.

64. **Correct answer: B**
Treatment of diabetes insipidus includes intravenous replacement with D_5W/ ½ NS with 20 mEq of potassium is titrated to replace hourly urine output. Other therapies include DDAVP (desmopressin) nasal spray or a pitressin infusion. Strict I&O and daily weights, monitoring electrolytes, and serum and urine osmolalities are also done.

65. **Correct answer: C**
Autonomic hyperreflexia, also known as autonomic dysreflexia, is caused by numerous stimuli such as bowel or bladder dysfunction, cool breezes, a clogged urinary catheter, and constipation.

66. **Correct answer: C**
A positive Babinski or plantar reflex is a sign of an upper motor neuron lesion. It is can be seen with spinal cord compression, head injury, and stroke. It is a pathologic sign.

67. **Correct answer: C**
Decerebrate posturing displays as both arms fully extended and internally rotated, legs fully extended with toes pointed. Decerebrate posturing demonstrates pressure on the midbrain and pons. It is a very poor neurologic sign, especially if it continues for more than 4 hours.

68. **Correct answer: B**
Ipsilateral, or same side, pupil dilation is the symptom seen with uncal herniation across the tentorium. The tentorium is a fold of dura mater that supports the temporal and occipital lobes. This herniation puts pressure directly on CN III, causing pupil dilation.

69. **Correct answer: C**
Personality changes and poor short-term memory are expected symptoms in a patient with left frontal lobe injury. The frontal lobe is responsible for personality, memory, motor function, Broca's area, and critical thinking skills.

70. **Correct answer: A**
TIAs typically last a very short time, sometimes less than an hour but no longer than 24 hours, and there are no neurologic deficits. With a RIND the symptoms last more than 24 hours but the patient still has a complete recovery. Both are possible precursors of a major stroke within a year.

71. **Correct answer: C**
400–800 ml of cerebrospinal fluid is produced daily by the choroid plexus in the third ventricle. There is approximately 125–150 ml circulating in the ventricular system and spinal column at one time.

72. **Correct answer: C**
Uncontrolled hypertension is the most common cause of stroke in the United States. More than 360,000 strokes per year are due to hypertension. Stroke can be the first symptom of hypertension for many patients. Diabetes mellitus can lead to cardiovascular disease and hypertension, but it is less common than hypertension alone.

73. **Correct answer: C**
Diabetes mellitus causes accelerated atherosclerosis in the large arteries of the cerebral circulation, thereby narrowing the lumen and increasing the risk for stroke.

74. **Correct answer: B**
Uncontrolled hypertension is most likely to cause a lacunar stroke. A lacunar infarction is due to thrombosis of the small arteries that penetrate the cerebrum. It causes facial, arm, and leg deficits.

75. **Correct answer: C**
In most people, the dominant side of the brain is the left cerebral hemisphere and is the most likely site for a cerebrovascular accident.

76. **Correct answer: B**
Prevention of aspiration should be the priority of the PCU nurse. Prevention of decubitus ulcers, contractures, and depression are also a part of caring for a patient with a cerebrovascular accident, but the ABCs (airway, breathing, circulation) are always the first priority.

77. **Correct answer: C**
A left temporal cerebrovascular accident will likely cause receptive aphasia. This patient has had a stroke affecting Wernicke's area in the temporal lobe, which affects verbal reception. This causes an inability to interpret speech and can also affect comprehension of written words.

78. **Correct answer: D**
Droplet precautions are indicated for suspected bacterial meningitis for the first 48 hours of antimicrobial therapy. This type of isolation is used for those types of infections spread when the patient talks, coughs, or sneezes. Reverse isolation is used to protect the immunocompromised patient. Contact isolation is for those patients with conditions such as MRSA or VRE.

79. **Correct answer: B**
Protein in the CSF is always increased with Guillain–Barré due to the destruction of the myelin sheath. Because Guillain–Barré is an autoimmune disorder, WBCs, abnormal glucose levels, and bacteria would not be present in the CSF.

80. **Correct answer: A**
Guillain–Barré patients experience motor weakness, impaired respiratory function, and acute pain. The pain is due to accentuated sympathetic response secondary to loss of parasympathetic counterbalance.

81. **Correct answer: C**
Autonomic dysfunction in Guillain–Barré is caused by lack of balance in the autonomic nervous system. The sympathetic nervous system is unopposed, causing heightened sensitivity and over-response to minor stimuli, causing pain.

82. **Correct answer: B**
Respiratory status and neurologic signs are the most important nursing management issues, especially during the early onset of the demylenating process.

83. **Correct answer: B**
Risk for impaired respiratory function is the most important nursing diagnosis. Other nursing diagnoses include acute pain, risk for impaired verbal communication, and potential for neuromuscular weakness related to demyelination.

84. **Correct answer: A**
Clipping of the aneurysm and endovascular coiling are the two common methods of managing aneurysms in the Circle of Willis. tPA is a thrombolytic and would not be given to this patient. Controlling the blood pressure involves maintaining a good cerebral perfusion pressure to reduce the risk of vasospasm. Amicar inhibits plasminogen activator, allowing fibrin production.

85. **Correct answer: C**
Panic attacks, transient ischemic attacks, cardiac arrhythmias, and syncope are some causes of seizures.

86. **Correct answer: A**
Cerebrospinal fluid results will show a negative syphilis (RPR), abnormal colloid gold curve, increased IgG, myelin debris, and slightly increased protein. Other tests include fluorescent treponomal antibody absorption (FTA-ABS), sedimentation rate, HTLV-1 serology, and check for vascular disorders. Neurologic testing includes evoked responses that are highly predicative for MS. MRI shows plaques as white spots in the brain.

87. **Correct answer: D**
Relapsing–remitting and progressive are the most common forms of multiple sclerosis. The frequency of relapsing–remitting episodes is related to stress and illness. Progressive may follow a continuous but slow route or it may advance quickly to the patient's death. Relapsing–remitting may worsen to progressive MS.

88. **Correct answer: B**
Myasthenia gravis is a pure motor disorder that occurs when an autoimmune response at the neuromuscular junction destroys acetylcholine receptors on the muscle membrane.

89. **Correct answer: C**
Most myasthenia gravis symptoms deal with the weakness caused by the lack of acetylcholine receptors at the neuromuscular junction. These symptoms include ptosis, diplopia, facial weakness, dysphagia, dysarthria, fatigue, neck weakness, proximal limb weakness, respiratory weakness, and generalized weakness.

90. Correct answer: A
Cholinergic crisis is a life-threatening problem with any overdose, accident or otherwise. It causes bradycardia, severe weakness, cardiac arrest, and occasionally respiratory arrest.

91. Correct answer: C
An abnormal response when testing for pronator drift indicates that the patient may have an upper motor neuron disease or weakness in the shoulder girdle. To elicit this response, have the patient stand for 20–30 seconds with both arms outstretched forward, palms up, and eyes closed. Tell the patient to hold that position while you tap the hands vigorously downward. The patient will not be able to maintain extension and supination and will drift into pronation.

92. Correct answer: A
When you attempt to passively flex your patient's neck and touch his chin to his chest, he complains of a stiff neck (nuchal rigidity) and pain. This response indicates meningeal irritation.

NEUROLOGY REFERENCES

Adeolu, A. A., & Akinbo, O. C. (2012). Gunshot injury as a cause of elevated skull fracture. *Journal of Neurosciences in Rural Practice, 3*(2), 219–220.

Ahrens, T., Prentice, D., & Kleinpell, R. M. (2011). *Progressive care nursing certification: Preparation, review and practice exams*. St. Louis, MO: McGraw-Hill.

Akopian, G., Gaspard, D. J., & Alexander, M. (2007). Outcomes of blunt head trauma without intracranial pressure monitoring. *American Surgeon, 73*(5), 447–450.

American Association of Critical-Care Nurses. (2006). *AACN core curriculum for critical care nursing*. St. Louis, MO: Saunders.

American Association of Critical-Care Nurses & Lynn-McHale Wiegand, D. J. (2011). *AACN procedure manual for critical care* (6th ed.). Maryland Heights, MO: Saunders.

Bader, M. K., & Littlejohns, L. R. (2004). *AANN core curriculum for neuroscience nursing* (4th ed.). St. Louis, MO: Saunders.

Bailey, M. J., Lacey, D. C., de Kok, B. V. A., Veith, P. D., Reynolds, E. C., & Hamilton, J. A. (2011). Extracellular proteomes of M-CSF (CSF-1) and GM-CSF-dependent macrophages. *Immunology & Cell Biology, 89*(2), 283–293.

Brabrand, M., Hosbond, S., & Folkestad, L. (2011). Capillary refill time: A study of interobserver reliability among nurses and nurse assistants. *European Journal of Emergency Medicine, 18*(1), 46–49.

Brorsen, A. (2012). *CEN examination review*. Burlington, MA: Jones & Bartlett Learning.

Brorsen, A., & Rogelet, K. (2009). *PCCN certification review*. Sudbury, MA: Jones and Bartlett.

Burns, S. M. (Ed.). (2007). *American Association of Critical-Care Nurses (AACN): AACN protocols for practice: Healing environments* (2nd ed.). Sudbury, MA: Jones and Bartlett.

Centers for Disease Control and Prevention. (2008). Spinal cord injuries: *Acute injury care*. Retrieved from http://www.cdc.gov/ncipc/dir/AcuteInjuryCare.htm

Chattopadhyay, S., & Tripathi, C. (2010). Skull fracture and haemorrhage pattern among fatal and nonfatal head injury assault victims—A critical analysis. *Journal of Injury & Violence Research, 2*(2), 99–103.

Cho, S. F., Liu, T. C., Lu, C. Y., & Chang, C. S. (2011). Epidural leukemic involvement and intracranial hemorrhage as initial manifestations in a newly diagnosed chronic myeloid leukemia patient. *Annals of Hematology, 90*(5), 607–609.

Chulay, M., & Burns, S. (2010). *Essentials of progressive care nursing* (2nd ed.). St. Louis, MO: McGraw-Hill.

Crespo-Ruiz, B., del-Ama, A. J., Jiminez-Diaz, F. J., Morgan, J., de la Peia-Gonzalez, A., & Gil-Agudo, Ã. M. (2012). Physical activity and transcutaneous oxygen pressure in men with spinal cord injury. *Journal of Rehabilitation Research & Development, 49*(6), 913–924.

Curley, M. A. Q. (2007). *Synergy: The unique relationship between nurses and patients*. St. Louis, MO: Saunders.

de Kruijk, J. R., Leffers, P., Meerhoff, S., Rutten, J., & Twijnstra, A. (2002). Effectiveness of bed rest after mild traumatic brain injury: A randomised trial of no versus six days of bed rest. *Journal of Neurology, Neurosurgery and Psychiatry, 73*(2), 167.

Dolbow, D. R., Gorgey, A. S., Daniels, J. A., Adler, R. A., Moore, J. R., & Gater, Jr., D. R. (2011). The effects of spinal cord injury and exercise on bone mass: A literature review. *Neuro Rehabilitation, 29*(3), 261–269.

Donohoe-Dennison, R. (2007). *Pass CCRN (*3rd ed.). St. Louis, MO: Mosby.

Dunning, M. B., & Fischbach, F. (2010). *Nurse's quick reference to common laboratory & diagnostic tests*. (5th ed.). Philadelphia, PA: Lippincott Williams & Wilkins.

Emergency Nurses Association, & Newberry, L. (2007). *Sheehy's emergency nursing: Principles and practice* (6th ed.). St. Louis, MO: Mosby/Elsevier.

Fehlings, M. G., Vaccaro, A., Wilson, J. R., Singh, A., Cadotte, D. W., Harrop, J. S., . . . Rampersaud, R. (2012). Early versus delayed decompression for traumatic cervical spinal cord injury: Results of the Surgical Timing in Acute Spinal Cord Injury Study. *PLoS ONE, 7*(2), 1–8.

Gasparis Vonfrolio, L., & Noone, J. (1997). *Emergency nursing examination review* (3rd ed.). Staten Island, NY: Power Publications.

Ghosh, S., Dey, S., Maltenfort, M., Vibbert, M., & Jallo, J. (2012). Relationship between serum and csf glucose in subarachnoid hemorrhage. *International Journal of Collaborative Research on Internal Medicine & Public Health, 4*(5), 813–824.

Grant, C., Briscoe, N., Mezei, M., & Krassioukov, A. (2011). Guillian–Barré syndrome in high tetraplegia following acute respiratory illness. *Spinal Cord, 49*(3), 480–481.

Green, J. S., Abeles, S. R., Uslan, D. Z., & Mehta, S. R. (2011). Persistent neutrophilic meningitis in an immunocompetent patient after basilar skull fracture: Case report. *BMC Infectious Diseases, 11*, 136.

Hardin, S. R., & Kaplow, R. (Eds.). (2008). *Synergy for clinical excellence: The AACN synergy model for patient care.* Sudbury, MA: Jones and Bartlett.

Hardin, S. R., & Kaplow, R. (2010). *Cardiac surgery essentials for critical care nursing.* Sudbury, MA: Jones & Bartlett Learning.

Hickey, J. V. (2002). *The clinical practice of neurological and neurosurgical nursing* (5th ed.). Philadelphia, PA: Lippincott Williams & Wilkins.

Holleran, R. S. (2005). *Emergency transport nursing* (4th ed.). St. Louis, MO: Mosby.

Jacobs, B. B., & Hoyt, K. S. (2007). *Trauma nursing core course provider manual* (6th ed.). Bedford, IL: Emergency Nurses Association.

Jones & Bartlett Learning. (2011). *2012 nurse's drug handbook. (*11th ed.). Sudbury, MA: Jones & Bartlett Learning.

Jyothi, B., Verma, H., Vaidya, N., & Shaikh, S. S. (2012). Perioperative management of term pregnant patient with Guillian–Barre syndrome. *Indian Journal of Anaesthesia, 56*(4), 409–411.

Kerman, M., & Senol, N. (2011). Interhemispheric subdural hematoma in an adult: Case report. *Journal of Neurological Sciences, 311*(2), 394–397.

Khan, F., Pallant, J. F., Ng, L., & Bhasker, A. (2010). Factors associated with long-term functional outcomes and psychological sequelae in Guillain–Barre syndrome. *Journal of Neurology, 257*(12), 2024–2031.

Kirkness, C. J., Burr, R. L., & Mitchell, P. H. (2009). Intracranial and blood pressure variability and long-term outcome after aneurysmal sub-arachnoid hemorrhage. *American Journal of Critical Care, 18*(3), 241–251.

Leen, W. G., Willemsen, M. A., Wevers, R. A., Verbeek, M. M., & Mendelson, J. E. (2012). Cerebrospinal fluid glucose and lactate: Age-specific reference values and implications for clinical practice. *PLoS ONE, 7*(8), 1–8.

Lichy, A. M., & Groah, S. (2012). Asymmetric lower-limb bone loss after spinal cord injury: Case report. *Journal of Rehabilitation Research & Development, 49*(2), 221–226.

Lilley, L. L., Rainforth Collins, S., & Snyder, J. S. (2012). *Pharmacology and the nursing process.* (7th ed.). Maryland Heights, MO: Mosby.

Lippincott. (2010). *Professional guide to signs and symptoms* (6th ed.). Philadelphia, PA: Lippincott.

Mallek, J. T., Inaba, K., Branco, B. C., Ives, C., Lam, L., Talving, P., . . . Demetriades, D. (2012). The incidence of neurogenic shock after spinal cord injury in patients admitted to a high-volume level I trauma center. *The American Surgeon, 78*(5), 623–626.

Manno, E. (Ed). (2012). *Emergency management in neurocritical care.* Hoboken, NJ: Wiley-Blackwell.

Mao, L., Wang, H. D., Pan, H., & Qiao, L. (2011). Sulphoraphane enhances aquaporin-4 expression and decreases spinal cord oedema following spinal cord injury. *Brain Injury, 25*(3), 300–306.

McMillan, T. M., McKenzie, P., Swann, I. J., Weir, C. J., & McAviney, A. (2009). Head injury attenders in the emergency department: The impact of advice and factors associated with early symptom outcome. *Brain Injury, 23*(6), 509–515.

McVeigh, K., Bhatt, V., Green, J., Monaghan, A., & Dover, M. S. (2012). The contemporary management of midface and craniofacial trauma. *Trauma, 14*(2), 128–138.

Medina, J., & Puntillo, K. (2006). *AACN protocols for practice: Palliative care and end-of-life issues in critical care.* Sudbury, MA: Jones and Bartlett.

Pellatt, G. C. (2010). Spinal surgery for acute traumatic spinal cord injury: Implications for nursing. *British Journal of Neuroscience Nursing, 6*(6), 271–275.

Ploumis, A., Yadlapalli, N., Fehlings, M. G., Kwon, B. K., & Vaccaro, A. R. (2010). A systematic review of the evidence supporting a role for vasopressor support in acute SCI. *Spinal Cord, 48*(5), 356–362.

Poletti-Muringaseril, S. C., Rufibach, K., Ruef, C., Holzmann, D., & Soyka, M. B. (2012). Low meningitis-incidence in primary spontaneous compared to secondary cerebrospinal fluid rhinorrhoea. *Rhinology, 50*(1), 73–79.

Porth, C. M., & Matfin, G. (2010). *Pathophysiology concepts of altered health states* (8th ed.). Philadelphia, PA: Lippincott Williams & Wilkins.

Proehl, J. A. (2008). *Emergency nursing procedures* (4th ed.). St. Louis, MO: Saunders.

Rynn, B., Pynn, T. P., & Sandor, G. K. S. (2006). Snowmobile accidents and facial fractures. *Oral Health, 96*(6), 33.

Seçer, M., Kalyoncu, N., Günal, M., & Kuruoğlu, E. (2012). Comparison of burr hole irrigation and closed system drainage methods after burr hole irrigation in the treatment of chronic subdural hematoma. *Journal of Neurological Sciences, 29*(2), 280–284.

Shin, J. C., Yoo, J. H., Lee, Y. S., Goo, H. R., & Kim, D. H. (2011). Dysphagia in cervical spinal cord injury. *Spinal Cord, 49*(9), 1008–1013.

Smeltzer, S., & Bare, B. G. (2003). *Brunner and Suddarth's textbook of medical-surgical nursing* (10th ed.). Philadelphia, PA: Lippincott Williams & Wilkins.

Smeltzer, S. C., Bare, B., Hinkle, J. L., & Cheever, K. H. (2010). *Brunner and Suddarth's textbook of medical-surgical nursing* (12th ed.). Philadelphia, PA: Lippincott Williams & Wilkins.

Smith, H. F., Peek-Asa, C., Nesheim, D., Nish, A., Normandin, P., & Sahr, S. (2012). Etiology, diagnosis, and characteristics of facial fracture at a Midwestern level I trauma center. *Journal of Trauma Nursing, 19*(1), 57–65.

Türedi, S., Gündüz, A., Türkmen, S., Patan, T., & Kalkan, A. (2010). Acute spontaneous spinal epidural hematoma complicating oral anticoagulant therapy. *Journal of Academic Emergency Medicine, 9*(2), 103–105.

Urdern, L. D., Stacy, K. M., & Lough, M. E. (2005). *Thelan's critical care nursing* (5th ed.). St. Louis, MO: Mosby.

Waninger, K. N., & Swartz, E. E. (2011). Cervical spine injury management in the helmeted athlete. *Current Sports Medicine Reports, 10*(1), 45–49.

Watcher, R. (2012). *Understanding patient safety* (2nd ed.). Los Altos, CA: Lange.

Watson, S., & Gorski, K. A. (2011). *Invasive cardiology* (3rd ed.). Sudbury, MA: Jones & Bartlett Learning.

Section 9

Gastrointestinal

SECTION 9: GASTROINTESTINAL QUESTIONS

1. **A drug that crosses the mucosal barrier and should be avoided in the treatment of a peptic ulcer is**
   A. Nicotine
   B. Indomethacin
   C. Corticosteroids
   D. Reglan

2. **A subjective sign of a peptic ulcer would be**
   A. Hyperactive bowel sounds
   B. Pallor
   C. Tarry stools
   D. Epigastric pain

3. **Which of the following lab values would be decreased in liver disease?**
   A. AST
   B. ALT
   C. Hgb
   D. LDH

4. **Which of the following levels is likely to be elevated in a patient with a peptic ulcer?**
   A. Total protein
   B. Albumin
   C. Transferrin
   D. Gastrin

5. **An absolute contraindication for providing tube feedings would include:**
   A. Intestinal obstructions
   B. Adhesions
   C. Bacteremia
   D. An enterocutaneous fistula

6. **A relative contraindication for providing tube feedings for a patient would not include:**
   A. Adhesions
   B. Bacteremia
   C. Severe malabsorption
   D. Pneumonia

7. **One way of confirming placement of a feeding tube is to sample the gastric aspirate. If the patient has not received any pH-altering medications, the pH of the aspirate should be in the range of**
   A. 5.2–6.0
   B. 2.5–4.0
   C. 1.0–3.0
   D. 3.5–4.8

8. **Which of the following nutrients supports function and growth of lymphocytes and macrophages?**
   A. Polyunsaturated fatty acids
   B. Saturated fatty acids
   C. Glutamine
   D. Nucleotides

9. **A gradual wasting of body fat and muscle, as well as the proteins contained in the internal organs (visceral protein), is known as**
   A. Somatosis
   B. Marasmus
   C. Somatic residual deficit
   D. Necrofascitis

10. **Amylase levels are usually elevated in patients with pancreatitis or pancreatic cancer. The normal range for amylase is**
    A. 150–215 units/L
    B. 12–15 units/L
    C. 30–45 units/L
    D. 56–190 units/L

11. **Your patient has cirrhosis, so you would expect his alinine transferase (ALT) to be elevated. The normal value for the ALT is in the range of**
    A. 5–36 units/ml
    B. 14–65 units/ml
    C. 45–65 units/ml
    D. 2–7.2 units/ml

12. **Your patient has been diagnosed with an intestinal obstruction. Which phosphorus level listed below would be indicative of this condition?**
    A. 2.2–2.9 mg/dL
    B. 3.0–4.2 mg/dL
    C. 3.7–4.9 mg/dL
    D. 3.0–4.5 mg/dL

13. **Ammonia levels are elevated in patients with heart failure, renal failure, and hepatic failure. A normal range for ammonia is**
    A. 5–60 mOsm/dL
    B. 15–110 mOsm/dL
    C. 50–200 mOsm/dL
    D. 170–240 mOsm/dL

14. **Your patient has had several bouts of diarrhea over the past 3 days. As a progressive care nurse you know this patient is likely to be low on magnesium. Which range of values listed below would indicate a lower than normal range for magnesium?**
    A. 3.5–4.2 mcg/dL
    B. 0.9–1.4 mEq/L
    C. 2.2–3.8 mmol/L
    D. 4.0–7.5 units/ml

15. **Total bilirubin levels may be elevated in patients suffering from profound hemolysis, a biliary obstruction, or hepatic disease. The normal range for total bilirubin is**
    A. 0.3–1.3 mg/dL
    B. 1.5:1 to 2.0:1 mmol/L
    C. 4.0–6.5 g/dL
    D. 2.4–4 units/ml

16. **Your patient is suffering from a biliary obstruction. As a progressive care nurse, you know his direct bilirubin levels will be affected. The normal value for a direct bilirubin level is**
    A. 0.1–0.3 mg/dL
    B. 10–30 mg/dL
    C. 1.3–3.0 mg/dL
    D. 0.3–1.3 mg/dL

17. **Indirect bilirubin levels are elevated in profound hemolysis and hepatic disease. An example of an elevated indirect bilirubin level is in the range of**
    A. 1.5:1 to 2.0:1 mmol/L
    B. 0.3–1.3 mg/dL
    C. 1.8 mg/dL
    D. 2.4–4 units/ml

18. **Which of the following statements is true about the appropriate use of a Miller–Abbott tube?**
    A. The tube is used for patients who are immediate surgical candidates
    B. The Miller–Abbott tube is used for proximal decompression of the bowel
    C. The Miller–Abbott tube is only used on patients when a bowel obstruction is believed to be irreversible
    D. The Miller–Abbott tube is used in patients to relieve a paralytic ileus

19. **Which of the following procedures is most likely to be performed on a patient with tumors of the descending or sigmoid colon?**
    A. A temporary colostomy
    B. A permanent colostomy
    C. A bowel resection
    D. A right hemicolectomy

20. **A low anterior resection is the likely surgical procedure for patients with**
    A. Malignant lesions of the lower sigmoid colon and anus
    B. Tumors of the mid or lower left transverse colon

C. Proximal and midrectal tumors
D. Tumors of the cecum

21. **While you are assessing a patient's abdomen, you note that on palpation of the left lower quadrant, the patient complains of pain in the right lower quadrant. This finding is known as**
A. McBurney's point
B. Rovsing's sign
C. Seat belt sign
D. Cullen's sign

22. **Which of the following actions will facilitate or confirm passage of a Miller–Abbott tube through the GI tract?**
A. Use aspirate pH
B. Place the patient on their right side for 4 hours
C. Do a chest X-ray within 1 hour after tube insertion
D. Tape the tube securely to the nose to measure length correctly

23. **Your patient fell out of bed at the end of the previous shift. Although an X-ray of his abdomen is negative, he is now complaining of pain in his left shoulder. You suspect the patient may be suffering from**
A. Splenic bleeding
B. A liver laceration
C. A dislocated shoulder
D. A rib fracture

24. **A major limitation of peritoneal lavage is**
A. Peritoneal lavage cannot be confirmed as positive without a microscopic examination
B. Peritoneal lavage is always inaccurate in cases of sepsis
C. Peritoneal lavage is only useful in detecting diaphragmatic injuries
D. Peritoneal lavage cannot diagnose retroperitoneal injuries

25. **When liver parenchymal cells are aggressively destroyed and replaced with fibrotic tissue, leading to impaired hepatic function, this condition is known as**
A. Cirrhosis
B. Ascites
C. Hepatic vein degradation
D. Budd–Chiari syndrome

26. **Which of the following medications is classified as a histamine H2 receptor antagonist?**
A. Calcium carbonate
B. Magnesium hydroxide
C. Aluminum hydroxide
D. Ranitidine

27. Three or more episodes of acute, midline abdominal pain lasting for 2 hours to several days with periods without symptoms is known as

A. An abdominal migraine
B. Chronic appendicitis
C. Functional dyspepsia
D. Esophagitis

28. Assessment of the abdomen should occur in which order?

A. Inspection, palpation, auscultation, percussion
B. Auscultation, inspection, palpation, percussion
C. Percussion, inspection, palpation, auscultation
D. Inspection, auscultation, percussion, palpation

29. Your patient has been diagnosed with gastroenteritis. The primary causative agent for this condition is

A. *Clostridium difficile*
B. *Salmonella typhi*
C. Cryptosporidium
D. A rotavirus

30. Your patient was admitted overnight to the PCU after a motor vehicle accident that left her only mildly bruised. Just prior to discharge, the patient complained of diffuse abdominal pain and described symptoms she has had during the past week. Which symptom probably indicates an early sign of appendicitis?

A. Flank pain
B. Pain while resting
C. Night waking
D. Pain after vomiting

31. Which of the following terms describes bleeding that is bright or dark red and that is passed from the rectum?

A. Melena
B. Occult
C. Hematemesis
D. Hematochezia

32. Hepatorenal syndrome is a complication of hepatic failure due to

A. Vasodilatation
B. Increased circulating plasma
C. Increased renal circulation
D. Release of mediators

33. Cullen's sign presents as

A. A marbled appearance to the abdomen
B. Bruising of the scrotum or labia

C. Bluish discoloration of the flanks
D. Bluish discoloration of the periumbilical area

34. Your patient is a recovering anorexic who attends group counseling sessions at your facility. The PCU was busy and the patient's discharge was delayed, so you ordered a lunch for the patient. Later in the afternoon, as you are preparing to discharge the patient, you note she has not touched her lunch. Your best therapeutic statement should be

A. "It's okay. I know that hospital food is not gourmet, but the cafeteria is more appetizing."
B. "If you don't eat, we will have to put a feeding tube in you."
C. "You need to eat to regain strength and prevent complications. We will work with you to find foods that you like."
D. "Food is not your enemy. Eating this is not going to make you fat."

35. Which of the following forms of hepatitis is often misdiagnosed as gastroenteritis?

A. Hepatitis A
B. Hepatitis B
C. Hepatitis C
D. Hepatitis E

36. Which form of hepatitis originates as a DNA virus?

A. Hepatitis A
B. Hepatitis B
C. Hepatitis C
D. Hepatitis D

37. You are preparing Frank for a paracentesis. Which of the following actions should be the first step in assisting with a paracentesis?

A. Have Frank void or insert a Foley catheter
B. Examine the abdomen for dullness
C. Order an upright X-ray of the abdomen
D. Position Frank with the affected side up

38. Your patient was diagnosed with Barrett's esophagus. Which of the following conditions is your patient at greatest risk for developing?

A. Esophageal varices
B. Gastritis
C. Esophageal cancer
D. GERD

39. Anastomotic leaks are common after bariatric surgeries. Symptoms can be subtle and may include hyperthermia, tachycardia, tachypnea, abdominal pain, and anxiety. If undiagnosed, all of the following complications may result except

A. Hyperoxia
B. Sepsis

C. MODS
D. Death

40. A patient was admitted to the PCU because of abdominal pain. She recently had knee surgery for which she received Tylenol #3 for pain control. She has no bowel sounds, her abdomen is firmly distended, and she is diffusely tender across the abdomen. What is the probable cause of this patient's symptoms?
A. Appendicitis from the pain meds
B. Paralytic ileus from the codeine
C. Gastroenteritis after eating undercooked chicken
D. Pancreatitis from lack of exercise

41. Common adverse reactions to cimetidine include
A. Elevated BUN and creatinine
B. Rash, nausea, and agitation
C. Decreased liver enzymes and anorexia
D. Jitteriness and mottled skin

42. Cimetidine, famotidine, and ranitidine belong to which class of medications?
A. Proton pump inhibitors (PPIs)
B. Antacids
C. H2 blockers
D. Antiemetics

43. Mr. Q. is a frequent patient in your unit for alcohol-induced comas. He has been in the ICU the past 2 days. Just before transfer from the gurney to the PCU bed, he begins projectile vomiting bright red blood. Your first action should be to
A. Position the patient flat
B. Obtain and insert a Linton–Nachlas tube
C. Make the patient NPO and verify IV access
D. Start dopamine at 5 μg/kg/min

44. A 20 year old college student had an appendectomy in another state while on spring break 1 week ago. He is admitted to the PCU with fever, nausea and vomiting, and abdominal pain with a red, swollen surgical incision. You anticipate his next treatment to include
A. Immediate surgery with IV antibiotics
B. Hydration and antibiotics
C. Bedside excision of abscess
D. Bedside wound debridement

45. Your patient was admitted for dehydration and malnutrition after collapsing in his bedroom. His wife reports he has been eating very bland, soft foods for 3 weeks because of reflux and difficulty swallowing. You suspect
A. Partial tongue paralysis
B. Gastric cancer

C. Tracheal neoplasm
D. Esophageal neoplasm

46. **Your patient is a post-gastric bypass patient experiencing dumping syndrome after eating any type of meal. Which of the following medications should she stop immediately?**
A. Nitroglycerin
B. Insulin
C. Pepcid
D. Reglan

47. **When patients have liver failure, fatty nodules may develop subcutaneously due to cholesterol accumulation. These nodules are called**
A. Asterixis
B. Factor hepaticus
C. Xanthomas
D. Telangiectasis

48. **Mr. J. is an Orthodox Jew who presents with an unintentional weight loss of 20 pounds. He also suffers from fatigue, anorexia, and chronic, watery diarrhea with bloody mucus. He is tachycardic, tachypneic, hyperthermic, with a Hgb of 7 g/dL and Hct of 21%. You suspect Mr. J. is suffering from**
A. Colonic diverticulitis
B. Ulcerative colitis
C. Pancreatitis
D. Cholecystitis

49. **Sandostatin is ordered for your patient with portal hypertension. Which of the following nursing actions is most important to perform when first starting this drug?**
A. Careful monitoring of input and output
B. Check nerve stimulation
C. Blood glucose checks
D. Check blood pressure every 5 minutes

50. **What is the drug of choice for treating gastroesophageal reflux?**
A. Metoclopramide
B. Questran
C. Regitine
D. Meperidine

51. **Your patient frequently eats at fast-food restaurants. He is now suffering with severe abdominal pain and diarrhea. The probable causative organism for his condition is**
A. *Giardia lamblia*
B. *E. coli*

C. *Staphylococcus aureus*
D. Norwalk virus

52. Which drug is classified as an ammonia detoxicant and a hyperosmotic laxative?
A. Lactulose
B. Cyclosporine
C. Tacrolimus
D. Muromonab

53. A side effect of erythromycin is
A. Tachycardia
B. Headache
C. Eosinophilia
D. Atrial arrhythmias

54. A patient was admitted to your unit with recurrent pneumonia and severe dysphagia. You are unable to pass an NG tube. You suspect this patient is suffering from
A. A tracheoesophageal fistula
B. Varices
C. Intestinal atresia
D. A diaphragmatic hernia

55. Your patient has cirrhosis, and he came to the unit today after a weekend party with alcohol, drugs, and smoking. His lab results are as follows:

ALT 245 U/L	AST 147 U/L
PT 24 sec	PLT 75 × 103/mm^3
Hgb 8.4 g/dl	Hct 31%
Bilirubin 10 mg/dl	

These results indicate this patient is at a high risk for
A. Variceal bleeding
B. Peptic ulcer disease
C. Gastritis
D. Boerhaave's syndrome

56. Ascites is a common finding in patients with chronic liver failure. Which of the following statements about ascites is true?
A. Ascites is a result of an increase in albumin
B. Ascites is the result of decreased hydrostatic pressure and increased oncotic pressures in the portal system
C. Ascites occurs secondary to aldosteronism
D. Ascites is due to an increased ventilation/perfusion (V/Q) ratio

57. During a Whipple procedure, which of the following organs is removed?
A. Esophagus
B. Gallbladder
C. Ascending colon
D. Jejunum

58. **Your patient underwent the Whipple procedure 10 days ago for pancreatic cancer. She was started on clear liquids and then advanced to a soft diet. She is now suffering from repetitive vomiting. She is sweating profusely, shaking, and confused as to place. On the monitor you note tachypnea and tachycardia. You suspect this patient is experiencing**
    A. An anxiety or panic attack
    B. Gastroesophageal reflux disease (GERD)
    C. Dumping syndrome
    D. Hypoglycemia

59. **Your patient underwent the Roux-en-Y gastric bypass procedure 2 days ago. Which nutritional complication is your patient most at risk for developing?**
    A. Hypercalcemia
    B. Vitamin C deficiency
    C. Vitamin B_{12} deficiency
    D. Hyperalbuminism

60. **The family of your patient with chronic liver failure would like to know what they can do to make him more comfortable after he is discharged tomorrow. You tell them that when they visit the patient in his long-term care facility, they can**
    A. Provide deep tissue massage every 2 hours
    B. Apply a moisturizing lotion when visiting
    C. Assist with rapid range of motion every 4 hours
    D. Limit visitation to once a day

61. **What is the most common means of infection with** ***Giardia lamblia*****?**
    A. Eating undercooked game such as rabbit
    B. Drinking water from a mountain stream
    C. Teens sharing food and soda
    D. Having venison steak at a restaurant

62. **What type of organism is** ***Giardia lamblia*****?**
    A. A spirochete
    B. A type of tape worm
    C. A protozoan parasite
    D. A flagellated bacterium

63. **Your patient has acute esophageal and gastric varices. Which esophagogastric tamponade tube is the best choice for differentiating bleeding from the esophagus or the stomach?**
    A. Minnesota tube
    B. Sengstaken–Blakemore tube
    C. Linton–Nachlas tube
    D. Standard nasogastric tube

64. Your patient is a 50 year old seen in the emergency department for abdominal pain and vomiting. On admission to the PCU, her heart rate is 150, respiratory rate is 30, blood pressure is 105/60, and temperature 100.4° F. She indicates that the pain began 6 hours ago with abdominal rigidity, and she has absent bowel tones when assessed. Which of the following symptoms supports a diagnosis of acute mesenteric artery occlusion?

A. Warm, flushed skin
B. Bruit noted in the left iliac fossa
C. Colicky periumbilical pain associated with explosive diarrhea
D. Pain is intermittent and localized

65. The stage of hepatitis characterized by jaundice, pallor, pale stool, dark urine, and pruritis is called the ________ stage.

A. Preicteric
B. Fulminant
C. Toxic
D. Icteric

66. Melena stools indicate bleeding from what body area?

A. Mouth
B. Upper gastrointestinal
C. Descending colon
D. Liver

67. The most common cause of death related to acute hepatic failure is

A. Pulmonary embolism
B. Anemia
C. Brainstem herniation
D. Pulmonary edema

68. Your patient is a model and weighs 95 pounds. She was found unconscious in the bathroom. She was admitted for severe dehydration and starvation. Which of the following symptoms would you expect to observe with this patient?

A. Decreased serum lactate
B. Normal urinary nitrogen excretion
C. Conservation of body fluids with third spacing
D. Decreased serum catecholamines, glucagon, and cortisol

69. Which of the following lab results would contraindicate performing a peritoneal lavage?

A. RBC 5.4 million/mm^3
B. PLT 78,000 mm^3/ml
C. PT 12.5 sec and PTT 75 sec
D. Hgb 14.5 g/dL and Hct 46%

70. **During gastric lavage for stress-related erosion syndrome (SRES) gastric bleeding, your patient becomes hyperthermic, tachycardic, complains of sudden abdominal pain, and has abdominal rigidity. As his nurse, you should**
    A. Continue with the lavage; the symptoms are normal
    B. Stop the infusion and contact the physician
    C. Stop the infusion and rewarm the fluid
    D. Slow the infusion and change the fluid

71. **Medications that are bound to protein may have which of the following effects?**
    A. Increased availability
    B. Rapid distribution
    C. Less available drug for the desired effect
    D. Idiosyncrasy

72. **Your patient has been diagnosed with chronic liver disease. In addition to a venous hum or murmur, you may also note which of the following findings during abdominal auscultation?**
    A. Aortic bruit
    B. Hepatic bruit
    C. Iliac artery bruit
    D. Renal artery bruit

73. **Your patient was involved in a motor vehicle accident with blunt abdominal trauma related to the seatbelt placement. He begins complaining of severe abdominal pain around the epigastric area that is knife-like and twisting. You also note a low-grade fever with diaphoresis, abdominal distension, decreased bowel tones, and rebound tenderness. You suspect this patient may be suffering from**
    A. Pancreatitis
    B. Acute liver failure
    C. Gastrointestinal bleeding
    D. Abdominal bruising

74. **A non-alcohol-abusing man was diagnosed with portal hypertension and direct variceal bleeding. His wedge hepatic venous pressure is less than portal pressure, due to portal vein thrombosis. His symptoms may be due to**
    A. Chronic active hepatitis
    B. Umbilical vein catheterization as a neonate
    C. Metastatic carcinoma
    D. Tuberculosis

75. **A patient with chronic pancreatitis was admitted for respiratory distress and pulmonary edema. These symptoms are due to**
    A. Pulmonary capillary endothelial damage related to phospholipase
    B. Bronchospasms related to stress
    C. Aspiration
    D. Atrial fibrillation

76. **You are admitting a patient after a head injury. As you perform your assessment, you note a stoma to the right iliac fossa in the lower abdomen. There are soft, scattered bowel tones. Output is loose, brownish-tinged, and without form. You document your findings as a(n)**
    A. Sigmoid colostomy
    B. Ileostomy
    C. Loop colostomy
    D. Ascending colostomy

77. **Which of the following types of bowel obstructions leads to infarction or strangulation?**
    A. Acute
    B. Subacute
    C. Chronic
    D. Intermittent

78. **A 56 year old male patient has been medically treated for GERD for the past 3 years. He is now being treated for aspiration pneumonia due to increasing difficulty swallowing and vomiting. He admits to noncompliance with his GERD medication regime and was diagnosed with Barrett's esophagus 6 months ago. He has also been diagnosed with esophageal cancer. Which surgical procedure will he likely undergo to remove his cancer?**
    A. Whipple
    B. Modified Whipple
    C. Esophagectomy
    D. Esophagastrectomy

79. **The most frequent cause of parasitic gastroenteritis in the United States is**
    A. *Giardia lamblia*
    B. *Clostridium difficile*
    C. *Entamoeba histolytica*
    D. Cryptosporidium

80. **An antimicrobial drug should improve diarrhea caused by**
    A. *E. coli*
    B. *Staphylococcus aureus*
    C. *Shigella*
    D. A rotavirus

81. **A glycoprotein produced in the stomach that is required for vitamin B_{12} absorption is**
    A. Hydrochloric acid
    B. Pepsinogen
    C. Secretin
    D. Intrinsic factor

82. Which of the following medications inhibits gastrin synthesis, gastric acid output, and decreases splanchnic circulation?

A. Vasopressin
B. Famotidine
C. Octreotide acetate
D. Ranitidine

83. A contraindication for use of magnesium hydroxide (Milk of Magnesia) is

A. Intestinal obstruction
B. Hyperacidity
C. Bowel evacuation
D. Depressed immune system

84. Your new patient initially presented to the ED with appendicitis. Morphine has controlled his symptoms during his stay in the ED, and the hospitalist plans to try to manage the appendicitis medically. As you are transferring him to his bed, he asks if the pain will ever come back. You tell him

A. "No. You should not ever have this problem again."
B. "Yes, but not for several years."
C. "Yes, but the pain will not be as severe."
D. "Possibly. About one-third of patients are readmitted and require surgery within 1 year."

85. A 36 year old female has severe Crohn's disease and an ileostomy. She is at greatest risk for which of the following complications?

A. Dehydration
B. Hypernatremia
C. Hemorrhage
D. Prolapsed stoma due to vigorous exercise once discharged

86. Patients considering gastric bypass for weight management control should begin bariatric education

A. Prior to the decision to have surgery
B. When the decision to have surgery is made
C. Bariatric surgery education is not necessary
D. After surgery

87. A young man is visiting his sister in the PCU. She was complaining to him about her severe stomach cramping. There is a familial history of polyposis and inflammatory bowel disease. He is worried about his risk of developing cancer, so in a quiet moment, he asks you about the possibility of his developing cancer. Which of the following statements is true regarding colorectal cancers?

A. Adenocarcinomas are the least common cancer
B. Right colon lesions are rare
C. Left colon tumors spread, ulcerate, and erode blood vessels
D. Rectal tumors are associated with localized metastasis

SECTION 9: GASTROINTESTINAL ANSWERS

1. **Correct answer: B**
   A drug that crosses the mucosal barrier and should be avoided in the treatment of a peptic ulcer is indomethacin. Other drugs that cross the mucosal barrier are aspirin, ibuprofen and NSAIDs. Nicotine increases stimulation.

2. **Correct answer: D**
   A subjective sign of a peptic ulcer would be epigastric pain. Pallor, tarry stools, and hyperactive bowel sounds are all objective signs.

3. **Correct answer: C**
   The Hgb and Hct would be decreased in liver disease. The liver exzymes (AST, ALT, and LDH) would be increased in liver failure.

4. **Correct answer: D**
   Gastrin and amylase are likely to be elevated in a patient with a peptic ulcer. Total proteins, albumin, and transferrin are likely to be decreased because the patient is often malnourished.

5. **Correct answer: A**
   Absolute contraindications for providing tube feedings would include intestinal obstructions, a paralytic ileus, tumors, an intestinal perforation, and adhesions.

6. **Correct answer: B**
   Relative contraindications for providing tube feedings for a patient would include bacteremia, severe malabsorption, and an enterocutaneous fistula.

7. **Correct answer: C**
   One way of confirming placement of a feeding tube is to sample the gastric aspirate. If the patient has not received any pH-altering medications, the pH of the aspirate should be in the range of 1.0–3.0.

8. **Correct answer: D**
   Nucleotides support the function and growth of lymphocytes and macrophages.

9. **Correct answer: B**
   A gradual wasting of body fat and muscle as well as the proteins contained in the internal organs (visceral protein) is known as marasmus. Patients with chronic illnesses and gradual starvation often exhibit marasmus.

10. **Correct answer: D**
    Amylase levels are usually elevated in patients with pancreatitis or pancreatic cancer. The normal range for amylase is 56–190 units/L.

11. **Correct answer: A**
    The normal value for the alinine transferase (ALT) is in the range of 5–36 units/ml. The ALT was formerly known as the SGPT.

12. **Correct answer:** C
In a patient diagnosed with an intestinal obstruction, the phosphorus would be elevated. A normal range for phosphorus would be about 3.0–4.5 mg/dL.

13. **Correct answer:** B
Ammonia levels are elevated in patients with heart failure, renal failure, and hepatic failure. A normal range for ammonia is 15 to 110 mOsm/dL. Since ammonia is a byproduct of protein metabolism, levels tend to be higher in conditions that interfere with this metabolism.

14. **Correct answer:** B
Your patient has had several bouts of diarrhea during the past 3 days. As a progressive care nurse, you know this patient is likely to be low on magnesium. The normal range for magnesium is 1.5–2.2 mEq/L, so a low level would correspond to answer B: 0.9–1.4 mEq/L.

15. **Correct answer:** A
Total bilirubin levels may be elevated in patients suffering from profound hemolysis, a biliary obstruction, or hepatic disease. The normal range for total bilirubin is 0.3–1.3 mg/dL.

16. **Correct answer:** A
Your patient is suffering from a biliary obstruction. As a progressive care nurse, you know his direct bilirubin levels will be affected. The normal value for a direct bilirubin level is 0.1–0.3 mg/dL.

17. **Correct answer:** C
Indirect bilirubin levels are elevated in profound hemolysis and hepatic disease. An example of an elevated indirect bilirubin level is 1.8 mg/dL.

18. **Correct answer:** B
The Miller–Abbott tube is used for proximal decompression of the bowel. This tube is not used for complete bowel obstruction or paralytic ileus.

19. **Correct answer:** D
A right hemicolectomy is most likely to be performed on a patient with tumors of the descending or sigmoid colon.

20. **Correct answer:** C
A low anterior resection is the likely surgical procedure for patients with proximal and midrectal tumors. Patients with malignant lesions of the lower sigmoid colon and anus will probably undergo an abdominoperineal resection. Tumors of the mid or lower left transverse colon usually result in a transverse colectomy.

21. **Correct answer:** B
While you are assessing a patient's abdomen, you note that on palpation of the left lower quadrant, the patient complains of pain in the right lower quadrant. This finding is known as a Rovsing's sign. This finding indicates peritoneal irritation and can also help in the diagnosis of appendicitis.

22. **Correct answer:** A
Using aspirate pH will facilitate or confirm passage of a Miller–Abbott tube through the GI tract. As the tube progresses, the pH of the stomach is acidotic. As the tube passes through the pylorus, the pH will become slightly more alkaline. The pH is alkaline in the intestine.

23. Correct answer: A
You should suspect the patient may be suffering from splenic bleeding. Your patient fell out of bed at the end of the previous shift. Although an X-ray of his abdomen is negative, he is now complaining of pain in his left shoulder. This finding is known as Kehr's sign and indicates bleeding occurring below the diaphragm that is irritating the phrenic nerve.

24. Correct answer: D
A major limitation of peritoneal lavage is that peritoneal lavage cannot diagnose retroperitoneal injuries or diaphragmatic injury/trauma.

25. Correct answer: A
When liver parenchymal cells are aggressively destroyed and replaced with fibrotic tissue, leading to impaired hepatic function, this condition is known as cirrhosis.

26. Correct answer: D
Ranitidine is classified as a histamine H2 receptor antagonist. Calcium carbonate, magnesium hydroxide, and aluminum hydroxide are all antacids.

27. Correct answer: A
Three or more episodes of acute, midline abdominal pain lasting for 2 hours to several days with periods without symptoms is known as an abdominal migraine.

28. Correct answer: D
This is another of those deceptively easy questions. Make absolutely certain you know the correct order for assessment. Inspection to determine landmarks and appearance, auscultation to establish location and quality of bowel tones, percussion notes or tones are different for various internal organs, and palpation to establish wall tone, tenderness, and size of organs. Percussion and palpation prior to inspection or auscultation could affect the assessment findings.

29. Correct answer: D
The primary causative agent for gastroenteritis is a rotavirus.

30. Correct answer: C
An early sign of appendicitis is night waking. The patient has nonspecific discomfort and wakes frequently.

31. Correct answer: D
Hematochezia describes bleeding that is bright or dark red blood that is passed from the rectum.

32. Correct answer: D
Hepatorenal syndrome is a complication of hepatic failure due to the release of mediators. The release of mediators results in vasoconstriction, which diverts blood flow to the kidneys. There is a decrease in circulating plasma as the patient develops ascites. Vasoconstriction, not vasodilatation, occurs in end-stage liver failure. There is a decrease in renal circulation due to plasma shifting and vasoconstriction.

33. Correct answer: D
Cullen's sign refers to the bluish discoloration of the periumbilical area as seen in pancreatitis and/or abdominal trauma. Marbled appearance is common with abdominal trauma. Coopernail's sign is bruising of the scrotum or labia. Turner's sign is bruising of the flanks.

34. **Correct answer:** C
The goal when working with bulimic and anorexic patients and their families is to support positive nutritional changes while acknowledging and supporting the psychological changes in body and food perception. By acknowledging the difficulties the patient has with food perception and willingness to providing support and counseling with a nutritionist, dietician, and psychologist, the patient will find foods that are both appealing and provide needed nutrition. The remaining answers are abrasive or do not address the physiologic or psychological struggle with eating.

35. **Correct answer:** A
Hepatitis A is often misdiagnosed initially as gastroenteritis because symptoms are usually self-limiting. Fecal–oral transmission may also be mistaken as food poisoning.

36. **Correct Answer:** B
Hepatitis B is the only DNA virus listed. The other forms of hepatitis are RNA viruses.

37. **Correct answer:** A
The correct order for these interventions when assisting with a paracentesis is to: have the patient void or insert a Foley catheter, order an upright X-ray of the abdomen, position the patient with the affected side up, and examine the abdomen for dullness.

38. **Correct answer:** C
Because of cellular changes in the esophageal lining, the patient is at increased risk for esophageal cancer. Barrett's esophagus is a result of mucosal changes in the esophagus after repeated and prolonged exposure to gastric secretions seen in untreated gastroesophageal reflux disease (GERD).

39. **Correct answer:** A
Patients who have had bariatric surgery are at risk for hypoxia, not hyperoxia.

40. **Correct answer:** B
This patient recently had knee surgery for which she received Tylenol #3 for pain control. She has no bowel sounds, her abdomen is firmly distended, and she is diffusely tender across the abdomen. The probable cause of her symptoms is a paralytic ileus from the codeine.

41. **Correct answer:** B
Common adverse reactions to cimetidine can include rash, nausea, agitation, vomiting, diarrhea, flushing, neutropenia, elevated liver enzymes, and drowsiness.

42. **Correct answer:** C
Cimetidine, famotidine, and ranitidine are H2 blockers. They inhibit gastric acid production by antagonism of the histamine H2 receptors. They are used for prevention of ulcers and in the treatment of GI bleeding.

43. **Correct answer:** C
This patient has likely ruptured varices. Priorities are to maintain airway, stop bleeding, and verify venous access for blood replacement, fluid management, and homeostasis. You want to position the patient upright to prevent aspiration, not flat. You would anticipate the placement of a Minnesota tube, not a Linton–Nachlas tube. Dopamine at 5 μg/kg/min would better support renal function, not blood pressure, as needed in this patient.

44. Correct answer: A
This patient is exhibiting signs and symptoms of an abscess after surgical intervention for appendicitis, which occurs in 5–33% of patients. Surgical debridement of the incision and IV antibiotics are appropriate immediate treatment to prevent sepsis. Hydration and antibiotics alone will not treat the abscess. Bedside excision of the abscess may reduce the amount of infected fluid and tissue at the site, but will not prevent further infection. Bedside wound debridement places a high risk of further contamination of the site. In approximately 2% of cases, the abscess may be intra-abdominal and may require surgical intervention under anesthesia as well as continued antibiotic treatment.

45. Correct answer: D
This patient is exhibiting classic progression of a developing esophageal neoplasm. Complications that coincide with this disease process are related to changes in nutritional intake. Narrowing of the esophageal lumen results in increasing difficulties and pain when swallowing, leading to a softer diet until the patient can swallow only liquids. Partial tongue paralysis would be supported if the patient also had difficulty speaking, but that symptom is not given. Gastric cancer is indicated with indigestion and fullness, not difficulty swallowing. Tracheal neoplasm would be exhibited with more respiratory distress.

46. Correct answer: D
Anyone experiencing dumping syndrome after gastric bypass surgery should stop taking reglan. Reglan increases gastric emptying by increasing peristalsis, thus increasing the effects of dumping syndrome. Reglan may be used after gastrectomy when gastroparesis is present, but once peristalsis has resumed it should be stopped.

47. Correct answer: C
When patients have liver failure, fatty nodules called xanthomas, may develop subcutaneously due to cholesterol accumulation.

48. Correct answer: B
Based on the presenting symptoms and ethnicity, Mr. J. probably has ulcerative colitis. He may also have leukocytosis and cachexia. Colonic diverticulitis presents with left upper quadrant pain, hyperthermia, vomiting, chills, diarrhea, and tenderness over the descending colon. Pancreatitis presents with left upper quadrant pain that radiates to the back or chest, hyperthermia, rigidity, rebound abdominal tenderness, nausea and vomiting, jaundice, Cullen's sign, Grey–Turner's sign, abdominal distention, and diminished bowel sounds. Cholecystitis presents with right upper quadrant or epigastric pain, pain that lasts up to 6 hours after a fatty meal, vomiting, and increased white blood cell counts.

49. Correct answer: C
Glycemic emergencies may occur with sandostatin, especially in the diabetic patient. It is important to monitor blood glucose to prevent hyperglycemia and/or hypoglycemia. Blood pressure and urinary function may also be impacted, but are not as quickly life-threatening as unstable glucose levels.

50. Correct answer: A
The drug of choice for treating gastroesophageal reflux is metoclopramide. Metoclopramide increases gastric emptying and motility, thereby reducing reflux symptoms. The patient should be monitored for diarrhea and neurologic signs such as tremors or muscle twitching.

51. Correct answer: B
E. coli is linked with abdominal pain and diarrhea from fast-food restaurants.

52. Correct answer: A
Lactulose is classified as an ammonia detoxicant and a hyperosmotic laxative.

53. Correct answer: C
Eosinophilia is a side effect of erythromycin. Additional side effects include bradycardia, abdominal pain, nausea, ventricular arrhythmias, and cholestatic jaundice.

54. Correct answer: A
When a patient has a tracheoesophageal fistula, the nurse will be unable to pass an NG tube.

55. Correct answer: A
These results indicate that this patient has a high risk for variceal bleeding. Fifty percent of deaths of patients with cirrhosis are from variceal bleeding. These lab tests are used to differentiate causes of bleeding. History and lab values lean toward varices. Although the Hgb and Hct are decreased in peptic ulcer disease and gastritis, the other lab changes would not be occurring. Boerhaave's syndrome is a full-thickness rupture or perforation of the esophageal wall due to prolonged and frequent vomiting related to eating disorders.

56. Correct answer: C
Ascites occurs secondary to aldosteronism. Aldosteronism initiates sodium retention, increasing portal hypertension. Low albumin levels with increased hydrostatic pressure and decreased oncotic pressures result in ascites. Because of fluid shifting there would be a decrease in ventilation/perfusion (V/Q) ratio.

57. Correct answer: B
The Whipple procedure removes the tip or head of the pancreas, the gallbladder, the duodenum, and part of the bile duct. Occasionally, part of the stomach may also be removed. The extent of the cancerous pancreatic tumor indicates the extent of removal.

58. Correct answer: C
This patient's symptoms are consistent with late dumping syndrome related to the partial gastrectomy during the Whipple procedure. With late dumping syndrome, symptoms occur 1 to 3 hours after meals. Additional symptoms include: weakness, fatigue, dizziness, anxiety, palpitations, and fainting. Patients may also exhibit early signs of dumping syndrome approximately 15–30 minutes after a meal with nausea, vomiting, cramps or abdominal pain, diarrhea, bloating, tachycardia, dysrhythmias, and dizziness. Although anxiety may be exhibited with dumping syndrome, an alteration in mental status with relation to food consumption and history supports a dumping syndrome diagnosis. Hypoglycemia is a greater risk for patients of just gastrectomy or bypass. GERD presents with heartburn and epigastric pain.

59. Correct answer: C
Because the gastric size is greatly reduced, there is less intrinsic factor to assist in vitamin B_{12} absorption to prevent pernicious anemia. Oral supplements are not recommended as they may not be absorbed quickly enough; sublingual or injected vitamin B_{12} may be required. Iron, thiamin, and calcium are all absorbed in the duodenum.

In gastric bypass, the duodenum is also bypassed greatly, limiting the absorption of these vitamins and minerals. Careful supplementation is mandatory to prevent malnutrition. Protein deficiencies are also common and supplementation is necessary, especially in early postoperative recovery to prevent muscle wasting during the rapid weight loss period.

60. Correct answer: B
Tell the family that when they visit the patient in his long-term care facility, they can apply a moisturizing lotion when visiting. Skin becomes very dry, and gentle application of a moisturizer may relieve discomfort. Deep tissue massage is contraindicated due to the decreased platelet count and increased bruising.

61. Correct answer: B
Drinking water from a mountain stream is not the only way to acquire giardiasis, because any contaminated water can lead to infection.

62. Correct answer: C
Giardia lamblia is a protozoan parasite that colonizes the small intestine, causing diarrhea.

63. Correct answer: A
The Minnesota tube is the best choice for differentiating bleeding from the esophagus or the stomach. The Minnesota tube has separate suction and balloons that can function independently. The Sengstaken–Blakemore tube has only three lumens with only one suction port. The Linton-Nachlas tube is for gastric varices only. The standard nasogastric tube has no balloon function to tamponade bleeding.

64. Correct answer: C
A diagnosis of acute mesenteric artery occlusion is supported by a history of colicky periumbilical pain associated with explosive diarrhea. Abdominal pain becomes constant and diffuse. As symptoms progress, the patient will become tachycardic, tachypneic, feverish and hypotensive with worsening abdominal pain and rigidity. Skin will become cold and clammy with shunting as compensatory mechanisms fail.

65. Correct answer: D
The stage of hepatitis characterized by jaundice, pallor, pale stool, dark urine, and pruritis is called the icteric stage.

66. Correct answer: B
Melena is black, tarry stool containing blood from the upper gastrointestinal area or ascending colon. Oral bleeding may result in hematemesis. Descending colon bleeding may lead to bright red stools. Iron, bismuth, and other foods may be mistaken for melena, but an occult blood test of the stool rules this out.

67. Correct answer: C
The most common cause of death related to acute hepatic failure is brainstem herniation. Brainstem herniation is the most common cause of death due to increased coagulation times, intracranial hemorrhaging, and hypoxia leading to cerebral edema. Anemia is a complication of prolonged bleeding times, but not the primary cause of death. Pulmonary impairment is the result of hemorrhaging, not embolism or edema.

68. **Correct answer:** C
Prolonged starvation and protein loss resulting in fluid shifting and third spacing are symptoms seen in a patient who is suffering from starvation and dehydration. Muscle wasting results in an increase in serum lactate levels, not a decrease. Initially, there is an increased urinary nitrogen excretion, which is followed by a decrease. There is also an increase in serum catecholamine, glucagons, and cortisal as the body releases elements to maintain energy and glucose available.

69. **Correct answer:** B
A patient with a platelet count of 78,000 mm^3/ml is thrombocytopenic and at risk for coagulation complications, which contraindicates performing a peritoneal lavage. Heparin is normally added to the solution to prevent clotting and can lead to further complications of bleeding. The other lab values are within normal range for either males or females.

70. **Correct answer:** B
The patient is exhibiting signs and symptoms of gastric perforation. This is a surgical emergency, and the lavage should be stopped, fluid aspirated, and the physician notified immediately. Additional actions include the placement of at least two large-bore IVs, preparing to administer IV fluid replacement if hypovolemic shock occurs, and preparing the patient for immediate surgery.

71. **Correct answer:** C
Medications that are bound to protein may have less available drug for the desired effect.

72. **Correct answer:** B
Hepatic bruits are heard over the liver and may also indicate primary liver cancer, alcoholic hepatitis, or vascular liver metastases. An aortic bruit over the epigastric area indicates a partial aortic occlusion. Iliac artery bruits are heard over the left/right inguinal areas. Renal artery bruits indicate renal artery stenosis.

73. **Correct answer:** A
Acute pancreatitis may occur as a result of seat-belt trauma to the pancreatic duct or abdominal ischemia. Acute liver failure is characterized by flu-like symptoms, jaundice, confusion, and enlarged liver. Gastrointestinal bleeding has a history of ulcers and/or esophageal varices with hemodynamic changes, narrowing pulse pressures, hematemesis, and hyperactive bowel tones. Abdominal trauma does not produce the knife-like and twisting pain, and tenderness and a marbled appearance would be noted.

74. **Correct answer:** B
This patient may have had an umbilical catheter placed when he was a neonate—a pre-hepatic factor. Pre-hepatic (pre-sinusoidal) factors lead to hepatic venous pressures less than portal pressures. Chronic active hepatitis is an intrahepatic (sinusoidal) factor. Wedge hepatic venous pressures are increased or equal to portal pressures. Metastatic carcinoma and cardiac diseases such as CHF can cause portal hypertension and may indirectly cause variceal bleeding.

75. **Correct answer:** A
A patient with chronic pancreatitis was admitted for respiratory distress and pulmonary edema. These symptoms are due to pulmonary capillary endothelial damage related to phospholipase. Pulmonary capillary endothelial damage allows fluid to leak into the interstitium.

76. Correct answer: B

An ileostomy is located at the right ileac fossa just before the colon. Because most water absorption occurs in the colon, stool from the small intestines is loose and unformed. Sigmoid colostomy stools more closely resemble normal stools, as most of the water has been absorbed. Loop, or transverse, and ascending colostomies have loose stools with more formation.

77. Correct answer: A

Acute bowel obstruction is the only type of obstruction that leads to infarction or strangulation. Obstruction occurs rapidly and may inhibit blood to a portion of the bowel. The other types of obstructions permit limited or intermittent blood flow that sustains but compromises tissue function.

78. Correct answer: C

This patient will probably undergo an esophagectomy. This procedure involves removal of the damaged esophagus to the proximal portion of the stomach. The stomach is then resectioned to form a new esophagus. If the stomach is also cancerous, the stomach is removed and the small bowel is resectioned to create a new esophagus.

79. Correct answer: A

Giardia lamblia is the most frequent cause of parasitic gastroenteritis in the United States.

80. Correct answer: C

An antimicrobial drug should improve diarrhea caused by *Shigella*.

81. Correct answer: D

Intrinsic factor is a glycoprotein produced in the stomach that is required for vitamin B_{12} absorption.

82. Correct answer: C

Octreotide acetate inhibits gastrin synthesis, gastric acid output, and decreases splanchnic circulation.

83. Correct answer: A

Intestinal obstruction is a contraindication for use of magnesium hydroxide (Milk of Magnesia). Additional contraindications include ileostomy, colostomy, and appendicitis.

84. Correct answer: D

This question requires honest communication with the patient regarding possible reoccurrence of symptoms. Approximately one-third of patients with appendicitis that are treated with antibiotics and pain management are readmitted and require appendectomies within 1 year. The remaining answers are stated as absolutes and are inappropriate for a nurse. If the appendix is not removed, the patient may have a reoccurrence of symptoms at a later date. There is no way to predict if and when an appendix may become infected or diseased. There is no way to predict the pain level of appendicitis, because pain is perceived differently for each patient.

85. Correct answer: A

Dehydration is a severe complication in patients with ileostomies. Water reabsorption is normally accomplished by the colon. This patient may have had a large portion or all of the large intestine removed related to the Crohn's disease process. Fluids should be encouraged and IV support maintained to prevent hypovolemic shock. Teaching should include signs and symptoms of shock and preventative home management. Although a stoma prolapse may occur after discharge home, the stoma can be reopened without major complications. Hyponatremia, not hypernatremia, is a serious complication as sodium uptake also occurs in the colon. Hemorrhage is not a concern unless the stoma is scratched or damaged during care. Light pressure should be applied until bleeding stops, but it is not a life-threatening complication.

86. **Correct answer: A**
Patients considering gastric bypass for weight management control should definitely begin bariatric education prior to the decision to have surgery. Gastric bypass surgery can lead to permanent gastric changes and places the obese patient at risk for both surgical- and anesthesia-related complications. For many bariatric patients, the initial gastric bypass surgery is not necessarily the only surgery required. Often, cosmetic surgery to remove loose skin around the stomach, back, thighs, arms, and chest is required to improve self-image. Each surgery has additional risk. Therefore, complete bariatric education should be provided to any patient considering bariatric surgery. Education should include preoperative changes in diet, nutritional consultation, psychological evaluation, and full medical evaluation including lab work and cardiovascular testing. Education and support for the bariatric surgery patient should continue throughout the surgical process with ongoing education, nutritional support, and physiological support for years after surgery.

87. **Correct answer: C**
Left colon (descending) lesions spread, ulcerate, and erode blood vessels within the colon. Obstruction is a very common complication with this type of lesion. Adenocarcinomas are the most common of the neoplasms. Right colon, or ascending colon, lesions are typically polypoid lesions and are associated with a familial history of polyps. Rectal lesions may spread to the vagina or prostate, but are known for systemic metastasis.

GASTROINTESTINAL REFERENCES

Ahrens, T., Prentice, D., & Kleinpell, R. M. (2011). *Progressive care nursing certification: Preparation, review and practice exams.* St. Louis, MO: McGraw-Hill.

Ajmera, V., Xia, G., Vaughan, G., Forbi, J. C., Ganova-Raeva, L. M., Khudyakov, Y., . . . Lee, W. M. (2011). What factors determine the severity of hepatitis A-related acute liver failure: Acute Liver Failure Study Group. *Journal of Viral Hepatitis, 18*(7), e167–e174.

Albilllos, A., & Garcia-Tsao, G. (2011). Classification of cirrhosis: The clinical use of HVPG measurements. *Disease Markers, 31*(3), 121–128.

Al-Hussaini, A., & Butzner, D. (2012). Therapeutic applications of octreotide in pediatric *patients. Saudi Journal of Gastroenterology, 18*(2), 87–94.

American Academy of Family Physicians. (2011). Cirrhosis and liver damage. *American Family Physician, 84*(12), 1360.

American Association of Critical-Care Nurses. (2006). *AACN core curriculum for critical care nursing.* St. Louis, MO: Saunders.

Appasani, S., Poornachandra, K. S., & Kochhar, R. (2012). Fluid replacement in acute pancreatitis. *Nutritional Therapy & Metabolism, 30*(2), 67–78.

Arheia, E. I. (2011). Current views on the hepatorenal syndrome. *Archives of Hellenic Medicine, 28*(3), 324–335.

Avard, B., & Fergusson, J. (2009). Necrotizing pancreatitis and antibiotic prophylaxis. To use or not to use . . . that is the question. *Journal of Gastroenterology and Hepatology, 24*(5), 710–711.

Bacher, A. (2011). Extracorporeal liver support with multipass albumin dialysis or plasmapheresis and filtering systems in acute liver failure. *Liver International, 31*(8), 16–18.

Bailey, K. (2009). Understanding Barrett's oesophagus, part 1: Surveillance and management. *Gastrointestinal Nursing, 7*(8), 28–35.

Banim, P. J., & Hart, A. R. (2010). Nutrition and diet in the aetiology and management of pancreatic cancer. *Gastrointestinal Nursing, 8*(8), 24–29.

Bashinskaya, B., Nahed, B. V., Redjal, N., Kahle, K. T., & Walcott, B. P. (2011). Trends in peptic ulcer disease and the identification of *Helicobacter Pylori* as a causative organism: Population-based estimates from the US Nationwide Inpatient Sample. *Journal of Global Infectious Diseases, 3*(4), 365–370.

Baumann, A., Audibert, G., Klein, O., & Mertes, P. M. (2009). Continuous intravenous lidocaine in the treatment of paralytic ileus due to severe spinal cord injury. *Acta Anaesthesiologica Scandinavica, 53*(1), 128–130.

Bayram, A., Eksi, F., Mehli, M., & Sözen, E. (2007). Prevalence of hepatitis E virus antibodies in patients with chronic hepatitis B and chronic hepatitis C. *Intervirology, 50*(4), 281–286.

Ben-David, K., Rosenthal, M., & Chauhan, S. S. (2012). A novel strategy for the management of acute hemorrhage from an atrio-esophageal fistula after atrial ablation. *The American Surgeon, 78*(5), E286–E287.

Blake, P. G. (2011). Should nonglucose-containing peritoneal dialysis solutions be used in all patients to avoid long-term membrane injury? *Seminars in Dialysis, 24*(4), 450–451.

Brorsen, A. (2012). *CEN examination review.* Burlington, MA: Jones & Bartlett Learning.

Brorsen, A., & Rogelet, K. (2009). *PCCN certification review.* Sudbury, MA: Jones and Bartlett.

Buti, M., Homs, M., Rodriguez-Frias, F., Funalleras, G., Jardi, R., Sauleda, S., . . . Esteban, R. (2011). Clinical outcome of acute and chronic hepatitis delta over time: A long-term follow-up study. *Journal of Viral Hepatitis, 18*(6), 434–442.

Cariati, A., & Piromalli, E. (2012). Conservative or operative management (open or laparoscopic) of acute appendicitis. *Canadian Journal of Surgery, 55*(3), 7–9.

Carlson, T. L., Plackett, T. P., Gagliano, R. A., & Smith, R. R. (2012). Methamphetamine-induced paralytic ileus. *Hawai'i Journal of Medicine & Public Health, 71*(2), 44–45.

Charrier, A. L., & Brigstock, D. R. (2010). Connective tissue growth factor production by activated pancreatic stellate cells in mouse alcoholic chronic pancreatitis. *Laboratory Investigation, 90*(8), 1179–1188.

Chiang, L. T., Yao, M., Ko, B. S., & Chen, C. H. (2011). Development of immunity against hepatitis B virus after donor lymphocyte infusion in a peripheral blood stem cell transplantation recipient with chronic hepatitis. *Infection, 39*(4), 363–365.

Chulay, M., & Burns, S. (2010). *Essentials of progressive care nursing* (2nd ed.). St. Louis, MO: McGraw-Hill.

Clark, K. L., Loscalzo, M., Trask, P. C., Zabora, J., & Philip, E. J. (2010). Psychological distress in patients with pancreatic cancer: An understudied group. *Psycho-Oncology, 19*(12), 1313–1320.

Craig, D. G., Lee, P., Pryde, E. A., Masterton, G. S., Hayes, P. C., & Simpson, K. J. Circulating apoptotic and necrotic cell death markers in patients with acute liver injury. (2011). *Liver International, 31*(8), 1127–1136.

Curley, M. A. Q. (2007). *Synergy: The unique relationship between nurses and patients*. St. Louis, MO: Saunders.

Danese, S., & Fiocchi, C. (2011). Ulcerative colitis. *The New England Journal of Medicine, 365*(18), 1713–1725.

Dapri, G., Cadière, G. B., & Himpens, J. (2011). Laparoscopic conversion of Roux-en-Y gastric bypass to distal gastric bypass for weight regain. *Journal of Laparoendoscopic & Advanced Surgical Techniques, 21*(1), 19–23.

Do, N., Wisniewski, P., Sarmiento, J., Vo, T., Aka, P. K., Hsu, J. H., & Tayyarah, M. (2010). Retrograde superior mesenteric artery stenting for acute mesenteric arterial thrombosis. *Vascular and Endovascular Surgery, 44*(6), 468–471.

Doklestic, K., Bajec, D., Stefanovic, B., Milic, N., Bumbasirevic, V., Sijacki, A., . . . Karamarkovic, A. (2012). Acute bowel obstruction: Risk factors of adverse outcomes following surgery. *HealthMed, 6*(5), 1846–1854.

Donohoe-Dennison, R. (2007). *Pass CCRN* (3rd ed.). St. Louis, MO: Mosby.

Englert, Z. P., White, M. A., Fitzgerald, T. L., Vadlamudi, A., Zervoudakis, G., & Zervos, E. E. (2012). Surgical management of malignant bowel obstruction: At what price palliation? *The American Surgeon, 78*(6), 647–652.

Ezzat, T. M., Dhar, D. K., Newsome, P. N., Malago, M., & Olde Damink, S. W. (2011). Use of hepatocyte and stem cells for treatment of post-resectional liver failure: Are we there yet? *Liver International, 31*(6), 773–784.

Fries, W., & Comunale, S. (2011). Ulcerative colitis: Pathogenesis. *Current Drug Targets, 12*(10), 1373–1382.

Fullwood, D. (2012). Portal hypertension and varices in patients with liver cirrhosis. *Nursing Standard, 26*(48), 52–57.

Furtado, L. C. (2010). Procedure and outcomes of Roux-en-Y gastric bypass. *British Journal of Nursing, 19*(5), 307–313.

García-Martínez, R., Simón-Talero, M., & Córdoba, J. (2011). Prognostic assessment in patients with hepatic encephalopathy. *Disease Markers, 31*(3), 171–179.

Gee, C. (2011). Pancreatic cancer: A whistle-stop tour. *Gastrointestinal Nursing, 9*(7), 41–45.

González, J. C. M., Mesejo, A., & Saris, A. B. (2011). Guidelines for specialized nutritional and metabolic support in the critically ill patient. Liver failure and liver transplantation. *Nutricion Hospitalaria*, 27–31.

Graziadei, I. W. (2011). The clinical challenges of acute on chronic liver failure. *Liver International, 31*(Suppl. 3), 24–26.

Green, B. R., Reddy, A., & Jha, M. (2012). Mesenteric fat necrosis after recent surgery causing bowel obstruction: A case report and review of the literature. *Journal of Postgraduate Medicine, 58*(1), 54–56.

Grönroos, J. M. (2011). Clinical suspicion of acute appendicitis: Is the time ripe for more conservative treatment? *Minimally Invasive Therapy & Allied Technologies, 20*(1), 42–45.

Grubina, R., Cha, Y., Bell, M. R., Sinak, L. J., & Asirvatham, S. J. (2010). Pneumopericardium following radiofrequency ablation for atrial fibrillation: Insights into the natural history of atrial esophageal fistula formation. *Journal of Cardiovascular Electrophysiology, 21*(9), 1046–1049.

Hardin, S., & Kaplow, R. (2005). *Synergy for clinical excellence: The AACN synergy model for patient care*. St. Louis, MO: Saunders.

Hasper, D., & Jorres, A. (2011). New insights into the management of hepato-renal syndrome. *Liver International, 31*(Suppl. 3), 27–30.

Hatzakis, A., Wait, S., Bruix, J., Buti, M., Carballo, M., Cavaleri, M., . . . Janssen, H. L. (2011). The state of hepatitis B and C in Europe: Report from the hepatitis B and C summit conference. *Journal of Viral Hepatitis, 18*(Suppl. 1), 1–16.

Hayes, C. (2011). The here and now of pancreatic cancer. *Gastrointestinal Nursing, 9*(10), 28–33.

Holcomb, S. S. (2007). Stopping the destruction of acute pancreatitis. *Nursing, 37*(6), 42–48.

Hryszko, T., Suchowierska, E., Rydzewska-Rosolowska, A., Brzosko, S., & Mysliwiec, M. (2012). Factors associated with early catheter-related complications in peritoneal dialysis. *Advances in Medical Sciences, 57*(1), 84–87.

Hsu, C. Y., Lee, F. Y., Huo, T. I., Chan, C. Y., Huang, H. C., Lin, H. C., . . . Lee, S. D. (2010). Lack of therapeutic effects of gabexate mesilate on the hepatic encephalopathy in rats with acute and chronic hepatic failure. *Journal of Gastroenterology and Hepatology, 25*(7), 1321–1328.

Huang, C., Lin, H., Chang, S., & Lee, W. (2011). Preoperative risk factors predict postoperative respiratory failure after liver transplantation. *PLoS ONE, 6*(8), 1–8.

Huang, Z. Q., Saluja, A. K., Dudeja, V., Vickers, S. M., & Buchsbaum, D. J. (2011). Molecular targeted approaches for treatment of pancreatic cancer. *Current Pharmaceutical Design, 17*(21), 2221–2238.

Isaksson, K., Weber, E., Andersson, R., & Tingstedt, B. (2011). Small bowel obstruction: Early parameters predicting the need for surgical intervention. *European Journal of Trauma & Emergency Surgery, 37*(2), 155–159.

Jin, H. T., Lamsa, T., Nordback, P. H., Hyvonen, M. T., Raty, S., Nordback, I., . . . Sand, J. (2011). Polyamine catabolism in relation to trypsin activation and apoptosis in experimental acute pancreatitis. *Pancreatology, 11*(2), 83–91.

Jones & Bartlett Learning. (2011.) *2012 nurse's drug handbook (*11th ed.). Sudbury, MA: Jones & Bartlett Learning.

Karvellas, C. J., Safinia, N., Auzinger, G., Heaton, N., Muiesan, P., O'Grady, J., . . . Bernal, W. (2010). Medical and psychiatric outcomes for patients transplanted for acetaminophen-induced acute liver failure: A case-control study. *Liver International, 30*(6), 826–833.

Keating, G. M. (2011). Intravenous esomeprazole: A pharmacoeconomic profile of its use in the prevention of recurrent peptic ulcer bleeding. *Pharmacoeconomics, 29*(6), 535–543.

Khan, A. S., Latif, S. U., & Eloubeidi, M. A. (2010). Controversies in the etiologies of acute pancreatitis. *Journal of the Pancreas, 11*(6), 545–552.

Kiss, L. S., & Lakatos, P. L. (2011). Natural history of ulcerative colitis: Current knowledge. *Current Drug Targets, 12*(10), 1390–1395.

Knezevich, E., Crnic, T., Kershaw, S., & Drincic, A. (2012). Liraglutide-associated acute pancreatitis. *American Journal of Health-System Pharmacy, 69*(5), 386–389.

Koliscak, L., & Maynor, L. (2012). Pharmacologic prophylaxis against venous thromboembolism in hospitalized patients with cirrhosis and associated coagulopathies. *American Journal of Health-System Pharmacy, 69*(8), 658–663.

Kramer, L., & Kodras, K. (2011). Detoxification as a treatment goal in hepatic failure. *Liver International, 31*(Suppl. 3), 1–4.

Kun-Chun, C., Chun-Nan, Y., & Chen, T. C. (2011). Vitamin D and pancreatic cancer: An update. *Cancers, 3*(1), 213–226.

Lal, A., & Lal, D. R. (2010). Hereditary pancreatitis. *Pediatric Surgery International, 26*(12), 1193–1199.

Lankisch, P. G., Breuer, N., Bruns, A., Weber-Dany, B., Lowenfels, A. B., & Maisonneuve, P. (2009). Natural history of acute pancreatitis: A long-term population-based study. *The American Journal of Gastroenterology, 104*(11), 2797–2805.

Lau, J. Y., Sung, J., Hill, C., Henderson, C., Howden, C. W., & Metz, D. C. (2011). Systematic review of the epidemiology of complicated peptic ulcer disease: Incidence, recurrence, risk factors and mortality. *Digestion, 84*(2), 102–113.

Lee, A., & Park, Y. (2012). Reducing peritoneal dialysis catheter exit site infections by implementing a standardised postoperative dressing protocol. *Renal Society of Australasia Journal, 8*(1), 18–22.

Lee, V., Cheng, H., Li, G., & Saif, M. W. (2012). Quality of life in patients with pancreatic cancer. *Journal of the Pancreas, 13*(2), 182–184.

Leithead, J. A., Ferguson, J. W., Bates, C. M., Davidson, J. S., Simpson, K. J., & Hayes, P. C. (2011). Chronic kidney disease after liver transplantation for acute liver failure is not associated with perioperative renal dysfunction. *American Journal of Transplantation, 11*(9), 1905–1915.

Letachowicz, K., Letachowicz, W., Weyde, W., Gołębiowski, T., Kusztal, M., Wątorek, E., & Klinger, M. (2012). Repair of damaged connectors of tunneled cuffed catheters with a two-piece adaptor for peritoneal dialysis. *The Journal of Vascular Access, 13*(2), 203–207.

Leung, A. M., & Vu, H. (2012). Factors predicting need for and delay in surgery in small bowel obstruction. *The American Surgeon, 78*(4), 403–407.

Li, T., Meng, Q. H., Zou, Z. Q., Fan, Y. C., Long, B., Guo, Y. M., . . . Wang, K. (2011). Correlation between promoter methylation of glutathione-S-tranferase P1 and oxidative stress in acute-on-chronic hepatitis B liver failure. *Journal of Viral Hepatitis, 18*(7), e226–e231.

Lockrey, G., & Lim, L. (2011). Peptic ulcer disease in older people. *Journal of Pharmacy Practice & Research, 41*(1), 58–61.

Luo, J. C., Huang, K. W., Leu, H. B., Chen, L. C., Hou, M. C., Li, C. P., . . . Lee, S. D. (2011). Randomized clinical trial: Rabeprazole plus aspirin is not inferior to rabeprazole plus clopidogrel for the healing of aspirin-related peptic ulcer. *Alimentary Pharmacology & Therapeutics, 34*(5), 519–525.

Lynn-McHale Wiegand, D. J. (Ed.). (2011). *AACN procedure manual for critical care* (6th ed.). St. Louis, MO: Saunders.

MacIntyre, J. (2011). Metastatic pancreatic cancer: What can nurses do? *Clinical Journal of Oncology Nursing, 15*(4), 424–428.

Magdalan, J., Zawadzki, M., & Sozanski, T. (2011). Fulminant hepatic failure in woman with iron and non-steroidal anti-inflammatory drug intoxication. *Human & Experimental Toxicology, 30*(8), 1106–1111.

Manjunath, H., Venkatesh, D., Jalihal, U., Prashanth, K. M., & Al, A. (2011). An altered pulmonary function—A cause or consequence of gastroesophageal reflux disease (GERD). *Journal of Medical Sciences, 4*(4), 391–395.

Mattioni, S., Zamy, M., Mechai, F., Raynaud, J. J., Chabrol, A., Aflalo, V., . . . Bouchaud, O. (2012). Isoniazid-induced recurrent pancreatitis. *Journal of the Pancreas, 13*(3), 314–316.

Milic, S., Mikolasevic, I., Radic, M., Hauser, G., & Stimac, D. (2011). Clinical utility of red cell distribution width in alcoholic and non-alcoholic liver cirrhosis. *Collegium Antropologicum, 35*(Suppl. 2), 335–338.

Mitlyng, B. L., & Ganz, R. A. (2012). Understanding the GERD. *Minnesota Medicine, 95*(4), 42–45.

Nahar, K., Jahan, M., Nessa, A., & Tabassum, S. (2011). Antibody responses after hepatitis B vaccination among maintenance haemodialysis patients. *Bangladesh Medical Research Council Bulletin, 37*(3), 88–91.

Nakayama, N., Oketani, M., Kawamura, Y., Inao, M., Nagoshi, S., Fujiwara, K., . . . Mochida, S. (2011). Novel classification of acute liver failure through clustering using a self-organizing map: Usefulness for prediction of the outcome. *Journal of Gastroenterology, 46*(9), 1127–1135.

Navarro, V. J., & Rossi, S. (2011). Drug-induced liver injury—Its pathophysiology and evolving diagnostic tools. [Review article.] *Alimentary Pharmacology & Therapeutics, 34*(1), 11–20.

Nayak, V., Chogtu, B., Devaramane, V., Vasudeva, S., & Bhandary, P. V. (2010). Clozapine-induced paralytic ileus. *Journal of Pharmaceutical Research & Health Care, 2*(4), 330–332.

Nicković, V., Nikolić, J., Djindjić, N., Ilić, M., Nicković, J., Mladenović, D., . . . Vojnosanitetski, P. (2012). Diagnostical significance of dimethylarginine in the development of hepatorenal syndrome in patients with alcoholic liver cirrhosis. *Military-Medical and Pharmaceutical Review, 69*(8), 686–691.

Okazaki, K., Uchida, K., Fukui, T., Takaoka, M., & Nishio, A. (2010). Autoimmune pancreatitis—A new evolving pancreatic disease? *Langenbeck's Archives of Surgery, 395*(8), 989–1000.

Paik, C. N., Choi, M. G., Lim, C. H., Park, J. M., Chung, W. C., Lee K. M., . . . Chung, I. S. (2011). The role of small intestinal bacterial overgrowth in postgastrectomy patients. *Neurogastroenterology & Motility, 23*(5), 191–196.

Pandol, S. J., Lugea, A., Mareninova, O. A., Smoot, D., Gorelick, F. S., Gukovskaya, A. S., & Gukovsky, I. (2011). Investigating the pathobiology of alcoholic pancreatitis. *Alcoholism, Clinical and Experimental Research, 35*(5), 830–837.

Pascarella, S., & Negro, F. (2011). Hepatitis D virus: An update. *Liver International, 31*(1), 7–21.

Patrick, L. (2011). Gastroesophageal reflux disease (GERD): A review of conventional and alternative treatments. *Alternative Medicine Review, 16*(2), 116–133.

Penny, S. M. (2012). Clinical signs of pancreatitis. *Radiologic Technology, 83*(6), 561–581.

Pezzilli, R., Zerbi, A., Di Carlo, V., Bassi, C., & Delle Fave, G. F. (2010). Practical guidelines for acute pancreatitis. Working Group of the Italian Association for the Study of the Pancreas on Acute Pancreatitis. *Pancreatology, 10*(5), 523–535.

Policha, A., Hu, C., Holmes, P., Cohn, J. R., & Martin, N. D. (2010). Acute perforated appendicitis secondary to sarcoidosis. *The American Surgeon, 78*(5), 616–619.

Prowant, B. F., Moore, H., Satalowich, R., & Twardowski, Z. J. (2010). Peritoneal dialysis survival in relation to patient body size and peritoneal transport characteristics. *Nephrology Nursing Journal, 37*(6), 641–646.

Puylaert, M., Kapural, L., Van Zundert, J., Peek, D., Lataster, A., Mekhail, N., . . . Keulemans, Y. C. A. (2011, September-October). Pain in chronic pancreatitis. *Pain Practice, 11*(5), 492–505.

Qahtani, A. A., Holcroft, C., Gordon, P. H., & Szilagyi, A. (2012). Clinical variables related to small bowel obstruction: Comparison of patients with and without Crohn's disease. *Gastroenterology Insights, 4*(2), 57–62.

Qu, W., Tokar, E. J., Kim, A. J., Bell, M. W., & Waalkes, M. P. (2012). Chronic cadmium exposure in vitro causes acquisition of multiple tumor cell characteristics in human pancreatic epithelial cells. *Environmental Health Perspectives, 120*(9), 1265–1271.

Rahbari, N. N., Schmidt, T., Falk, C. S., Hinz, U., Herber, M., Bork, U., . . . Koch, M. (2011). Expression and prognostic value of circulating angiogenic cytokines in pancreatic cancer. *BMC Cancer, 11*, 286.

Richardson, J. F., Lee, J. G., Smith, B. R., Nguyen, B., Pham, K. P., & Nguyen, N. T. (2012). Laparoscopic transgastric endoscopy after Roux-en-Y gastric bypass: Case series and review of the literature. *American Surgeon, 78*(10), 1182–1186.

Saif, M. W. (2012). Revising you the staging for pancreatic cancer in 2012. *Journal of the Pancreas, 13*(2), 128–130.

Sargent, S. (2010). An overview of acute liver failure: Managing rapid deterioration. *Gastrointestinal Nursing, 8*(9), 36–42.

Saugel, B., Gaa, J., Phillip, V., Schmid, R. M., & Huber, W. (2010). Splenic artery embolization in a woman with bleeding gastric varices and splenic vein thrombosis: A case report. *Journal of Medical Case Reports, 4*(1), 1–3.

Schaffler, A., Hamer, O. W., Dickopf, J., Goetz, A., Landfried, K., Voelk, M., . . . Brunnler, T. (2011, May 1). Admission visfatin levels predict pancreatic and peripancreatic necrosis in acute pancreatitis and correlate with clinical severity. *The American Journal of Gastroenterology, 106*(5), 957–967.

Seliman, A. M. A., El-Soussi, A. H., Sultan, M. A. A., & Othman, S. Y. (2011). Effect of implementing nursing guidelines for tube feeding on the occurrence of aspiration among critically ill patients. *Nature & Science, 9*(11), 164–175.

Sephton, M. (2010). Nursing management of patients with severe ulcerative colitis. *Nursing Standard, 24*(15–17), 48–58.

Slack, A., & Wendon, J. (2011). Acute liver failure. *Clinical Medicine, 11*(3), 254–258.

Srivastava, B., & Alexander, G. J. (2011). Renal failure in chronic liver disease and the hepatorenal syndrome. *British Journal of Hospital Medicine, 72*(9), 497–503.

Starr, S. P., & Raines, D. (2011). Cirrhosis: Diagnosis, management, and prevention. *American Family Physician, 84*(12), 1353–1359.

Stepter, C. R. (2012). Maintaining placement of temporary enteral feeding tubes in adults: A critical appraisal of the evidence. *MEDSURG Nursing, 21*(2), 61–102.

Suda, K., Takase, M., Fukumura, Y., & Kashiwagi, S. (2007). Pathology of autoimmune pancreatitis and tumor-forming pancreatitis. *Journal of Gastroenterology, 42*(Suppl. 18), 22–27.

Tanweer, S., Pervez, T., Taseer, I., Khan, A. Q., & Arshad, M. (2011). Hepatic cirrhosis: Association of platelet count, splenomegaly, and esophegeal varices in patients. *Professional Medical Journal, 18*(3), 426–429.

Thng, C., Babiker, Z. O., Brown, B., & Babu, C. (2012). The perils of relying on anti-hepatitis B total core antibody in screening individuals infected with HIV. *International Journal of STD & AIDS, 23*(2), 149–150.

Toshikuni, N., Izumi, A., Nishino, K., Inada, N., Sakanoue, R., Yamato, R., . . . Yamada, G. (2009). Comparison of outcomes between patients with alcoholic cirrhosis and those with hepatitis C virus-related cirrhosis. *Journal of Gastroenterology and Hepatology, 24*(7), 1276–1283.

Tranah, G. J., Holly, E. A., Wang, F., & Bracci, P. M. (2011). Cigarette, cigar, and pipe smoking, passive smoke exposure, and risk of pancreatic cancer: A population-based study in the San Francisco Bay Area. *BMC Cancer, 11*, 138.

Tuñón, M. J., San Miguel, B., Crespo, I., Jorquera, F., Santamaría, E., Alvarez, M., . . . González-Gallego, J. (2011). Melatonin attenuates apoptotic liver damage in fulminant hepatic failure induced by the rabbit hemorrhagic disease virus. *Journal of Pineal Research, 50*(1), 38–45.

Turgay, A. S., & Khorshid, L. (2010). Effectiveness of the auscultatory and pH methods in predicting feeding tube placement. *Journal of Clinical Nursing, 19*(11/12), 1553–1559.

Tursi, T. (2010). Use of ß-blocker therapy to prevent primary bleeding of esophageal varices. *Journal of the American Academy of Nurse Practitioners, 22*(12), 640–647.

Twilla, J. D., & Mancell, J. (2012). Hypertriglyceridemia-induced acute pancreatitis treated with insulin and heparin. *American Journal of Health-System Pharmacy, 69*(3), 213–216.

Vassileva, C. M., Shawgo, T., Shabosky, J., Soliman, S., & Hazelrigg, S. (2011). Repair of left atrial-esophageal fistula following percutaneous radiofrequency ablation for atrial fibrillation. *Journal of Cardiac Surgery, 26*(5), 556–558.

Vela, M. F., Craft, B. M., Sharma, N., Freeman, J., & Hazen-Martin, D. (2011). Refractory heartburn: Comparison of intercellular space diameter in documented GERD vs. functional heartburn. *The American Journal of Gastroenterology, 106*(5), 844–850.

Verrill, C., Markham, H., Templeton, A., Carr, N. J., & Sheron, N. (2009). Alcohol-related cirrhosis: Early abstinence is a key factor in prognosis, even in the most severe cases. *Addiction, 104*(5), 768–774.

Wang, G. J., Gao, C. F., Wei, D., Wang, C., & Ding, S. Q. (2009). Acute pancreatitis: Etiology and common pathogenesis. *World Journal of Gastroenterology, 15*(12), 1427–1430.

Wang, J., Zhou, B., Lai, Q., Wang, Y., Shen, G., Wang, Z., . . . Hou, J. (2011). Clinical and virological characteristics of chronic hepatitis B with concurrent hepatitis E antigen and antibody detection. *Journal of Viral Hepatitis, 18*(9), 646–652.

Watcher, R. (2012). *Understanding patient safety* (2nd ed.). New York: Lange.

Werner, R. (2011). Pathology perspectives. The ABCs of hepatitis: Know the basics of contagious liver infections. *Massage & Bodywork, 26*(6), 100–105.

Wiklund, M., Olsén, M. F., & Willén, C. (2011). Physical activity as viewed by adults with severe obesity, awaiting gastric bypass surgery. *Physiotherapy Research International, 16*(3), 179–186.

World Health Organization [WHO]. (2012). WHO position paper on hepatitis A vaccines--June 2012. *Weekly Epidemiological Record, 87*(28/29), 261–276.

Wright, S., Ali, M., Robinson, A., Ramanathan, K., & Parker, R. B. (2011). Paralytic ileus associated with use of diltiazem. *American Journal of Health-System Pharmacy, 68*(15), 1426–1429.

Xu, Z., Ren, X., Liu, Y., Li, X., Bai, S., Zhong, Y., . . . Xu, D. (2011). Association of hepatitis B virus mutations in basal core promoter and precore regions with severity of liver disease: An investigation of 793 Chinese patients with mild and severe chronic hepatitis B and acute-on-chronic liver failure. *Journal of Gastroenterology, 46*(3), 391–400.

Yamada, H., Shinohara, T., Yokoyama, K., Takasu, K., Fujimori, Y., & Yamagishi, K. (2011). Thoracoscopic enucleation of esophageal gastrointestinal stromal tumor using prone positioning in a patient with severe chronic obstructive lung disease. *Journal of Laparoendoscopic & Advanced Surgical Techniques, 21*(7), 635–639.

Yashima, Y., Isayama, H., Tsujino, T., Nagano, R., Yamamoto, K., Mizuno, S., . . . Omata, M. (2011). A large volume of visceral adipose tissue leads to severe acute pancreatitis. *Journal of Gastroenterology, 46*(10), 1213–1218.

Yatsuji, S., Hashimoto, E., Tobari, M., Taniai, M., Tokushige, K., & Shiratori, K. (2009). Clinical features and outcomes of cirrhosis due to non-alcoholic steatohepatitis compared with cirrhosis caused by chronic hepatitis C. *Journal of Gastroenterology and Hepatology, 24*(2), 248–254.

Yeh, C. C., Wu, S. C., Liao, C. C., Su, L. T., Hsieh, C. H., & Li, T. C. (2011). Laparoscopic appendectomy for acute appendicitis is more favorable for patients with comorbidities, the elderly, and those with complicated appendicitis: A nationwide population-based study. *Surgical Endoscopy, 25*(9), 2932–2942.

Zelickson, M. S., Bronder, C. M., Johnson, B. L., Camunas, J. A., Smith, D. E., Rawlinson, D., . . . Taylor, S. M. (2011). *Helicobacter pylori* is not the predominant etiology for peptic ulcers requiring operation. *The American Surgeon, 77*(8), 1054–1060.

Zmora, O., Kori, Y., Samuels, D., Kessler, A., Schulman, C. I., Klausner, J. M., & Soffer, D. (2009). Proximal splenic artery embolization in blunt splenic trauma. *European Journal of Trauma & Emergency Surgery, 35*(2), 108–114.

Section 10

Renal

SECTION 10: RENAL QUESTIONS

1. **Use of the colloid Hetastarch may affect your patient in which of the following ways?**
   A. Hetastarch may elevate serum amylase levels
   B. Hetastarch may decrease serum potassium levels
   C. Hetastarch will increase capillary permeability
   D. Hetastarch will cause acute tubular necrosis
2. **The normal adult glomerular filtration rate (GFR) is**
   A. 180 L/day
   B. 600 ml/min
   C. 250 ml/hr
   D. 75 L/day
3. **Which of the following fluids can accelerate systemic inflammation in trauma patients by activating neutrophils?**
   A. Colloids
   B. Crystalloids
   C. Osmotic diuretics
   D. Hypertonic saline
4. **Which of the following IV fluids actually suppresses inflammation?**
   A. Hypertonic saline
   B. Normal saline
   C. Hetastarch
   D. D_5W
5. **A type of IV fluid used to create volume expansion would be**
   A. Hypotonic
   B. A crystalloid
   C. A colloid
   D. 0.45% normal saline
6. **An IV fluid not considered to be a colloid would be**
   A. 0.2% normal saline
   B. Mannitol
   C. Dextran
   D. Hetastarch

7. **Which IV fluid listed below is least likely to be used for resuscitation?**
   A. 5% albumin
   B. 25% albumin
   C. Dextrose 5% in water (D_5W)
   D. Lactated Ringer's

8. **If water shifts out of the vascular bed and into the cells by osmosis, an IV fluid causing that effect would be**
   A. 25% albumin
   B. Mannitol
   C. 0.9% normal saline
   D. 0.45% NS

9. **Which of the following statements is true regarding the administration of colloids?**
   A. As hydrostatic pressure decreases, pores increase in size to let particles through
   B. You can give smaller amounts of fluid (about 250 ml) and achieve the same effect you would with 4 liters of crystalloids
   C. Edema takes a much shorter time to resolve
   D. Colloids are neuroprotective

10. **The two most commonly used isotonic fluids are**
    A. 0.45% NS and 0.2% NS
    B. Normal saline (0.9%) and lactated Ringer's
    C. 0.45% NS and 0.9% NS
    D. 5% albumin and 0.2% NS

11. **Which drug is known to cause nephrogenic diabetes insipidus?**
    A. Demeclocycline
    B. Morphine
    C. Lactulose
    D. Vasopressin

12. **One of the most common causes for the symptoms of hyponatremia is**
    A. Adrenal gland tumors
    B. An impaired thirst impulse
    C. Lung muscle paralysis
    D. Brain swelling

13. **The definition of euvolemic hyponatremia is**
    A. Water intake is sufficient to meet the body's needs
    B. Sodium and water are lost from the body to neutralize sodium content
    C. As total body water increases, the body's sodium content stays the same
    D. Sodium and water are both lost from the body, but the sodium loss is greater

14. **When sodium and water are both lost from the body and the sodium loss is greater, this condition is known as**
    A. Hypovolemic hyponatremia
    B. Hyponatremia valgus

C. Water intoxication
D. Hyponatremic gravidarum

15. Your patient is suffering from a condition where both sodium and water content in the body increase. However, the water gain is greater and the patient is developing pulmonary edema. This patient's condition is called
A. Hypervolemic hyponatremia
B. Hyperphosphatemia
C. Manheim syndrome
D. Hyponatremia valgus

16. Causes of hyponatremia include
A. Confusion
B. Muscle spasms
C. Burns
D. Convulsions

17. The normal range for serum osmolality in a healthy adult is
A. 163 to 240 mOsm/kg
B. 275 to 295 mOsm/kg
C. 55 to 110 mOsm/kg
D. 120 to 195 mOsm/kg

18. Causes of SIADH may include
A. Stupor
B. Guillain–Barré syndrome
C. Seizures
D. Hallucinations

19. Urinary calculi most often form in the
A. Ureters
B. Glomerulus
C. Bladder
D. Renal pelvis

20. Hypertonic hyponatremia may occur as a result of
A. Mannitol administration
B. Hypoglycemia
C. Myocardial infarction
D. Hormonal medication from the pituitary gland

21. Which of the following statements is false regarding water and sodium regulation in the elderly?
A. The sensation of thirst, renal function, concentration, and hormonal modulators of salt and water balance are often impaired in the elderly patient
B. Elderly patients have fewer problems with sodium and water balance secondary to nutritional deficits
C. Elderly patients are highly susceptible to iatrogenic events involving salt and water
D. Age-related changes, chronic diseases, and lapses in care are often associated with impairment of sodium and water metabolism in elderly patients

22. **Which of the following statements about creatinine is true?**
    A. A normal range is 0.8 to 1.4 mg/dl
    B. Creatinine levels are higher in females
    C. Lower than normal levels may indicate pyelonephritis
    D. Low levels are a precursor to eclampsia

23. **Sudden anuria may be due to**
    A. An embolic event
    B. Congestive heart failure
    C. Prostate enlargement
    D. Azotemia

24. **BUN may be elevated in patients**
    A. Undergoing steroid treatments
    B. Taking streptomycin
    C. Taking chloramphenicol
    D. With a low protein intake

25. **The current definition of acute renal failure is**
    A. Trauma to one or both kidneys
    B. Decrease in renal perfusion from shock or anaphylaxis
    C. A sudden or rapid decline in renal filtration function
    D. An obstruction to passage of urine

26. **Postrenal AKI may be caused by**
    A. Malignant hypertension
    B. Transplant rejection
    C. Neurogenic bladder
    D. Preeclampsia

27. **Anuria is defined as a urine output of**
    A. Less than 30 ml/h
    B. 200 ml/d
    C. 300 ml/d
    D. Less than 100 ml/d

28. **Nephrotoxicity may be caused by**
    A. Furosemide
    B. Aspirin
    C. Thioguanine
    D. Acyclovir

29. **Allergic nephritis may be caused by**
    A. Inadequate protein consumption
    B. Weight loss
    C. Cimetidine
    D. Water intoxication

30. **The primary site for urea synthesis is in the**
    A. Kidneys
    B. Liver

C. Lungs
D. Pancreas

31. Increased production of urea may be due to
A. GI bleeding
B. Low protein diet
C. Congenital kidney disease
D. Hypothermia

32. You notice your patient's hand spasming when the automatic blood pressure cuff inflates. When you attempt a manual blood pressure measurement, the same thing happens when you inflate just past the systolic pressure and keep the pressure in place. This carpopedal spasm is indicative of
A. Hypokalemia
B. Hyperphosphatemia
C. Hypocalcemia
D. Hypernatremia

33. While assessing your patient, you notice significant pretibial and pedal edema. When the patient is weighed, you note he stated he has gained 1.2 kilograms of weight in 24 hours. This is equal to at least __________ml of excess fluid.
A. 2,000
B. 1,200
C. 3,000
D. 500

34. One way to check for low calcium levels is to tap over a branch of the facial nerve. If the patient is hypocalcemic, the upper lip on the same side (ipsilateral) will twitch. This is known as
A. Trousseau's sign
B. Chvostek's sign
C. Grey–Turner's sign
D. Homan's sign

35. Your patient is a 66 year old diabetic with congestive heart failure. After 4 days of no contact, her daughter found her in bed, unresponsive. She has a red, dry, swollen tongue, temperature of 102° F, and flushed dry skin. She is tachycardic, hypotensive, and has decreased reflexes. Her urine specific gravity is 1.050. You suspect this patient is suffering from
A. Hypernatremia
B. Hypocalcemia
C. Hypermagnesemia
D. Hypokalemia

36. What percentage of the body's potassium may be found in the extracellular fluid?
A. 2%
B. 5%
C. 10%
D. 98%

37. Potassium is reabsorbed in the

A. Proximal tubules
B. Distal tubules
C. Ascending colon
D. Descending colon

38. Hypokalemia may cause

A. Respiratory alkalosis only
B. Metabolic alkalosis only
C. Both respiratory and metabolic alkalosis
D. Metabolic acidosis only

39. Hypokalemia due to excessive urinary excretion would not be caused by

A. Oliguria
B. Renal disease
C. Lasix
D. Increased adrenal cortical hormones

40. It is recommended that adults consume approximately ______ mg of potassium daily.

A. 500
B. 1,000
C. 2,000
D. 3,500

41. Normal magnesium levels for an adult are in the range of

A. 0.5–1.5 mg/dl
B. 1.5–2 mg/dl
C. 2–3 mg/dl
D. 4–5 mg/dl

42. Magnesium is most prevalent in which of the following areas of the body?

A. Extracellular fluid
B. In the liver
C. In the bone
D. In the spleen

43. As part of his discharge teaching, you are helping your patient determine what foods are rich in magnesium. He asks you what the recommended daily intake of magnesium is for an adult. Your answer is

A. 50–100 mg per day
B. 100–200 mg per day
C. 200–350 mg per day
D. 350–420 mg per day

44. Your patient had gastric bypass surgery 2 weeks ago. Which of the following electrolytes is she at most risk for an imbalance?

A. Potassium
B. Magnesium

C. Calcium
D. Sodium

45. Your patient eats a diet high in calcium because her family has a history of osteoporosis. She was admitted to the PCU for a fractured pelvis and pulmonary embolism suffered when she fell down her stairs. She has been experiencing increasing weakness and muscle tremors. She has noted an increase of "skipping" beats. She stated she was very dizzy and disoriented just before she fell. Based on the symptoms, which of the following labs should you assess immediately?
A. Calcium level
B. Sodium level
C. Hemoglobin and hematocrit
D. Magnesium level

46. Your new patient was diagnosed with breast cancer 8 years ago. The cancer has now metastasized to the bone. She came to the ED because her current pain medication is ineffective and her physician could not be reached by phone. She was transferred to the PCU about an hour ago. You would expect to see which changes in her electrolyte levels?
A. Decrease in magnesium and increase in calcium levels
B. Decrease in both magnesium and calcium levels
C. Increase in both magnesium and calcium levels
D. Increase in magnesium and a decrease in calcium levels

47. Your patient is in cardiac arrest. Magnesium replacement is ordered. What is the usual dose of magnesium for a patient in cardiac arrest?
A. 0.5 grams
B. 1–2 grams
C. 3–4 grams
D. 4–5 grams

48. Magnesium is ordered for your patient. During the infusion, you note flaccidity, absent patellar reflexes, shallow respirations, and a flushed face. Your first nursing action should be
A. Give the magnesium—the patient is just sleeping
B. Hold the dose for 1 hour
C. Give the dose over 3 hours
D. Hold the dose, contact the physician, and obtain a magnesium level

49. The family of your patient with hypermagnesemia asks why his face is flushed. You answer,
A. "He has a temperature."
B. "His magnesium level is a little high and causes his face to look flushed."
C. "He is embarrassed because the hospital gown does not provide enough coverage."
D. "He just completed his physical therapy."

50. Which of the following statements about calcium is true?
A. Approximately 40% of calcium is ionized in the serum
B. Calcium levels cannot be correlated with albumin levels

C. Calcium bonded to protein cannot pass the capillary wall
D. Calcium is not necessary for coagulation

51. **You are testing for hypocalcemia by trying to elicit Trousseau's sign. You elicit this response by**
A. Tapping the cheek
B. Lifting the left leg up and looking for head movement toward the chest
C. Inflating a BP cuff to greater than the systolic pressure for 3 minutes and waiting for a carpal spasm
D. Taking a sharp object up from the heel to the toes and watching for the toes to spread

52. **Your patient is scheduled to undergo continuous renal replacement therapy (CRRT) this week. Your patient teaching should include which of the following drugs that need to be stopped 2–3 days prior to therapy?**
A. Beta-blockers
B. ACE inhibitors
C. Heparin
D. Calcium channel blockers

53. **Your patient has renal failure and will be undergoing continuous renal replacement therapy (CRRT). She asks if she can have visitors during the procedure. You tell her**
A. "Of course. There are no restrictions."
B. "No. They would be in the way of the equipment."
C. "No. They will increase your risk of infection."
D. "Probably, but if they are sensitive to the sight of blood, they may want to wait until after the procedure."

54. **Your patient is in renal failure after cardiac arrest. He has continued cardiovascular instability. The best method for removal of his extra fluid is by using**
A. Hemodialysis
B. Peritoneal dialysis
C. Continuous renal replacement therapy
D. Plasmapheresis

55. **Hemodialysis is used to treat many metabolic abnormalities as well as renal failure. One possible use for hemodialysis is to administer**
A. Vitamin C and calcium carbonate for patients with osteoporosis
B. Erythropoietin for excessive iron
C. Phosphate binders for hyperphosphatemia
D. Glucose for hyperglycemia

56. **Communication among all staff is vital. When transferring your patient with a graft, which of the following information is a priority to communicate to all staff that may come in contact with this patient?**
A. Last dialysis date
B. Location of the graft
C. Type of dialysis machine used
D. Total fluid removed with last dialysis

57. **Which of the following is the correct fluid exchange sequence in peritoneal dialysis?**
    A. Dump, dwell, and drain
    B. Instillation, dwell, and drain
    C. Drain, instillation, and dwell
    D. Instillation, drain, and dwell

58. **Peritoneal dialysis functions by using which two principles?**
    A. Diffusion and ultrafiltration
    B. Osmotic pressure and osmosis
    C. Ultrafiltration and oncotic pressure
    D. Diffusion and osmosis

59. **During the drain phase you note only 50% return in the collection bag. Your next action should be to**
    A. Position the patient prone
    B. Check for kinks, bends, or cracks in the tubing
    C. Double check the amount installed
    D. Assess for subcutaneous fluid

60. **Apheresis is best defined as**
    A. The removal of plasma and/or proteins from the blood
    B. The selective removal of cells, plasma, and substances from the blood
    C. The selective removal of cellular components from the blood
    D. The removal of an antigen in the blood

61. **A male patient has been diagnosed with hypertension. He states that to control his blood pressure, he "will never eat another thing with salt." You should tell him**
    A. "That is not easy. Most fresh vegetables and fruit have tons of sodium."
    B. "Great. Sodium only plays a minor part in water balance and cellular activity, so your body won't know the difference."
    C. "You cannot completely eliminate sodium from your diet. Your body has an intricate system of safety measures to protect the level of sodium in your body."
    D. "Good idea. That should work fine."

62. **The recommended sodium daily intake for someone limiting sodium in their diet ranges between**
    A. 100 and 900 mg
    B. 1,000 and 2,000 mg
    C. 3,000 and 5,000 mg
    D. 4,000 and 6,000 mg

63. **Your patient was put on a limited sodium diet and has been working with a nutritionist. He was admitted to your PCU for chest pain and pulmonary edema. He reports that he had stopped all additional sodium intake, has been following his diet regimen closely, stopped eating out, and is drinking 8–10 8-ounce glasses of tap water every day. He also states he is voiding sufficient amounts. His sodium level is 155 mEq/L. What is the likely cause of this patient's hypernatremia?**
    A. Renal failure
    B. Hypotonic fluids

C. Diabetes mellitus
D. His water softener system

64. **Your patient was having chest pain while lifting boxes into his attic. The symptoms abated immediately when he stopped lifting the weight. His wife brought him to the ED anyway. The EKG and tests were normal, so he was transferred to the PCU. The patient's wife says he does not eat a good diet and that it may cause a heart attack. The patient loves cheese, but wants to limit his sodium intake. Which of the following cheeses has the highest sodium per 3.5 ounces?**
   A. Swiss cheese
   B. Mozzarella cheese
   C. Cheddar cheese
   D. Parmesan cheese

65. **A common cause of hyponatremia is**
   A. Salt water drowning
   B. Over-hydration
   C. Administration of hypertonic solutions
   D. Hyperoxia

66. **An elderly patient has a fever, chills, dysuria, frequency, and pain at the costovertebral angle. It is likely this patient is suffering from**
   A. Pyelonephritis
   B. Urinary calculi
   C. A lower urinary tract infection
   D. Prerenal AKI

67. **The primary causative organism for urinary tract infections is**
   A. *Escherichia coli*
   B. *Staphylococcus aureus*
   C. *Proteus* species
   D. *Klebsiella*

68. **An elderly male patient requires urinary catheterization. As you attempt to advance the catheter, you meet resistance and cannot advance the catheter more than about 3 inches into the urethra. The probable cause of this blockage is**
   A. A urinary calculus
   B. Benign prostatic hyperplasia
   C. A large catheter
   D. A small catheter that has curled on itself

69. **What symptoms would you expect in a patient with genital herpes?**
   A. Dysuria, myalgia, and burning pain
   B. Dyspareunia, pustules, and itching
   C. Single, crusted lesion that is painful
   D. Fever, groin pain, and lymphadenopathy

70. **Which of the following drugs would be used for an initial outbreak of genital herpes?**
   A. Penicillin VK 500 mg every 8 hours for 10 days
   B. Acyclovir 400 mg every 8 hours for 10 days

C. Septra DS 160/800 mg every 12 hours for 10 days
D. Doxycycline 100 mg every 12 hours for 10 days

71. Intrinsic AKI is most commonly caused by
A. Arteriolar vasoconstriction
B. Acute ischemic or cytotoxic injury
C. Amphotericin
D. Hypercalcemia

72. You are receiving report on a patient who was injured when he suffered a seizure while working on his roof. His sodium level on admission was 130 mEq/L. What symptoms of hyponatremia would you expect this patient to exhibit?
A. Twitching
B. Tachypnea
C. Lethargy
D. Flattened T waves

73. Your female patient has a fever, chills, pain on urination, moderate burning at the supra pubic area, and diarrhea. This patient is most likely suffering from
A. Acute renal failure
B. A kidney infection
C. A lower urinary tract infection
D. An upper urinary tract infection

74. A renal transplant that results from humoral rejection or acute cellular rejection may be definitively diagnosed only via
A. Ultrasound
B. Nuclear scan
C. Doppler scan
D. Renal biopsy

75. In the polyuric phase of AKI, it is important for the nurse to carefully monitor
A. Nitrogen balance
B. Potassium and phosphorus
C. Dopamine and mannitol levels
D. Desmopressin levels

76. Oliguria is a urine output of 100–400 ml/d and is usually the result of
A. Pyelonephritis
B. Rhabdomyolysis
C. Pre-renal syndrome
D. Potassium levels

77. Mrs. G. was sent to the PCU directly from her physician's office. She had been complaining of fatigue and generalized pain. Her lab work indicated a rapidly rising BUN, and she is now undergoing further tests. While assessing Mrs. G., you note she has severe acne around the face and neck. You suspect that the rise in BUN may be due to
A. Tetracycline
B. HCTZ

C. Bumetanide
D. Mannitol

78. **Mannitol and loop diuretics may be used in the treatment of AKI. Mannitol is nontoxic but must be used with caution because**
A. Mannitol may damage the eighth cranial nerve
B. Mannitol may cause vestibular impairment
C. Mannitol may produce a hyperosmolar state
D. Mannitol may bind with proteins in the renal tubule

79. **NSAIDs may cause**
A. Prerenal AKI
B. Intrinsic AKI
C. Postrenal AKI
D. Increased urine osmolality

80. **Medications that can decrease BUN levels include**
A. Neomycin and rifampin
B. Chloral hydrate and furosemide
C. Bacitracin and gentamicin
D. Chloramphenicol and streptomycin

81. **Your patient is becoming confused, is lethargic, and has muscle weakness. A review of her lab reports shows a calcium level of 11.7. A common way to treat this condition is to use**
A. D_5W and a Kayexalate enema
B. Normal saline and a loop diuretic
C. Glucose followed by insulin
D. Nothing. This is a normal value.

82. **Your patient has a calcium level of 7.8. You would expect which of the following changes to be observed on the EKG tracing?**
A. Tall, peaked T waves
B. A prominent U wave
C. A first-degree AV block
D. A prolonged QT interval

83. **What is the primary acid–base disturbance exhibited by patients with AKI?**
A. Metabolic acidosis
B. Respiratory acidosis
C. Metabolic alkalosis
D. Respiratory alkalosis

84. **Your patient came to the PCU with severe abdominal pain. It was determined that she has peritonitis and had a J-tube placed while waiting for an ICU bed. This patient is at risk for which of the following electrolyte deficits?**
A. Sodium
B. Magnesium

C. Manganese
D. Phosphorus

85. __________ is the major extracellular cation, and ________ is the major intracellular cation.
A. Calcium, magnesium
B. Sodium, calcium
C. Potassium, sodium
D. Sodium, potassium

86. If your patient is hypokalemic, what changes would you expect to see on an EKG tracing?
A. Peaked T waves
B. U waves
C. Shortened QT intervals
D. Absent P waves

87. The food listed below that has the lowest amount of potassium is
A. Avocados
B. Raisins
C. Potatoes
D. Carrots

88. Mr. H. originally came to the ED for exercise intolerance and shortness of breath. It was determined he had excess fluid retention secondary to mild CHF. Mr. H. was placed on diuretics, then transferred to the PCU, where you have been educating him about dietary issues. You discussed cooking methods for vegetables with your patient and his wife. Which of the following cooking techniques leaches out the greatest amount of potassium from vegetables?
A. Boiling
B. Baking
C. Steaming
D. Microwaving

89. Your patient is receiving potassium in his IV fluid, and the physician has ordered a potassium rider. What is the maximum rate of infusion for potassium solutions in a peripheral IV line?
A. 2 mEq/hour
B. 4 mEq/hour
C. 10 mEq/hour
D. 15 mEq/hour

90. All of the following are treatments for hyperkalemia except
A. Glucose and insulin
B. Kaon
C. Calcium gluconate
D. Bicarbonate administration

91. Your patient has congestive heart failure and was prescribed Lasix for water retention by her nurse practitioner. The patient's feet and legs continued to swell, so she took an extra Lasix this morning. She became dizzy and nauseous and then was admitted to the PCU. Now she has profound muscle weakness and flat T waves. You would expect this patient's potassium level this morning to be approximately

A. 1.8 mEq/L
B. 3.8 mEq/L
C. 4.2 mEq/L
D. 6.1 mEq/L

92. Magnesium is required for all of the following physiologic functions except

A. To act as an antagonist to calcium
B. Enzyme activation
C. Synthesis of nucleic acid and proteins
D. Sodium–potassium pump operation

93. Your patient was admitted and treated for Torsades de pointes. You are teaching about adding foods to his diet that are rich in magnesium. Your patient asks which of the following foods on his favorite food list is a poor source of magnesium.

A. Honey
B. Broccoli
C. Almonds
D. Chocolate

94. The most common cause of hypermagnesemia is

A. Gastrointestinal bypass
B. Gastrointestinal fistulas
C. Renal failure
D. Overdose

95. What percentage of calcium is stored in the bone?

A. 99%
B. 85%
C. 80%
D. 75%

96. Serum calcium is increased by

A. Increases in vitamin D
B. Renal tubular excretion
C. Gastrointestinal excretion
D. Bone demineralization

97. Your patient is undergoing hemodialysis in your PCU for acute renal failure as a result of uncontrolled type 2 diabetes. His wife asks how you know the hemodialysis is effective. Adequacy of dialysis is measured by

A. Urine creatinine clearance
B. Sodium, chloride, and potassium levels

C. Blood pressure
D. Urea clearance

98. You are assessing your patient's existing shunt prior to emergency hemodialysis. You note there is no thrill or bruit at the shunt site. Your next nursing action is to
A. Call the surgeon to do a new graft
B. Use a Doppler to determine graft patency
C. Administer a bolus of heparin
D. Continue with the hemodialysis, as there is nothing wrong

99. The usual amount of dialysate used in peritoneal dialysis is
A. 0.5–1 L
B. 1–2 L
C. 2–3 L
D. 3–4 L

100. You are preparing to teach your patient about peritoneal dialysis. It is important to tell the patient that which one of the following findings is normal?
A. During the instillation phase the insertion site may leak
B. During the dwell phase you may feel abdominal fullness and shortness of breath
C. During the dwell phase subcutaneous fluid may be seen in the groin
D. During the drain phase you will feel dizzy and have palpitations

101. You are providing discharge teaching to the family of a patient who received peritoneal dialysis. The patient will undergo at least three more treatments at a rural outpatient clinic. As part of the discharge teaching, you give the patient a home glucometer. The daughter questions this action because her mother is not a diabetic. You should tell the daughter
A. Peritoneal dialysis can cause diabetes
B. Her mother was just diagnosed with diabetes
C. The dialysate contains glucose and can lead to hyperglycemia
D. Peritoneal dialysis may lead to pancreatitis

102. Which of the following fruits has the lowest sodium content per 3.5-ounce serving?
A. Cantaloupe
B. Grapes
C. Peaches
D. Blackberries

103. Your patient is trying to limit his salt intake. Which of the following meat products would you recommend for him to eat?
A. Chicken without the skin
B. Canned beef hash
C. Fresh pike
D. Canned crab

SECTION 10: RENAL ANSWERS

1. **Correct answer: A**
Hetastarch may elevate serum amylase levels, but the levels will return to normal within a week after administration. Hetastarch will not increase serum potassium levels or increase capillary permeability. Hetastarch must be used with caution in patients in anaphylactic or septic shock because capillary permeability is already increased. Dextran may cause acute tubular necrosis.

2. **Correct answer: A**
The normal adult glomerular filtration rate (GFR) is 180 L/day or 125 ml/min. Normal adult urine volume is about 1–2 L/day.

3. **Correct answer: B**
Crystalloids, particularly lactated Ringer's solution, can accelerate systemic inflammation in trauma patients by activating neutrophils. These neutrophils destroy surrounding tissue by way of oxidative burst, then release hydrogen peroxide into the tissue, leading to acute respiratory distress syndrome (ARDS) and multiple organ failure (MOF/MODS).

4. **Correct answer: A**
Hypertonic saline suppresses inflammation, helps correct electrolyte imbalances, and pulls water back to the intravascular space from the cells and interstitial spaces.

5. **Correct answer: C**
Colloids are used for volume expansion. Particles suspended in colloids don't break down into smaller pieces in water and most won't fit through most capillary pores, so therefore they stay in the vascular bed.

6. **Correct answer: A**
An IV fluid not considered to be a colloid would be 0.2% normal saline. Colloids include human albumin (a natural protein that's separated from plasma) and hetastarch (HES), a synthetic starch derived from hydroxyethyl glucose. Additional colloids include mannitol (an alcohol sugar) and dextran (a polysaccharide).

7. **Correct answer: C**
Dextrose 5% in water (D_5W) is not used for resuscitation because its glucose is metabolized and quickly becomes hypotonic. In fact, D_5W is a good source of free water.

8. **Correct answer: D**
If water shifts out of the vascular bed and into the cells by osmosis, an IV fluid causing that effect would be 0.45% NS.

9. **Correct answer: B**
You can give smaller amounts of fluid (about 250 ml) and achieve the same effect you would with four liters of crystalloids. As hydrostatic pressure rises in the capillaries, the pores stretch. This phenomenon causes edema that takes longer to resolve.

10. **Correct answer: B**
The two most commonly used isotonic fluids are normal saline (0.9%) and lactated Ringer's. All the other solutions listed are hypotonic or hypertonic.

11. **Correct answer: A**
    Demeclocycline is known to cause nephrogenic diabetes insipidus.

12. **Correct answer: D**
    Brain swelling causes most of the symptoms of hyponatremia. Sodium is found mostly in the body fluids outside the cells. When the amount of sodium in fluids outside cells drops, water moves into the cells to balance the levels. This causes the cells to swell with too much water. Although most cells can handle this swelling, brain cells cannot because the skull is essentially a closed space. An impaired thirst impulse and lung muscle paralysis are symptoms of hypernatremia.

13. **Correct answer: C**
    The definition of euvolemia is the state that exists when as total body water increases, the body's sodium content stays the same.

14. **Correct answer: A**
    When sodium and water are both lost from the body and the sodium loss is greater, this condition is known as hypovolemic hyponatremia.

15. **Correct answer: A**
    If your patient is suffering from a condition where both sodium and water content in the body increase and the water gain is greater, this condition is called hypervolemic hyponatremia.

16. **Correct answer: C**
    Causes of hyponatremia may include burns, CHF, diuretics, SIADH, cirrhosis, kidney disease, vomiting, diarrhea, and sweating. The other answers presented (confusion, muscle spasms, and convulsions) are symptoms of hyponatremia, not causes.

17. **Correct answer: B**
    The normal range for serum osmolality in a healthy adult is from 275 to 295 mOsm/kg.

18. **Correct answer: B**
    Causes of SIADH may include Guillain-Barré syndrome, meningitis, encephalitis, brain tumors, head trauma, medications, psychoses and damage to the hypothalamus or pituitary gland during surgery. Stupor, hallucinations, and seizures are symptoms of SIADH, not causes.

19. **Correct answer: D**
    Urinary calculi most often form in the renal pelvis. Patients who consume a diet high in proteins, calcium, or fruit juices are at risk, as are patients with a sedentary lifestyle and a history of gout or previous calculi.

20. **Correct answer: A**
    Hypertonic hyponatremia can occur after the administration of mannitol or glycerol. The osmotically active non-electrolytes in the extracellular fluid create an osmotic gradient that draws water out of the cells and into the extracellular space. This results in a dilutional hyponatremia. Hyperglycemia is an additional cause of hypertonic hyponatremia. The large sugar molecules draw water from the cells.

21. **Correct answer: B**
"Elderly patients have fewer problems with sodium and water balance secondary to nutritional deficits" is a false statement.

True statements include:

"The sensation of thirst, renal function, concentration, and hormonal modulators of salt and water balance are often impaired in the elderly patient."
"Elderly patients are highly susceptible to iatrogenic events involving salt and water."
"Age-related changes, chronic diseases, and lapses in care are often associated with impairment of sodium and water metabolism in elderly patients."

22. **Correct answer: A**
A normal range for creatinine is 0.8 to 1.4 mg/dl. Females have less muscle mass than males, so they have lower levels of creatinine. Higher levels than normal may indicate pyelonephritis or eclampsia.

23. **Correct answer: A**
Sudden anuria is usually due to postrenal AKI, such as from an embolic event. Mechanical obstruction of the urinary collection system is involved. The collection system is comprised of the renal pelvis, the ureters, the bladder, and the urethra.

24. **Correct answer: A**
The BUN may be elevated in patients undergoing steroid treatments. The BUN may also be elevated in cases of GI or mucosal bleeding or excessive protein intake.

25. **Correct answer: C**
The current definition of acute renal failure is a sudden or rapid decline in renal filtration function. Acute renal failure is now known as acute renal injury (AKI) and can be classified as prerenal, intrinsic, or postrenal. Because material covered on the PCCN exam reflects practice up to about 6 months ago, the new terminology should be added. Some item writers may use this new terminology on the exam.

26. **Correct answer: C**
Postrenal AKI may be caused by a neurogenic bladder. Other causes include tumor, tricyclic antidepressants, fibrosis, BPH, prostate CA, urethral obstruction, stone disease, and ligation during surgery. Malignant hypertension, transplant rejection, DIC, and preeclampsia are causes of intrinsic failure/injury.

27. **Correct answer: D**
Anuria is defined as a urine output less than 100 ml/d.

28. **Correct answer: D**
Acyclovir is nephrotoxic and can crystallize in the kidney and cause AKI. It is important for the nurse to carefully monitor the infusion time and the amount of fluid used to dilute intravenous drugs. Additional drugs that can crystallize in the kidney are sulfonamides, idinivir, and triamterine.

29. **Correct answer: C**
Allergic nephritis may be caused by cimetidine. Cimetidine interferes with creatinine excretion in the renal tubule. Renal function does not decrease, but the creatinine does rise. If diminished renal function exists, an allergic nephritis may develop.

30. **Correct answer: B**
Over 99% of urea synthesis occurs in the liver. Dietary protein is converted into amino acids and peptides. About 90% of these molecules are absorbed and transferred to the liver. Any excess nitrogen is converted into urea.

31. **Correct answer: A**
Increased production of urea may be due to GI bleeding. Approximately 500 ml of whole blood equals 100 grams of protein. The extra protein must be converted to urea.

32. **Correct answer: C**
The carpopedal spasm is indicative of hypocalcemia and is known as Trousseau's sign. You can also elicit this response by having the patient hyperventilate. When the patient becomes alkalotic, the serum calcium level decreases and a carpopedal spasm occurs.

33. **Correct answer: B**
1 kilogram = 2.2 pounds = 1,000 ml. Thus, 1.2 kilograms equals 1,200 ml. Although you may believe this is too basic a piece of information for a PCCN exam, it is the little pieces of information like this that trip people up on the exam.

34. **Correct answer: B**
One way to check for low calcium is to tap over a branch of the facial nerve. If the patient is hypocalcemic, the upper lip on the same side (ipsilateral) will twitch. This is known as Chvostek's sign. Trousseau's sign utilizes a BP cuff to elicit a carpopedal spasm indicative of hypocalcemia. Grey–Turner's sign is ecchymosis around the umbilicus, indicating abdominal issues, and Homan's sign may indicate DVT.

35. **Correct answer: A**
Because of her diabetes, this patient was unable to drink sufficient fluids, leading to dehydration, hemoconcentration, and resultant hypernatremia. Due to her diabetes she may have additional renal injury. Because of the decreased blood flow through the kidneys from the CHF, the kidneys were unable to filter the excess sodium from her body.

36. **Correct answer: A**
Approximately 2% of potassium is extracellular, whereas the remaining 98% is intracellular. Intracellular electrolytes cannot be directly measured, but extracellular levels can be measured. Normal extracellular values range from 3.5 to 5.0 mEq/L.

37. **Correct answer: B**
Regulated excretion (absorption) of potassium is in the distal tubules.

38. **Correct answer: C**
Potassium and hydrogen move opposite of each other. When a patient is hypokalemic, hydrogen moves into the extracellular fluid, leading to both respiratory and metabolic alkalosis.

39. **Correct answer: A**
Hypokalemia due to excessive urinary excretion is not caused by oliguria. Oliguria is a result of hyperkalemia. Renal disease, Lasix, and increased adrenal cortical hormones lead to hypokalemia.

40. **Correct answer: C**
It is recommended that adults consume approximately 2,000 mg of potassium daily.

41. **Correct answer:** C
The current recommended serum magnesium level is 2–3 mg/dl. This level may be higher for patients with cardiac disease or in their third trimester of pregnancy to treat pregnancy-induced hypertension and to control premature contractions.

42. **Correct answer:** C
Approximately 50% of the body's magnesium is within the bone marrow. The measured serum magnesium only reflects approximately 1% of the body's magnesium and the remaining 49% is found in the intracellular space.

43. **Correct answer:** D
Currently, the recommended adult intake for magnesium is 350–420 mg per day. For pregnant women, the preferred intake is at the higher end of the range. Children's intake should be less, based on age.

44. **Correct answer:** B
Because magnesium is absorbed in the small intestines, surgeries, such as gastric bypass, that remove or alter the small intestines place the patient at risk for hypomagnesemia. Gastric surgeries also impact water reabsorption, time processing in the intestines, calcium level, and amount of lactose in the diet.

45. **Correct answer:** D
This patient is exhibiting signs and symptoms of hypomagnesemia. This is related to the high calcium intake. Calcium and magnesium are absorbed in the small intestines. Calcium consumed in extremely high doses competes with magnesium absorption. The patient needs nutritional teaching to balance her diet.

46. **Correct answer:** A
As cancer spreads through bone, calcium is released into the serum. In a hypercalcemic state, magnesium secretion decreases, thus leading to hypomagnesemia.

47. **Correct answer:** B
Only if a patient is in cardiopulmonary arrest would you infuse 1 to 2 grams of magnesium. IV infusions of magnesium should run no faster than 30 mg per minute. Careful monitoring should be done for further EKG changes.

48. **Correct answer:** D
The patient is exhibiting the signs and symptoms of hypermagnesemia. The dose should be held, the physician contacted, and the magnesium level evaluated.

49. **Correct answer:** B
The best answer from the choices listed is, "His magnesium level is a little high and causes his face to look flushed." Magnesium levels greater than 5 mEq/L lead to vasodilation of the facial vessels.

50. **Correct answer:** C
If calcium is bonded with protein, the molecule is too large to pass from the extracellular fluid into intracellular due to restrictive capillary permeability. Fifty to 70% of serum calcium is ionized in the serum. Because of the protein binding ability of calcium, albumin and calcium levels can be directly correlated. Calcium plays a major role in coagulation.

51. **Correct answer: C**
The technique for eliciting a Trousseau's sign is to inflate a blood pressure cuff greater than the systolic blood pressure for 3 minutes. A positive sign is if the carpal nerve spasms, causing the hand to curve inward with all fingers touching.

52. **Correct answer: A**
Beta-blockers may cause an anaphylactic reaction with the membranes or the filter in the CRRT. Bradykinins are released as a result, causing the systemic anaphylaxis.

53. **Correct answer: D**
Some individuals do not tolerate the sight of blood. Because CRRT occurs outside the body, blood is in full sight. To improve communication between both patient and visitors, it is best for the patient to let visitors know when procedures are occurring so they may visit at a time when a CRRT procedure is not occurring. There are some restrictions to how many people may fit in one room with the equipment. This will vary by facility. The more people in a room, the higher the risk that the equipment could be touched and/or disconnected.

54. **Correct answer: C**
The best method for removal of this patient's extra fluid is by using continuous renal replacement therapy. CRRT results in slower volume regulation to avoid rapid shifts in volume. This method results in continuous removal and/or regulation of solutes and volume.

55. **Correct answer: C**
Hemodialysis is used to administer phosphate binders for patients with hyperphosphatemia. In addition, it may be used to provide vitamin D and calcium carbonate for osteoporosis, erythropoietin for iron deficiencies (anemia), and glucose for hypoglycemia.

56. **Correct answer: B**
It is imperative that all staff members are made aware of graft site location. This includes lab techs, nursing assistants, student nurses, medical staff, physical therapy, and respiratory therapy. You want to avoid any lab or blood draws, blood pressures, or occlusions in the grafted limb.

57. **Correct answer: B**
The correct sequence for fluid exchange in peritoneal dialysis is to first instill the dialysate, allow the fluid to dwell within the abdomen for a predetermined time, and drain the fluid. The number of exchanges is determined by the physician and the desired outcomes.

58. **Correct answer: D**
Peritoneal dialysis functions by the principles of diffusion and osmosis. Diffusion is the passive movement of solutes across a membrane. The direction of diffusion is based on concentration (from higher to lower), heat, and pressure. The speed at which diffusion occurs is based on the grade or steepness of the differences in concentrations on each side of the membrane and the molecule moving across the membrane (size, polarity). Osmosis is the passive movement of solvents (i.e., water) over a permeable membrane. Movement of the solvent depends on the permeability of the membrane—the more permeable the membrane, the more passive the movement of solutes and solvents. Permeability may impact the type of solutes able to unintentionally cross the membrane.

59. Correct answer: B
Kinking, bends, and cracks in the tubing are the most likely causes of a decreased dialysate return. If that does not correct fluid flow, then reposition the patient, assess for any subcutaneous fluid or fluid within the groin, double check the amount of fluid installed, and complete an assessment before reporting the situation to the physician.

60. Correct answer: B
Apheresis is the general term used for all pheresis techniques and encompasses any selective removal of cells, plasma, and substances from blood with the return of remaining components and volume to the patient. Plasmapheresis is the removal of plasma and/or proteins from the blood or as a plasma exchange. Cytapheresis is the selective removal of cellular components from the blood (i.e., WBC). Leukocytopheresis is the specific removal of WBCs. Erythrocytopheresis is the removal of RBCs. Plateletpheresis is the removal of platelets. Plasma adsorption/perfusion is the filtering and treatment of plasma via adsorptive fiber filters. Immunoadsorption is the removal of an antigen via an antibody filter. Photopheresis is the removal and return of blood after exposure to ultraviolet light to destroy specific cells (in solid organ transplant rejection).

61. Correct answer: C
Sodium cannot be completely eliminated from the diet. Sodium is a major cation in the extracellular fluid within the body. Sodium plays a key part in the sodium–potassium pump, stabilizing polarization of cells, and water balance. The body protects sodium levels by titrating aldosterone and antidiuretic hormone (ADH), and changing filtration within the kidneys. Fresh fruits and vegetables contain minimal amounts of salt. Canned vegetables use sodium to preserve flavor and have the highest sodium levels.

62. Correct answer: B
The daily recommended sodium intake for someone limiting sodium from their diet should be between 1,000 and 2,000 mg per day. This challenges the body to use sodium efficiently without overstressing the body's systems. A low-sodium diet aims for daily sodium intake less than 1,000 mg.

63. Correct answer: D
Many water-softening systems filter out calcium and magnesium (these minerals make water hard) and replace them with sodium. The longer the filter has been in place, the greater the sodium content of the water. Not all water softeners use sodium, so recommend to patients to check their system type. Possibly, instead of drinking the tap water, Ben should drink and food should be prepared with distilled or bottled water. He may also consider replacing the water filter with a reverse osmosis system. The patient is following his diet as prescribed and does not exhibit any signs of renal failure. Hypertonic fluids would lead to higher sodium levels. Diabetes insipidus would lead to elevated sodium levels due to the lack of ADH.

64. Correct answer: D
Parmesan cheese has a sodium level of 1,862 mg, whereas Swiss has 260 mg, cheddar has 620 mg, and mozzarella has 373 mg.

65. Correct answer: B
Overhydration is a common cause of hyponatremia. The level is below normal due to dilution and not a disease process or injury. Intake of fluids orally or intravenously

has caused an artificial drop in sodium. Correction is done through fluid restriction or decreasing IV rates. Other causes of hyponatremia include loss of sodium through sweating or vomiting, shock, bleeding, SIADH, renal failure (inability to save sodium), hypoxia, freshwater drowning, or an over-administration of hypotonic fluids.

66. **Correct answer: A**
A patient presenting with fever, chills, dysuria, frequency, and pain at the costovertebral angle is likely suffering from pyelonephritis. The patient will also likely present with orthostatic vital signs and pain on palpation or urination that may radiate toward the umbilicus or lower abdomen.

67. **Correct answer: A**
The primary causative organism for urinary tract infections is *Escherichia coli*. Newer studies have shown that adenovirus-related hemorrhagic cystitis is becoming a more frequently diagnosed cause of UTIs.

68. **Correct answer: B**
Benign prostatic hyperplasia is common in elderly men. The prostate gland enlarges and impinges on the urethra.

69. **Correct answer: A**
Dysuria, myalgia, and burning pain are common symptoms of genital herpes. Genital herpes (herpes simplex II) may have no symptoms for years. The most common symptoms of an initial outbreak include fever, malaise, dysuria, dyspareunia, and vesicles anywhere boxer shorts fit. Most of the vesicles occur on the labia for a female and the penis, glans, or scrotum for the male.

70. **Correct answer: B**
Acyclovir (Zovirax), valacyclovir (Valtrex), or famciclovir (Famvir) are the three antiviral medications used for herpes outbreaks.

71. **Correct answer: B**
Intrinsic AKI is most commonly caused by acute ischemic or cytotoxic injury. Other causes include cell detachment, dilatation of the lumen, and injury to the distal nephron. Arteriolar vasoconstriction, amphotericin, and hypercalcemia are causes of prerenal AKI.

72. **Correct answer: A**
With hyponatremia, sodium levels drop below 135 mEq/L. Twitching and seizures are common, as well as apnea (not tachypnea), irritability (lethargy is seen with hypernatremia), and generalized muscle weakness (late sign). Flattened T waves are seen with hypokalemia.

73. **Correct answer: C**
This patient has fever, chills, pain on urination, moderate burning at the supra pubic area, and diarrhea. This patient is most likely suffering from a lower urinary tract infection. Females are more likely to have urinary tract infections than men because they have shorter urethras and bacteria can easily ascend the tract.

74. **Correct answer: A**
A renal transplant that results from humoral rejection or acute cellular rejection may be definitively diagnosed only via ultrasound. Ultrasound may be difficult to obtain or interpret due to ascites, obesity, or fluid in the retroperitoneal area. Doppler scans

measure blood flow, and the flow is diminished due to prerenal and intrinsic AKI. Nuclear scans are of limited value because the excretion rates may be slowed by disease. The renal biopsy is the gold standard for diagnosing rejection.

75. **Correct answer: B**
Potassium and phosphorus must be diligently monitored during the polyuric phase of AKI because of the potential for dysrhythmias.

76. **Correct answer: C**
Oliguria is a urine output of 100–400 ml/d and is usually the result of prerenal syndrome or hepatorenal syndrome. Pyelonephritis, rhabdomyolysis, and acute glomerular nephritis are causes of non-oliguria (>400 ml/d of urine output).

77. **Correct answer: A**
While assessing Mrs. G., you note she has severe acne around the face and neck. You suspect that the rise in BUN may be due to tetracycline. Tetracycline decreases anabolism and thereby increases the BUN.

78. **Correct answer: C**
Mannitol is nontoxic but must be used with caution because it may produce a hyperosmolar state. Damage to the eighth cranial nerve, vestibular impairment, and renal tubule binding of proteins are characteristics of loop diuretics. Loop diuretics include furosemide, bumetadine, and torsemide.

79. **Correct answer: A**
NSAIDs block prostaglandin production, which alters glomerular arteriolar perfusion and may cause prerenal AKI.

80. **Correct answer: D**
Medications that can decrease BUN levels include chloramphenicol and streptomycin. Chloral hydrate, furosemide neomycin, rifampin, bacitracin, and gentamicin are medications that increase BUN levels.

81. **Correct answer: B**
The patient has hypercalcemia, as evidenced by the calcium level of 11.7. A loop diuretic prevents reabsorption of calcium, and normal saline is used to increase the patient's glomerular filtration rate. If you were to administer a thiazide diuretic, it would actually decrease calcium excretion. Use of glucose, insulin, and Kayexalate are not indicated because they are treatments for hyperkalemia.

82. **Correct answer: D**
This patient is hypocalcemic. Lack of calcium slows cardiac contractility (the prolonged QT) and the patient might develop Torsades de pointes (polymorphic ventricular tachycardia). Torsades is also caused by hypomagnesmia.

83. **Correct answer: A**
The primary acid–base disturbance exhibited by patients with AKI is metabolic acidosis. The AKI patient cannot excrete ammonium or acid ions in quantities that are necessary to aid in the excretion of hydrogen. The buildup of the hydrogen causes the acidosis.

84. **Correct answer: A**
This patient is at risk for hyponatremia. Large amounts of extracellular fluids are in the peritoneal cavity. If sodium is lost in here, then the calcium is no longer available to be absorbed into the vasculature.

85. **Correct answer: D**
Sodium is the major extracellular cation, and potassium is the major intracellular cation.

86. **Correct answer: B**
A U wave is seen in patients who are hypokalemic. A peaked T wave, a shortened QT interval, and an absent P wave are seen with hyperkalemia.

87. **Correct answer: D**
Carrots have the lowest amount of potassium at 233 mg. Avocados have about 1,484 mg, raisins 751 mg, and potatoes 610 mg.

88. **Correct answer: A**
Boiling leaches out most of the nutrients into the water. Baking is the best method, allowing the vegetables to retain most of their potassium and other nutrients.

89. **Correct answer: C**
Potassium should not be infused at any rate greater than 10 mEq/hour to prevent extravasations, pain, or spasms related to rapid electrolyte changes.

90. **Correct answer: B**
Kaon is not a treatment for hyperkalemia. Kaon is another name for potassium gluconate, a common potassium replacement medication. Glucose and insulin, calcium gluconate, and bicarbonate all bind or push the potassium back into the cell from the intravascular space and reduce extracellular potassium levels.

91. **Correct answer: A**
This patient is exhibiting signs and symptoms of hypokalemia. Hypokalemia is defined as any potassium level under 3.5 mEq/L. It is important to reinforce teaching patients how diuretics impact electrolyte levels and the underlying condition.

92. **Correct answer: A**
Magnesium does not act as an antagonist to calcium. Magnesium is required for enzyme activation, synthesis of nucleic acid and proteins, and sodium–potassium pump operation. Magnesium is usually synergistic with calcium to control neuromuscular function within all muscle groups.

93. **Correct answer: A**
Honey has the lowest amount of magnesium. It is better to recommend foods such as leafy vegetables that have a deep, green color, whole grains, nuts, legumes, seafood, cocoa, and chocolate.

94. **Correct answer: C**
Renal failure is one of the most common causes of hypermagnesemia. The patient is unable to excrete excess magnesium via the urine. Gastrointestinal bypass and fistulas lead to hypomagnesemia.

95. **Correct answer: A**
99% of the body's calcium is stored in the bone.

96. **Correct answer: A**
Vitamin D increases serum calcium levels.

97. **Correct answer: D**
Urea clearance in the blood is the best indicator for monitoring dialysis effectiveness. Electrolytes may be altered due to fluid shifting and the distillate used. Blood pressure

may fluctuate with fluid removal and is not the best measurement method. Urine creatinine clearance indicates residual renal function.

98. **Correct answer: B**
Lack of thrill and/or bruit may indicate that the graft has occluded and dialysis is not possible. It is best to use a Doppler to determine graft patency prior to any calls or administration of any medication. Although you may not hear or feel the thrill and bruit, the graft may still be patent. The surgeon should be notified if the Doppler study is negative. Heparin will not lyse an existing clot.

99. **Correct answer: C**
Two to 3 L of dialysate are commonly used for peritoneal dialysis.

100. **Correct answer: B**
It is common for patients to have a feeling of abdominal fullness related to the 2–3 L of dialysate installed in the abdomen and allowed to dwell. Leaking at the insertion site must be reported to the physician, as the patient may develop peritonitis, and the patient should be monitored closely. Dialysis cannot continue until the insert site is repaired. If fluid is felt or seen in the groin, this indicates a hernia and may lead to strangulation of any bowel that enters the groin during the dwell phase and is trapped there when the dialysate is drained. If a patient feels dizzy or has palpitations during the drain phase, this indicates a too-rapid fluid shift or triggering of the vagal nerve. The drain time may need to be lengthened.

101. **Correct answer: C**
The daughter questions the use of a glucometer because her mother is not a diabetic. You should tell the daughter the dialysate contains glucose and can lead to hyperglycemia. During diffusion, glucose may cross the membranes and cause hyperglycemia. It is important for the patient to monitor this complication at home. Careful education will assist the family in managing any complications and when to notify the physician. Some smaller, rural settings are performing outpatient peritoneal dialysis or hiring dialysis nurses to perform this function.

102. **Correct answer: D**
Blackberries have 1 mg of sodium per 3.5 ounce serving. Peaches have 2 mg, grapes have 3 mg, and cantaloupe has 12 mg.

103. **Correct answer: C**
To reduce sodium intake, suggest that the patient eat fresh pike. Most fresh fish is low in sodium. Pike has only 51 mg sodium per 3.5 ounce serving, compared with chicken at 60–80 mg, canned beef hash at 540 mg, and canned crab at 1000 mg. Any canned or processed meat contains some preservative. For most people, eating fresh or fresh frozen meats, vegetables, and fruits will aid in limiting sodium, fat, and sugar intake.

RENAL REFERENCES

Ahrens, T., Prentice, D., & Kleinpell, R. M. (2011). *Progressive care nursing certification: Preparation, review and practice exams.* St. Louis, MO: McGraw-Hill.

Allison, S. O., & Lev-Toaff, A. S. (2010). Acute pelvic pain: What we have learned from the ER. *Ultrasound Quarterly, 26*(4), 211–218.

American Association of Critical-Care Nurses. (2006). *AACN core curriculum for critical care nursing.* St. Louis, MO: Saunders.

Anderson, B., & Khadra, A. (2006). Acute urinary retention: Developing an A&E management pathway. *British Journal of Nursing, 15*(8), 434–438.

Avihingsanon, Y., & Hirankarn, N. (2010). Major lupus organ involvement: Severe lupus nephritis. *Lupus, 19*(12), 1391–1398.

Babel, N., Sakpal, S. V., & Chamberlain, R. S. (2010). The Page kidney phenomenon secondary to a traumatic fall. *European Journal of Emergency Medicine, 17*(1), 24–26.

Betz, T. G., Lee, P., & Victor, J. C. (2008). Hepatitis A vaccine versus immune globulin for postexposure prophylaxis. *New England Journal of Medicine, 358*(5), 531–532.

Bhatnagar, R., & Alexiev, B. A. (2012). Renal-cell carcinomas in end-stage kidneys: A clinicopathological study with emphasis on clear-cell papillary renal-cell carcinoma and acquired cystic kidney disease-associated carcinoma. *International Journal of Surgical Pathology, 20*(1), 19–28.

Bielawska, H., & Epstein, N. L. (2010). A stone down below: A urethral stone causing acute urinary retention and renal failure. *Canadian Journal of Emergency Medical Care, 12*(4), 377–380.

Bisan, S. (2008). How to recognize the top three STDs in women: Elusive and often misleading, these infections can have serious consequences if not caught in time. Here's how to diagnose and treat them. *Clinician Reviews, 18*(8), 39.

Bolmers, M. D. M., Linthorst, G. E., Soeters, M. R., Nio, Y. C., & van Lieshout, J. J. (2009). Green urine, but no infection. *Lancet, 374*(9700), 1566.

Bradway, C., & Rodgers, J. (2009). Evaluation and management of genitourinary emergencies. *Nurse Practitioner, 34*(5), 36–43.

Brorsen, A. (2012). *CEN examination review.* Burlington, MA: Jones & Bartlett Learning.

Brorsen, A., & Rogelet, K. (2009). *PCCN certification review.* Sudbury, MA: Jones and Bartlett.

Brown, A. S. (2010). Renal tubular acidosis. *Dimensions of Critical Care Nursing, 29*(3), 112–119.

Burns, S. M. (Ed.). (2007). *American Association of Critical-Care Nurses (AACN): AACN protocols for practice: Healing environments* (2nd ed.). Sudbury, MA: Jones and Bartlett.

Chapagain, A., Dobbie, H., Sheaff, M., & Yaqoob, M. M. (2011). Presentation, diagnosis, and treatment outcome of tuberculous-mediated tubulointerstitial nephritis. *Kidney International, 79*(6), 671–677.

Chulay, M., & Burns, S. (2010). *Essentials of progressive care nursing* (2nd ed.). St. Louis, MO: McGraw-Hill.

Cohen, M. J., Serkova, N. J., Wiener-Kronish, J., Pittet, J. F., & Niemann, C. U. (2010). 1H-NMR-based metabolic signatures of clinical outcomes in trauma patients beyond lactate and base deficit. *Journal of Trauma-Injury Infection and Critical Care, 69*(1), 31–40.

Curley, M. A. Q. (2007). *Synergy: The unique relationship between nurses and patients.* St. Louis, MO: Saunders.

Davis, A. D., & Calvet, H. M. (2003). Sexually transmitted diseases in the emergency department. *Topics in Emergency Medicine, 25*(3), 247–255.

Decloedt, E., & Maartens, G. (2011). Rus-induced renal injury. *Continuing Medical Education Journal, 29*(6), 252–255.

Desilva, M. B., & Mueller, P. S. (2009). Renal consequences of long-term, low-dose intentional ingestion of ethylene glycol. *Renal Failure, 31*(7), 586–588.

Doi, K., Leelahavanichkul, A., Hu, X., Sidransky, K. L., Zhou, H., Qin, Y., . . . Star, R. A. (2008). Preexisting renal disease promotes sepsis-induced acute kidney injury and worsens outcome. *Kidney International, 74*(8), 1017–1025.

Donohoe-Dennison, R. (2007). *Pass CCRN* (3rd ed.). St. Louis, MO: Mosby.

Eisengart, L. J., MacVicar, G. R., & Yang, X. J. (2012). Predictors of response to targeted therapy in renal cell carcinoma. *Archives of Pathology & Laboratory Medicine, 136*(5), 490–495.

Emergency Nurses Association, Newberry, L., & Criddle, L. M. (2007). *Sheehy's manual of emergency care* (6th ed.). St. Louis, MO: Mosby.

Fisher, E. M., & Brown, D. K. (2010). Hepatorenal syndrome: Beyond liver failure. *AACN Advanced Critical Care, 21*(2), 165–184.

Gadler, T., Keedy, M., & Rivas, N. (2010). A case of hematuria. *Advanced Emergency Nursing Journal, 32*(1), 30–41.

Gupta, A., Rohrscheib, M., & Tzamaloukas, A. H. (2008). Extreme hyperglycemia with ketoacidosis and hyperkalemia in a patient on chronic hemodialysis. *Hemodialysis International, 12*(S2), S43–437.

Guthrie, P. S. (2010). Combining herbal remedies and prescription drugs. *American Journal of Nursing, 110*(7), 18–19.

Haase, M., Haase-Fielitz, A., Bellomo, R., & Mertens, P. R. (2011). Neutrophil gelatinase-associated lipocalin as a marker of acute renal disease. *Current Opinion in Hematology, 18*(1), 11–18.

Hardin, S. R., & Kaplow, R. (Eds.). (2008). *Synergy for clinical excellence: The AACN synergy model for patient care.* Sudbury, MA: Jones and Bartlett.

Hardin, S., & Kaplow, R. (2005). *Synergy for Clinical Excellence: The AACN Synergy Model for Patient Care.* St. Louis, MO: Saunders.

Hernandez, J. O., Norstrom, J., & Wysock, G. (2009). Acyclovir-induced renal failure in an obese patient. *American Journal of Health-System Pharmacy, 66*(14), 1288.

Indu, K., Lakshminarayana, G., Anil, M., Rajesh, R., George, K., Ginil, K., . . . V. Sanjeevan, K. (2012). Is early removal of prophylactic ureteric stents beneficial in live donor renal transplantation? *Indian Journal of Nephrology, 22*(4), 275–279.

Jones & Bartlett Learning. (2011). *2012 nurse's drug handbook.* (11th ed.). Sudbury, MA: Jones & Bartlett Learning.

Joshi, B., Jones, D., Rochford, A., & Giblin, L. (2009). Hypothyroidism and associated acute renal failure. *Journal of the Royal Society of Medicine, 102*(5), 199–200.

Kawamoto, S., Horton, K., & Fishman, E. K. (2008). Detection of renal calculi on late arterial phase computed tomography images: Are noncontrast scans always needed to detect renal calculi? *Journal of Computer Assisted Tomography, 32*(6), 859–864.

King, J., & Rosner, M. H. (2010). Osmotic demyelination syndrome. *American Journal of the Medical Sciences, 339*(6), 561–567.

Koirala, S., Penagaluri, P., Smith, C., & Lippmann, S. (2009). Priapism and risperidone. *Southern Medical Journal, 102*(12), 1266–1268.

Krost, W. S., Mistovich, J. J., & Limmer, D. D. (2009). Beyond the basics: Electrolyte disturbances. *EMS Magazine, 38*(4), 47–50, 52–55.

Kuhn, L., Wang, C., Tsai, W., Wright, T. C., & Denny, L. (2010). Efficacy of human papillomavirus-based screen-and-treat for cervical cancer prevention among HIV-infected women. *AIDS, 24*(16), 2553–2561.

Laouad, I., Bretagnol, A., Fabre, E., Halimi, J. M., Al-Najjar, A., Boutin, J. M., . . . Bachler, M. (2012). Kidney transplant with multiple renal artery grafts from deceased donors: Are long-term graft and patient survival compromised? *Progress in Transplantation, 22*(1), 102–109.

Lippincott. (2010). *Professional guide to signs and symptoms* (6th ed.). Philadelphia, PA: Lippincott.

Lynn-McHale Wiegand, D. J. (Ed.). (2011). *AACN procedure manual for critical care* (6th ed.). St. Louis, MO: Saunders.

Medina, J., & Puntillo, K. (2006). *AACN protocols for practice: Palliative care and end-of-life issues in critical care*. Sudbury, MA: Jones and Bartlett.

Mehta, R. L. (2011). Biomarker explorations in acute kidney injury: The journey continues. *Kidney International, 80*(4), 332–334.

Merchant, R. C., Depalo, D. M., Stein, M. D., & Rich, J. D. (2009). Adequacy of testing, empiric treatment, and referral for adult male emergency department patients with possible chlamydia and/or gonorrhoea urethritis. *International Journal of STD & AIDS, 20*(8), 534–539.

Miano, R., Germani, S., & Vespasiani, G. (2007). Stones and urinary tract infections. *Urologia Internationalis, 79*(S1), 32–36.

Murphy, F., & Byrne, G. (2010). The role of the nurse in the management of acute kidney injury. *British Journal of Nursing, 19*(3), 146–152.

Noble, H., & Page, K. (2012). Renal cell cancer: Nurses' role in prevention and management. *British Journal of Nursing, 21*, S18–S22.

Ortega, L. M., Schultz, D. R., Lenz, O., Pardo, V., & Contreras, G. N. (2010). Review: Lupus nephritis: Pathologic features, epidemiology and a guide to therapeutic decisions. *Lupus, 19*(5), 557–574.

Pace, R. C. (2007). Fluid management in patients on hemodialysis. *Nephrology Nursing Journal, 34*(5), 557–559.

Park, M., Coca, S. G., Nigwekar, S. U., Garg, A. X., Garwood, S., & Parikh, C. R. (2010). Prevention and treatment of acute kidney injury in patients undergoing cardiac surgery: A systematic review. *American Journal of Nephrology, 31*(5), 408–418.

Phillips, E., Kieley, S., Johnson, E. B., & Monga, M. (2009). Emergency room management of ureteral calculi: Current practices. *Journal of Endourology, 23*(6), 1021.

Powell, H. R. F., & Almeyda, J. (2009). An immunocompetent patient presenting with severe nasal herpes simplex: A case report. *Cases Journal, 2*, 9079.

Praga, M., & González, E. (2010). Acute interstitial nephritis. *Kidney International, 77*(11), 956–961.

Prescott, A. M., Lewington, A., & O'donoghue, D. (2012). Acute kidney injury: Top ten tips. *Clinical Medicine, 12*(4), 328–332.

Proehl, J. A. (2008). *Emergency nursing procedures* (4th ed.). St. Louis, MO: Saunders.

Ramsey, S., & McIlhenny, C. (2011). Evidence-based management of upper tract urolithiasis in the spinal cord-injured patient. *Spinal Cord, 49*(9), 948–954.

Salman, I. M., Ameer, O. Z., Sattar, M. A., Abdullah, N. A., Yam, M. F., Najim, H. S., . . . Johns, E. J. (2011). Characterization of renal hemodynamic and structural alterations in rat models of renal impairment: Role of renal sympathoexcitation. *Journal of Nephrology, 24*(1), 68–77.

Seo, W., & Oh, H. (2010). Alterations in serum osmolality, sodium, and potassium levels after repeated mannitol. *Journal of Neuroscience Nursing, 42*(4), 201–207.

Shirey, T. L. (2011). Identification of acute kidney injury. *Critical Care Medicine, 39*(1), 200–201.

Smeltzer, S., & Bare, B. G. (2003). *Brunner and Suddarth's textbook of medical-surgical nursing* (10th ed.). Philadelphia, PA: Lippincott Williams & Wilkins.

Soper, D. E. (2010). Pelvic inflammatory disease. *Obstetrics & Gynecology, 116*(2), 419–428.

Stroup, S. P., & Auge, B. K. (2008). Important military role for medical expulsion therapy of urolithiasis. *Military Medicine, 173*(4), 393–398.

Stuart, C., & Rodger, R. (2012). Approach to the management of end-stage renal disease. *Clinical Medicine, 12*(5), 472–475.

Takumi, T., Mathew, V., Barsness, G. W., Kataoka, T., Rubinshtein, R., Rihal, C. S., . . . Lerman, A. (2011). The association between renal atherosclerotic plaque characteristics and renal function before and after renal artery intervention. *Mayo Clinic Proceedings, 86*(12), 1165–1172.

Urdern, L. D., Stacy, K. M., & Lough, M. E. (2005). *Thelan's critical care nursing* (5th ed.). St. Louis, MO: Mosby.

Venzin, R. M., Cohen, C. D., Maggiorini, M., & Wüthrich, R. P. (2009). Aliskiren-associated acute renal failure with hyperkalemia. *Clinical Nephrology, 71*(3), 326–328.

Watcher, R. (2012). *Understanding patient safety* (2nd ed.). Los Altos, CA: Lange.

Williams, P. T. (2008). Effects of running distance and performance on incident benign prostatic hyperplasia. *Medicine & Science in Sports & Exercise, 40*(10), 1733–1739.

Wirk, B. (2011). Renal failure in multiple myeloma: A medical emergency. *Bone Marrow Transplantation, 46*(6), 771–783.

Yaklin, K. M. (2011). Acute kidney injury: An overview of pathophysiology and treatments. *Nephrology Nursing Journal, 38*(1), 13–19.

Section 11

Multisystem

This section contains questions on diverse topics.

It is imperative you know the following criteria for systemic inflammatory response syndrome:

In 1992, the American College of Chest Physicians (ACCP) and the Society of Critical Care Medicine (SCCM) introduced definitions for systemic inflammatory response syndrome (SIRS), and clarified definitions for sepsis and multiple organ dysfunction syndrome.

SIRS is defined as 2 or more of the following variables:

1. Fever of more than 38° C (100.4° F) or less than 36° C (96.8° F)
2. Heart rate of more than 90 beats per minute
3. Respiratory rate of more than 20 breaths per minute or arterial carbon dioxide tension ($PaCO_2$) of less than 32 mmHg
4. Abnormal white blood cell count (>12,000/µL or <4,000/µL or >10% immature [band] forms)

SECTION 11: MULTISYSTEM QUESTIONS

1. **The antidote for digoxin overdose is**
   A. Calcium gluconate
   B. Digoxin immune Fab
   C. Glucagon
   D. Potassium chloride

2. **If a patient sustains an injury from electromagnetic waves, such as those from an X-ray, the type of energy involved is**
   A. Mechanical
   B. Electrical
   C. Chemical
   D. Radiant

3. **When energy is transferred from a bullet to an individual, the type of energy transferred is called**
   A. Mechanical energy
   B. Kinematic energy
   C. Physical energy
   D. Thermal energy

4. **The systemic response to infection defined as the presence of SIRS in addition to a documented or presumed infection is known as**
   A. A SIRS sustained response
   B. Sepsis

C. Bacteremia
D. A mediated response

5. **The presence of bacteria within the bloodstream is known as**
   A. Bacteremia
   B. An inflammatory response
   C. Septic shock
   D. Septicemia

6. **A state of physiologic dysfunction in which two or more organ systems are not capable of maintaining homeostasis is known as**
   A. Cell-mediated sepsis
   B. Cellular ischemia
   C. End-organ hypoperfusion
   D. Multiple organ dysfunction syndrome

7. **A sepsis-induced state with hypotension, despite adequate fluid resuscitation, is called**
   A. Secondary sepsis-induced hypotension
   B. Severe sepsis
   C. Primary sepsis-induced hypotension
   D. Septic shock

8. **The Progressive Care unit director has tasked you with representing your department in a risk management task force. The purpose of risk management is to**
   A. Identify healthcare staff who are negligent
   B. Collect and store records regarding potential and actual injuries in the hospital
   C. Monitor staff competency
   D. Determine scope of practice within the hospital based on financial liability

9. **Which type of isolation is required for vancomycin-resistant enterococci (VRE) infections?**
   A. Standard or universal precautions
   B. Reverse isolation
   C. Contact isolation
   D. Droplet isolation

10. **Signs and symptoms of heat stroke include**
    A. Slow pulse
    B. Hot, dry skin
    C. Muscle cramps
    D. Fatigue

11. **Signs of vitamin D toxicity include**
    A. Seizures
    B. Increased susceptibility to respiratory diseases
    C. Azotemia
    D. Hypocalcemia

12. **A microbial phenomenon characterized by an inflammatory response to the microorganisms or the invasion of normally sterile tissue by those organisms is known as**
    A. Septicemia
    B. SIRS
    C. MODS
    D. Infection

13. **The presence of a systolic blood pressure of less than 90 mmHg or a reduction of more than 40 mmHg from baseline in the absence of other causes of hypotension is known as**
    A. Septic shock
    B. Secondary hypotension
    C. Sepsis-induced hypotension
    D. End-organ hypoperfusion

14. **Your patient was admitted to the PCU with recurrent *Pneumocystis carinii.* She is currently taking protease inhibitors and a non-nucleoside reverse transcriptase inhibitor. Which of the following herbals may be contributing to her recurrent** *Pneumocystis carinii*?
    A. Ginkgo biloba
    B. Ginseng
    C. St. John's Wort
    D. Thyme

15. **Your patient, a victim of a black widow spider bite, became obtunded, bradycardic, apneic, and hypotensive soon after arrival in the PCU. Your first action should be to**
    A. Administer morphine 2 mg IV
    B. Administer antivenin
    C. Tie a tourniquet around the leg
    D. Prepare to intubate

16. **Your patient is preparing to go home after treatment with antivenin for a black widow spider bite. Which of the following discharge instructions is appropriate?**
    A. "You may experience muscle spasms for only a few days."
    B. "You may experience tingling and weakness for several years."
    C. "Call your doctor immediately if you have joint or abdominal pain or begin to have trouble breathing."
    D. "It is normal to have a rash or fever in the next 3 days."

17. **Many people are adding "exotic" herbs and supplements into their food and diets. Many may be very harmful and interact with medicines a child is taking or may result in serious or deadly complications of existing diseases. Your patient is experimenting with flavorings. She made a roast with Scotch Broom on it the night prior to admission to the PCU. After ingesting the soup she began to feel light-headed and experienced palpitations and weakness. A priority of treatment is to**
    A. Insert a nasogastric tube and provide gastric lavage with activated charcoal
    B. Insert a Foley catheter

C. Continue quinidine medications taken at home
D. Continue the amiodarone infusion started for PVCs

18. **A college student was helping a friend clean out a garage yesterday. He developed a raised area that initially looked like a mosquito bite but is now red, pus-filled, and inflamed. He is admitted to the unit with a necrotizing wound. You suspect a brown recluse spider bite. This patient should not exhibit which of the following signs and symptoms?**
    A. Dyspnea
    B. Nausea and vomiting
    C. DIC
    D. Hemolysis and thrombocytopenia

19. **A 38 year old woman was admitted to your unit after experiencing abdominal cramping, nausea, and severe diarrhea. Her EKG shows sinus tachycardia with frequent PVCs. She is currently on an amiodarone infusion. The only significant history was that the patient ate at a seafood restaurant 3 days ago. This patient is probably suffering from**
    A. Irritable bowel syndrome
    B. Hypokalemia
    C. Celiac disease
    D. Shellfish poisoning

20. **Cadmium accumulates in the lungs, liver, and kidneys by exposure to**
    A. Cigarette smoke
    B. Asbestos
    C. Lead paint
    D. Freshwater fish

21. **What is the incubation period for inhalation anthrax?**
    A. 7–10 days
    B. 5–7 days
    C. 7–60 days
    D. 20–30 days

22. **What are the initial symptoms for inhaled anthrax?**
    A. Mild, flu-like symptoms
    B. Severe dyspnea and productive cough
    C. High fever, cough, and stridor
    D. Cutaneous lesions, cough, and high fever

23. **Your patient works at a fast food restaurant. She found an envelope that was torn and had white powder falling out of the tear. She and her fellow employees were sent to the hospital and are being evaluated for possible inhalation anthrax. What is the treatment of choice for this patient?**
    A. Penicillin G 2 million units intravenously every 6 hours
    B. Ciprofloxacin 400 mg intravenously every 12 hours
    C. Doxycycline 500 mg intravenously every 12 hours
    D. Augmentin 875/125 mg intravenously every 12 hours

24. **What form of isolation should be used for the patient with inhalation anthrax?**
    A. Full isolation with laminar air flow
    B. Droplet precautions
    C. Standard contact precautions
    D. Reverse isolation

25. **Your hospital is put on an external disaster notice after a ricin poisoning incident at a local train station. Your PCU prepares to accept casualties. What makes ricin so toxic to humans?**
    A. Ricin causes respiratory failure
    B. Ricin causes renal failure
    C. Ricin inhibits protein synthesis, leading to cell death
    D. Ricin destroys the mitochondria in the cell, causing cell death

26. **A male patient was pumping gas when a spark ignited the fumes. He suffered full thickness burns of the right arm. He has been a patient on your unit for 4 hours. During your initial assessment you note that eschar is present and the right radial pulse is not palpable. A Doppler pulse is also not discernible. Which of the following actions is appropriate at this time?**
    A. Move the arm away from the torso and elevate it on a pillow
    B. Escharotomy
    C. Morphine 4 mg IV
    D. Ice packs to reduce swelling

27. **A 40 year old man was admitted to your PCU after a burn injury. He was helping his friend barbeque in the back yard and a sudden flame-up burned his chest, right shoulder, and chin. What finding would be indicative of probable smoke inhalation in this patient?**
    A. PaO_2 81, met HgB level of 2%
    B. PaO_2 76, pCO_2 26
    C. Increased CO_2
    D. A carboxyhemoglobin of 18%, burned chin

28. **During the immediate postburn period, which of the following fluids would be most beneficial?**
    A. Normal saline
    B. 0.45% normal saline
    C. Lactated Ringer's
    D. Albumin

29. **Your patient was burned over the anterior chest, right forearm, anterior neck, and the lateral aspect of the right leg. The burns on his right forearm have a white, leather-like appearance, and the patient has no sensation in that area. What classification of burn are these injuries to the right forearm?**
    A. First degree
    B. Second-degree partial thickness
    C. Third-degree full thickness
    D. Fourth-degree full thickness

30. Which of the following medications would you anticipate using to improve the pumping action of the heart when a patient is developing cardiogenic shock?

A. Dobutamine
B. Epinephrine
C. Diltiazem
D. Isoproterenol

31. Your patient lived in the country at a camp all summer and ate large quantities of deer and fish. He was admitted to the PCU for respiratory distress, weight loss, vomiting, and numbness around the mouth. He is also suffering from mouth sores and he drools constantly. His probable diagnosis is

A. Botulism
B. Chlamydia infection
C. Difficile infection
D. Mercury poisoning

32. Your patient was very anxious prior to a bronchoscopy. He received an IM injection of Versed. His blood pressure dropped from 142/80 to 88/56 and he became bradycardic. To counter this reaction, he should be given

A. Xanax
B. Ativan
C. Valium
D. Romazicon

33. Which of the following vasodilators should not be mixed with Ringer's lactate?

A. Nesiritide
B. Captopril
C. Cardene
D. Epinephrine

34. Your patient lives on a ranch. Yesterday he complained of a stiff neck and was very lethargic. Last night he was found unconscious and had apparently vomited and possibly aspirated. He was immediately transported to your ED. After a preliminary evaluation, he was admitted to the PCU. This patient probably has

A. Pneumonia
B. West Nile virus
C. Western equine encephalitis
D. A brain tumor

35. Which statement about plague is incorrect?

A. Plague is caused by *Yersinia pestis*
B. Aerosol droplets may spread plague person to person
C. Plague is usually transmitted by rats
D. Plague may be used as a biological weapon

36. Which of the following choices is not a form of anthrax?

A. Nonspecific
B. Cutaneous
C. Pulmonary
D. Gastrointestinal

37. The type of chemical agent that can cause blistering is called a

A. Vesicant
B. Contaminant
C. Intoxicant
D. Nerve agent

38. The type of device made by combining radioactive materials and an explosive is known as a(n)

A. Improved nuclear device
B. Radiologic dispersal device
C. Simple radiological device
D. Improved explosive device

39. Today you were floated to the ED. An ambulance brought in a patient from an incident at a bus station. The patient is irritable, confused, and has paresthesias around the mouth. He is having watery, rice-like diarrhea, nausea, and vomiting. These symptoms are indicative of

A. Arsenic poisoning
B. Digoxin toxicity
C. Methanol poisoning
D. Insecticide poisoning

40. A blast injury that occurs when a body is hurled though the air and struck by another object is known as

A. A primary blast injury
B. A compound blast injury
C. A secondary blast injury
D. A tertiary blast injury

41. An example of a primary blast injury is

A. Hemorrhagic contusion
B. Fractured femur
C. An arm impaled by a stick
D. Gunshot wound

42. A burn that involves muscle, fat, or bone is classified as a

A. First-degree partial thickness burn
B. Second-degree partial thickness burn
C. Third-degree full thickness burn
D. Fourth-degree full thickness burn

43. Use of 0.5% silver nitrate solution is a good treatment for burns because of its broad-spectrum antibacterial action. As a PCU nurse, you know a disadvantage of using this medication is

A. Metabolic acidosis
B. Hypochloremia and hyponatremia
C. Transient leucopenia
D. Limited penetration of eschar

44. **The area of a burn that has the closest contact with the heat source and sustains the most damage is the**
   A. Zone of stasis
   B. Zone of hyperemia
   C. Zone of erythema
   D. Zone of coagulation

45. **After a patient ingests toxic levels of iron, there is a latent asymptomatic phase. This phase may cause caregivers to underestimate the continuing risk to the patient. This latent phase usually occurs _______ hours after ingestion.**
   A. 1–4
   B. 2–12
   C. 8–16
   D. 12–24

46. **The toxic ingredient in automobile antifreeze is**
   A. Freon
   B. Ethanol
   C. Methanol
   D. Ethylene glycol

47. **An acid that is absorbed even through intact skin, causing local and systemic effects, is**
   A. Ethylene glycol
   B. Hydrofluoric acid
   C. Carbonic acid
   D. Acetic acid

48. **High-dose epinephrine was started for your patient after resuscitation from a cardiac arrest due to beta-blocker overdose. Which of the following lab results should you monitor closely?**
   A. Glucose levels
   B. Calcium levels
   C. Chloride levels
   D. Sodium levels

49. **Which statement is true regarding alkaline substances?**
   A. The pH is lower than 2
   B. Vascular thrombosis may result
   C. Eschar forms over the burned area
   D. Alkalines dehydrate tissues

50. **Which of the following substances contain large amounts of alkali?**
   A. Toilet bowl cleaners
   B. Swimming pool chemicals
   C. Oven cleaners
   D. Metal cleaners

51. **Symptoms of salicylate poisoning include**
   A. Respiratory acidosis and bradycardia
   B. Lethargy and hypotension

C. Abdominal cramping and hyperglycemia
D. Tachycardia and hyperthermia

52. The antidote for iron poisoning is
A. No antidote is available, treat symptoms only
B. Chelation
C. Deferoxamine
D. Activated charcoal

53. The acid–base imbalance likely to be seen with an iron overdose is
A. Respiratory acidosis
B. Metabolic alkalosis
C. Metabolic acidosis
D. Respiratory alkalosis

54. You just discovered your patient is being treated at home for MRSA. She has been receiving vancomycin. You are able to check a trough level and the result was >20 μg/ml. This level
A. May cause ototoxicity
B. May cause nephrotoxicity
C. Is therapeutic
D. Indicates the current dosage is too low

55. Poisoning by arsenic may cause which of the following symptoms?
A. Pneumonia, renal dysfunction
B. Tachycardia, hypertension
C. Paresthesia, cerebral edema
D. Convulsions

56. Your patient overdosed on metoprolol. As a progressive care nurse you know an appropriate nursing action would be to
A. Prepare for cardioversion
B. Administer activated charcoal
C. Have a pacer at the bedside
D. Prepare to administer beta-blockers

57. The burn on your patient's right arm is pink and blistered. When touched the patient screams with pain. This classification of burn is
A. First degree
B. Second-degree partial thickness
C. Third-degree full thickness
D. Fourth-degree full thickness

58. Initially, a burned area can be estimated by the Rule of Nines, or using the palm as 1% of the body surface area. There are many ways to calculate the body surface area involved. If your patient was burned over 30% of his body and weighs 70 kg, calculate the total fluid requirements during the first 24 hours using the Parkland formula for burn resuscitation
A. 2,100 ml
B. 6,300 ml
C. 4,500 ml
D. 8,400 ml

59. Using the Parkland formula for burn resuscitation, calculate the fluid requirements (first 24 hours) for a patient who weighs 65 kg and is burned over 45% of his body

A. 29,250 ml
B. 11,700 ml
C. 26,000 ml
D. 10,300 ml

60. When utilizing the Parkland formula to calculate fluid needs, the preferred fluid for burn resuscitation is

A. Normal saline
B. D_5/Isolyte M
C. Lactated Ringer's
D. D_5W

61. To minimize inflammation in burns, which of the following therapies may be used?

A. Vitamin C
B. Hyperbaric therapy
C. Prednisone
D. Burns open to air

62. Which of the following is not considered a direct source of energy that would lead to a patient's injury?

A. Electrical
B. Oxygen deprivation
C. Chemical
D. Thermal

63. Rocky Mountain spotted fever is caused by

A. A parasite
B. Fleas
C. Rotavirus
D. Fungi

64. Your patient was a spectator at a soccer tournament when he was struck by lightning. He was thrown about 10 feet into a tree. He suffered a fractured left radius and ulna, a concussion, and burns on his left arm, chest, and right leg. He has been somewhat confused since the accident. Which of the following statements about lightning injuries is true?

A. Internal burns are common
B. Barotrauma is rare
C. Myoglobinuria is rarely seen
D. DC current will most likely cause ventricular fibrillation

65. Your new patient lives on a farm. She frequently helps her sister home-prepare meat and vegetables and preserve them by canning. She was admitted to the PCU with profound weakness, double vision, slurred speech, and dysphagia. Her initial

diagnosis is Guillain–Barré syndrome. While you are interviewing her sister, you learn that a few days ago your patient ingested some home-canned green beans that were several years old. No other family members ate the beans because the color was odd. What do you do with this information?

A. Do nothing, it is of no consequence
B. Notify the physician immediately, the patient may have botulism
C. Tell the physician tomorrow during rounds
D. Continue the interview

66. **A possible adverse effect with the use of fentanyl is**
A. Neutropenia
B. Chest wall rigidity
C. Hyperthyroidism
D. Tachypnea

67. **A possible adverse effect of morphine is**
A. Ileus
B. Hyperactive bowel tones
C. Ototoxicity
D. Increased venous capacitance

68. **Fentanyl administered intravenously is incompatible with**
A. Piperacillin
B. Phenytoin
C. Esmolol
D. Morphine

69. **A contraindication for the use of fentanyl is**
A. Asthma
B. A urinary tract infection
C. Concomitant use of penicillin
D. Open heart surgery

70. **Your patient tells you she uses witch hazel. Your first question after hearing this should be**
A. "Why did you take witch hazel?"
B. "How did you obtain the witch hazel?"
C. "How much and how often did you use witch hazel?"
D. "Does your family know you use witch hazel?"

71. **Your new patient was brought into the emergency room after collapsing at a party. Her cardiac and neurologic work-up is negative. Her preliminary urine drug screen is also negative, so she was transferred to the PCU. What do you suspect caused her collapse?**
A. GHB
B. Dehydration
C. Ecstasy
D. Metoprolol

72. **Which of the following statements is false regarding the use of activated charcoal for suspected or confirmed poisoning?**
   A. Activated charcoal adsorbs most poisons
   B. Activated charcoal adsorbs metals
   C. Activated charcoal cannot be mixed with ice cream
   D. Single doses of activated charcoal are indicated for serious poison exposures

73. **Multiple doses of activated charcoal should be used for ingestion of**
   A. Theophylline
   B. Gentamicin
   C. Aspirin
   D. Acetaminophen

74. **By definition, systemic inflammatory response syndrome (SIRS) must be comprised of two or more variables identified by the American College of Chest Physicians (ACCP) and the Society of Critical Care Medicine (SCCM). Which of the following variables was not identified in the definition of SIRS?**
   A. Fever of more than 38° C (100.4° F) or less than 36° C (96.8° F)
   B. Respiratory rate of more than 20 breaths per minute or arterial carbon dioxide tension ($PaCO_2$) of less than 32 mmHg
   C. Abnormal white blood cell count (>12,000/μL or <4,000/μL or >10% immature [band] forms)
   D. A heart rate of more than 80 beats per minute

75. **Ketamine is contraindicated in a patient with**
   A. Bronchospasm
   B. Altered intracranial pressure
   C. Barbiturate overdose
   D. Opioid overdose

76. **Which of the following statements is true regarding the administration of propofol?**
   A. Propofol is used for long-term procedures
   B. Propofol is not indicated for use in a patient with bronchospasm
   C. Propofol is made from eggs and soybeans
   D. Propofol increases cerebral blood flow

77. **Which of the following statements about superficial frostbite is true?**
   A. Use heavy blankets to help rewarm the entire patient
   B. The skin will be bright pink and feel cold to the touch
   C. Rewarm the affected part using warm water at 104° to 110° F
   D. Keep the affected part dependent

78. **Your patient was admitted directly to the PCU with deep frostbite. Which of the following actions should not be performed ASAP for this patient?**
   A. Remove the patient's wet clothing
   B. Administer warm, noncaffeinated fluids

C. Administer narcotic analgesics
D. Amputate tissue that is black in color

79. What is the hallmark symptom of primary syphilis?
A. Painful vesicular lesions on genitalia
B. Painless chancre or lesion at the site of inoculation
C. Painless maculopapular lesions on the groin
D. Painful papules on genitalia

80. A 19 year old man is admitted complaining of a rash on his penis he has had for the past 3 days. The rash looks like blisters in a small cluster on the shaft of the penis. This patient's symptoms are suspicious for which sexually transmitted infection?
A. Herpes zoster
B. Syphilis
C. *Molluscum contagiosum*
D. Herpes simplex I or II

81. A 63 year old, retired school teacher presented initially to the ED for cocaine intoxication. After admission to the PCU, he begins to complain of severe epigastric pain. Labs are as follows: WBC 17.5 with 76% neutrophils, hematocrit 41%, LDH 341, platelets 226, BUN 7, creatinine 1.0. Urine analysis shows trace of proteins, few RBCs, and + urine toxicology for cocaine. What is the likely cause of his pain?
A. Peptic ulcer disease
B. Renal infarction
C. Gastroenteritis
D. Infarcted mesenteric artery

82. If muscle is burned, what classification is this type of burn?
A. First degree
B. Second-degree partial thickness
C. Third-degree full thickness
D. Fourth-degree full thickness

83. Your patient has burns on the right arm that are circumferential (all the way around the arm). What is the highest immediate risk with this type of burn?
A. Infection into the bone
B. Difficulty removing dead tissue
C. Compartment syndrome
D. Escharotomy

84. This morning a fire broke out in your patient's home. The patient's bed was covered in wool blankets and wool clothing was in the closet. She did not suffer any burns but did inhale large quantities of smoke. What would be the most potent toxin she might have inhaled?
A. Carbon monoxide
B. Smoke
C. Inhaled nitrates
D. Cyanide

85. **A 73 year old female is admitted to your unit with tachycardia (HR 136), RR 34, BP 90/60, T 96.4° F. Her white count is 17,000. The patient states she was treated for a "kidney infection" 2 weeks ago. She denies pain at this time. This patient probably has**
    A. MODS
    B. A kidney stone
    C. SIRS
    D. Appendicitis

86. **Your patient, age 19, was admitted to your unit because of increased respiratory effort and possible pneumonia. The blood culture revealed the presence of *E. coli*. Which of the following antibiotics would have the best effect on the bacteria?**
    A. Ganciclovir
    B. Gentamycin
    C. Cytarabine
    D. Cefoxitin

87. **Your patient had a root canal. He has developed Ludwig's angina. This type of angina can be defined as**
    A. A type of painful bradycardia in which the QT interval is lengthened
    B. An infectious process
    C. A dysrhythmia with severe pain secondary to inhalation of noxious gases
    D. Cardiac ischemia post-code syndrome

88. **In sepsis, endotoxins stimulate production of tumor necrosis factor (TNF). The TNF, in turn, stimulates**
    A. Neutrophil activation and platelet aggregation
    B. Parathyroid hormone production
    C. Increased CO_2 retention
    D. Increased CPP

89. **Patients who have oral amphetamine overdoses should receive which of the following as part of their treatment regimen?**
    A. Ammonium chloride
    B. Ipecac
    C. Caffeine
    D. Theophylline

90. **A 68 year old victim of a brown recluse spider bite is leaving your unit. As part of his discharge teaching, you include ways to prevent future bites. Recommendations should not include**
    A. Shaking out all clothing prior to getting dressed
    B. Always wearing gloves when touching wood products or rocks and when working in basements or attics
    C. Changing all storage boxes to cardboard
    D. Installing yellow or sodium vapor light bulbs outdoors

91. You are treating a patient with long QT syndrome. Which of the following herbs should he avoid?
A. Ginseng
B. Ginkgo biloba
C. Marijuana
D. Oregano

92. Your 28 year old male patient has been prescribed ergotamine. This drug was probably prescribed for
A. Erectile dysfunction
B. Headaches
C. Pruritis
D. Nausea

93. Patients who are stung by bees numerous times are in danger of developing
A. Kidney failure
B. Anemia
C. Long QT interval
D. Hydrocephalus

94. A possible side effect of cocaine is
A. Malignant hyperthermia
B. Cherry red skin
C. Paralytic ileus
D. Constricted pupils

95. Your patient is a recovering alcoholic started on pantoprazole sodium (Protonix) for GERD. The IV push injection should be administered over what period of time?
A. Rapid push
B. 2 minutes
C. 4 minutes
D. Protonix should not be given as an IV push

96. Your patient underwent PTCA therapy yesterday. Integrilin 0.5 mcg/kg/min is infusing via IV. You would anticipate
A. Change over to PO administration today
B. Discontinue the medication and switch to another platelet aggregation inhibitor today
C. Increase dosage to 0.75 mcg/mg/min today to maximize effect
D. Wean to 0.25 mcg/kg/min in anticipation of discontinuing the medication in the morning

97. Which of the following drugs should be held while your patient is receiving diltiazem hydrochloride?
A. Nitroglycerin
B. Digoxin

C. Insulin
D. Rifampin

98. **Your patient was stabbed in the chest 2 weeks ago. The damage done to the heart required a prosthetic mitral valve replacement. The patient is now experiencing transient chest pain and syncopal episodes. A TEE is ordered. You anticipate performing which of the following actions prior to the procedure?**
A. Holding all medications 8 hours prior to procedure
B. Allowing the patient to keep dentures in
C. Administering prophylactic antibiotics
D. Positioning the patient on the right side

99. **Contraindications for a pulmonary angiogram would include**
A. Perfusion deficits
B. Vascular filling defects
C. Pulmonary thromboembolism
D. Pregnancy

100. **Acetaminophen overdose may take as long as 2 weeks to resolve. From 72 to 96 hours after ingestion, the patient's symptoms will include**
A. Pallor, lethargy, and metabolic acidosis
B. Increased renal function
C. Right upper quadrant pain and increased serum hepatic enzymes
D. Jaundice, confusion, and coagulation disorders

101. **Which of the following statements about cocaine is false?**
A. Cocaine use, even just one time, can cause rhabdomyolysis
B. Cocaine and tobacco use are associated with spontaneous abortion
C. Laboratory specimens should be kept on ice
D. Cocaine causes the placenta to shrink

102. **Patient and family teaching for digital subtraction angiography includes**
A. The length of the procedure is approximately 90 minutes
B. Women who are breastfeeding should substitute formula for breast milk for one or more days after the procedure
C. The patient will be able to change position frequently during the procedure
D. The patient will be free to move around during the procedure

103. **Your patient has a history of cluster migraine headaches and has been treated with lithium. Her lithium level on admission was 1.7 mmol/L. This value would correspond with which of the following symptoms?**
A. Somnolence and coma
B. Ataxia and diarrhea
C. Seizures and flattened T wave
D. Manic-depressive behavior

104. Your patient, post-PTCA, is receiving eptifibatide (Integrilin) therapy. Which of the following lab results represents effective therapeutic management?

A. An aPTT 52 seconds

B. An aPTT 89 seconds

C. Platelet level of 89,000/mm^3

D. ACT 221 seconds

105. Your patient underwent pulmonary function testing. The respiratory therapist tells you the preliminary result is a low peak expiratory flow rate (PEFR). This might indicate

A. Asthma

B. Pneumothorax

C. Pulmonary cysts

D. Heart failure

106. What is the causative organism for Lyme disease?

A. *Escherichia coli*

B. *Klebsiella pneumonia*

C. *Serratia marcescens*

D. *Borrelia burgdorferi*

107. Your patient is a 40 year old construction worker who was seen in the ED after falling into a trench. He sustained a left fractured tibia and fibula and a fractured left scapula. He required a splenectomy and was just admitted to your care. The nursing supervisor tried to get a bed in the ICU, but none was available. Your initial assessment results are as follows:

EKG: ST at 126 with isolated PVC

BP 84/50

Skin pale, cool, clammy

RR 26, breath sounds clear, slightly diminished RLL

O_2 2 L/min via NC

Mentation: Responds to questions slowly, oriented to self and time

CVP 4

Which of the following conditions do you believe this patient is developing?

A. Cardiogenic shock

B. Hypovolemic shock

C. Septic shock

D. Left ventricular failure

108. Which of the following is not an action of diltiazem (Cardizem)?

A. Blocks calcium channels

B. Relaxes coronary vessels

C. Increases peripheral vascular resistance

D. Prolongs AV conduction

109. Which of the following is not an action of octreotide acetate (Sandostatin)?
A. Increases gastrointestinal motility
B. Inhibits serotonin secretion
C. Decreases pancreatic secretion
D. Decreases hepatic venous pressure

110. Which of the following is a side effect of concurrent administration of carvedilol and clonidine?
A. Hypotension and bradycardia
B. Hypoglycemia
C. Heart blocks and bradycardia
D. Tachycardia and hypertension

111. Which electrolyte should be monitored closely while the patient is receiving valsartan (Diovan)?
A. Potassium
B. Phosphate
C. Calcium
D. Magnesium

112. Your patient received spinal Duramorph with general anesthesia for surgery. As you are transferring the patient from the gurney to the bed, you note that the patient has periodic apnea and audible wheezing. What other adverse reactions can you anticipate in this situation?
A. Hypotension and decreased intracranial pressures
B. Bradycardia and increased libido
C. Palpitations and anemia
D. Rapid capillary refill and bounding pulses

113. Your patient is going home on olmesartan for hypertension. Which of the following patient teaching elements is false?
A. Drink 2–3 L of fluid daily
B. Exercising during any part of the day is acceptable
C. Avoid alcohol consumption
D. Monitor urine output and notify your physician if urine becomes dark in color

114. Your patient is a computer programmer being treated for DVT. Enoxaparin sodium was ordered. Which of the following key points for patient teaching is true?
A. Rub the injection site to increase absorption and avoid nodule formation
B. Injection sites should be rotated between the abdomen, bilateral thighs, and bilateral underarms
C. Injections should be administered with the patient lying down
D. Expel the air bubble in the syringe prior to administration to prevent air embolism

115. You are admitting a patient from the ER with a fractured femur, mild concussion, and multiple facial lacerations after a motor vehicle accident. His blood alcohol level was elevated despite his report of only drinking one standard-sized beer while with friends at a bar 3 hours prior to driving. His stated medical history includes OTC Pepcid use to treat GERD. What factor is most likely to have contributed to the patient's elevated blood alcohol level?

A. The patient is not being honest and consumed more than one beer before driving
B. The Pepcid increased blood alcohol level by delaying metabolism
C. The patient consumed a larger than standard size beer
D. The patient's report of waiting 3 hours prior to driving

116. What are the primary actions of milrinone?
A. Vasodilation and positive inotropy
B. Vasodilation and positive chronotropy
C. Positive chronotropy and vasodilation
D. Beta and alpha receptor inhibitor

117. Your patient with hyperthyroidism is being started on metoprolol for angina. What would happen if the patient suddenly stops taking this drug?
A. No effect
B. Leukopenia
C. Thyroid storm
D. Bradycardia

118. Metoprolol is prescribed for hypertension. If dosing exceeds 400 mg daily, the patient should be monitored closely for
A. Bronchospasms
B. Agitation
C. Increased HDL
D. Flushing

Please note: As of this writing, Pradaxa has been reported to cause fatal bleeding and is under investigation by the FDA. We have included questions on this drug to help you with other key points for the PCCN exam if the drug is still in use.

119. It is late evening and you are admitting a patient from the ED for observation after a syncopal episode due to atrial fibrillation. She reports that she missed her dose of Pradaxa this morning. The patient tells you that she has a dose with her and says she will take it if you bring her water. You should
A. Allow her to take the dose since pharmacy may not have Pradaxa in stock
B. Tell her to take two doses since she missed this morning's dose
C. Tell her to take her dose now and you will provide the evening dose when arrives it from pharmacy
D. Tell her to send her medications home and you will administer just the evening dose when available from pharmacy

120. During your history and physical assessment of a 50 year old female admitted for chest pain, she reports a history of shingles outbreak 3 months ago. You would question which physician order for clarification?
A. Aspirin 160 mg daily
B. Morphine 2 mg IV PRN
C. Nitroglycerin 2 sprays every 3–5 min for chest pain
D. Oxygen via nasal cannula PRN

121. Which lab value is critical when dosing dabigatran etexilate (Pradaxa)?
A. INR
B. Creatinine clearance

C. APTT
D. ECT

122. Which of the following is a true statement regarding the administration of bivalirudin (Angiomax)?
A. Bivalirudin binds to fibrinogen to prevent clot formation
B. Bivalirudin is available in 75 mg tablets for home administration
C. The aPTT should be monitored during administration of bivalirudin
D. Administer vitamin K and protamine if bivalirudin overdose occurs

123. Your patient with unstable angina weighs 110 lbs. What is an appropriate dose of Effient for this patient?
A. 1 mg PO bid
B. 3 mg IV daily
C. 5 mg PO daily
D. 10 mg IV daily

124. Your 38 year old patient has suffered from chronic neck pain since a car accident 4 years ago. He underwent cervical fusion yesterday and is complaining of cervical neck pain. Your order is for "Fentanyl 0.5 mg IM every 1–2 hours for pain." You should
A. Administer as ordered via a rapid push
B. Administer over 10 minutes to prevent apnea
C. Notify the physician for clarification as the ordered frequency should be every 3–4 hours
D. Notify the physician for clarification as the ordered amount should be 0.05 mg IM

125. Your patient is being started on digoxin for paroxysmal atrial tachycardia. Which patient teaching statement is inappropriate with regard to digoxin?
A. Avoid eating grapefruit or drinking grapefruit juice
B. Avoid taking digoxin with high fiber foods
C. Take the medication at the same time every day
D. Check your pulse prior to taking the medication and do not take it if your heart rate is <60 bpm

126. Why would immediately stopping Effient administration when life-threatening bleeding occurs not improve patient condition?
A. Effient onset is 2 hours
B. Effient binds to thrombin systemically
C. Effient half-life is 7 hours
D. Effient irreversibly binds with platelets for the life of the platelet

127. Your patient with chronic pain has transitioned to transdermal fentanyl administration in anticipation of discharge home. You note skin irritation under the patch when changing sites. You should
A. Do nothing, this is expected and the patient is not complaining of irritation
B. Notify the physician and request an order for Kenalog administration

C. Advise the patient to rotate patch sites every 24 hours for a total of 72 hours using the same patch
D. Advise the patient to cut the patch into 4 pieces and place the pieces in multiple locations

128. Your 75 kg patient is to receive midazolam prior to a bronchoscopy. Which of the following is an appropriate order for this patient?
A. Versed 2.5 mg IVP over 2 min just prior to procedure
B. Ativan 3.75 mg IV x1 15 to 20 min prior to procedure
C. Valium 20 mg IV x1 30 minutes prior to procedure
D. Precedex 75 mcg IV x1 prior to procedure

129. The appropriate potency conversion from morphine to fentanyl is
A. 100 mcg of fentanyl equals 10 mg of morphine
B. 10 mg of fentanyl equals 1 mg of morphine
C. 1,000 mcg of fentanyl equals 100 mcg of morphine
D. 1 mg of fentanyl equals 10 mg of morphine

130. Aspirin inhibits platelet aggregation by
A. Inhibiting thrombin
B. Inhibiting fibrin
C. Inhibiting thromboxane
D. Inhibiting fibrinogen

131. Your diabetic patient with chronic pain is being started on Duragesic patches. You would anticipate what changes to the patient's insulin dosing?
A. No change is anticipated
B. The amount of insulin administered to this patient will increase
C. The amount of insulin administration to this patient will decrease
D. The amount of insulin administration will only decrease during the first 24 hours of administration of a Duragesic patch

132. Guidelines are available for aspirin administration to patients to prevent or have had MIs, TIAs, and strokes. You would anticipate your patient admitted for a lateral MI to be started on aspirin therapy at
A. 81 mg daily
B. 160 mg daily for 30 days
C. 325 mg daily
D. 325 mg BID

133. A disadvantage of using negative pressure wound care devices is
A. NPWC cannot be used on wounds associated with malignancies
B. NPWC removes interstitial fluid
C. NPWC promotes a moist healing environment
D. NPWC removes barriers to cell migration and proliferation

SECTION 11: MULTISYSTEM ANSWERS

1. **Correct answer: B**
   The antidote for digoxin overdose is digoxin immune Fab. Digoxin immune Fab reverses hyperkalemia and most dysrhythmias. Patients in renal failure may require dialysis to remove the digoxin immune Fab.

2. **Correct answer: D**
   If a patient sustains an injury from electromagnetic waves such as those from an X-ray, the type of energy involved is radiant. Other sources of radiant energy are sunlight, sound waves, and radioactive emissions.

3. **Correct answer: A**
   When energy is transferred from a bullet to an individual, the type of energy transferred is called mechanical energy. Energy is loaded onto the patient, and if the load overcomes the body's ability to tolerate it, injury to one or more of the body's tissues occurs.

4. **Correct answer: B**
   The systemic response to infection defined as the presence of SIRS in addition to a documented or presumed infection is known as sepsis.

5. **Correct answer: A**
   The presence of bacteria within the bloodstream is known as bacteremia. An individual with bacteremia does not necessarily develop sepsis or SIRS.

6. **Correct answer: D**
   A state of physiologic dysfunction in which two or more organ systems are not capable of maintaining homeostasis is known as multiple organ dysfunction syndrome (MODS).

7. **Correct answer: D**
   A sepsis-induced state with hypotension despite adequate fluid resuscitation is called septic shock.

8. **Correct answer: B**
   Risk management plays a role in the collection, analysis, and storage of records regarding potential and actual injuries in the hospital, as well as court filings. It also identifies situations or actions of potential liability and analyzes techniques to prevent future injuries, medication errors, and accidents.

9. **Correct answer: C**
   Vancomycin-resistant enterococci isolation requires contact isolation. The VRE can survive on surfaces such as your stethoscope for 1 hour and up, to 6 days on countertops.

10. **Correct answer: B**
    Signs and symptoms of heat stroke include hot, dry skin, flushed face, high body temperature (>40° C or 104° F), dyspnea, tachycardia, mental status changes, and absence of sweating (unless engaged in activity). This is a medical emergency as the patient's body can no longer maintain thermoregulation.

11. **Correct answer: C**
Signs of vitamin D toxicity include azotemia, hypercalcemia, vomiting, and nephrocalcinosis. Vitamin D deficiency will result in hypocalcemia, increased susceptibility to respiratory diseases, lethargy, and seizures.

12. **Correct answer: D**
A microbial phenomenon characterized by an inflammatory response to the microorganisms or the invasion of normally sterile tissue by those organisms is known as infection.

13. **Correct answer: C**
The presence of a systolic blood pressure of less than 90 mmHg or a reduction of more than 40 mmHg from baseline in the absence of other causes of hypotension is known as sepsis-induced hypotension.

14. **Correct answer: C**
St. John's Wort is contraindicated in patients with HIV/AIDS because the herb interferes with the metabolism of protease inhibitors and non-nucleoside reverse transcriptase inhibitors.

15. **Correct answer: D**
This patient is having a severe reaction to the black widow bite. He is apneic and bradycardic. Priorities are to maintain the airway to provide ventilation and oxygen therapy. The next step is to administer antivenin as soon as available. Morphine may help with pain but will worsen the bradycardia and hypotension. It is a myth that tying a tourniquet around the affected limb will stop the venom from reaching the bloodstream or lymphatic system. At this point, the venom is already systemic. In minor cases involving healthy patients, symptoms may be managed with pain control, muscle relaxants, and comfort measures. Symptoms should dissipate during the first 3 days after exposure.

16. **Correct answer: C**
This patient suffered a black widow spider bite. Her discharge instructions should include contacting her physician immediately if she has joint or abdominal pain or difficulty breathing. Joint and abdominal pain (pain related to splenomegaly), as well as dyspnea, may be signs of anaphylaxis or serum sickness up to 2 to 4 weeks after antivenin administration. Patients should be taught to contact their physicians immediately so early treatment can be initiated to prevent complications. Administration of corticosteroids and antihistamines will aid in combating the inflammatory response to the animal proteins in the antivenin. The neurotoxin may cause residual muscle spasms, tingling, weakness, and nervousness for weeks to months after the exposure to the venom. Patients may need to slowly increase activity during their recovery.

17. **Correct answer: A**
The priority of care is to insert a nasogastric tube and provide gastric lavage with activated charcoal. Scotch Broom contains sparteine, which has very powerful cardiovascular effects. Arrhythmias, blood pressure changes (increased or decreased), coagulation changes, and vision changes are possible side effects of this herb. The best action listed is to lavage the stomach to remove any un- or partially digested Scotch Broom. You will need to insert a Foley catheter, as Scotch broom does have diuretic properties,

but it is not a priority. Quinidine and amiodarone should be stopped immediately because they will interact with the Scotch Broom to cause further cardiovascular collapse by increasing the toxicity of the Scotch Broom.

18. **Correct answer: A**
Patients suffering from a brown recluse spider bite will not present with dyspnea. Patients may not initially know they were bitten and will seek medical help 12 to 36 hours after the initial bite. Because treatment is delayed, symptoms may be difficult to treat. Most patients may present with flu-like symptoms such as nausea and vomiting. DIC, hemolysis, and thrombocytopenia are severe symptoms. Treatment includes ice to control inflammation, keeping the area clean and protected, and treating symptoms. No specific treatment has been proven to be 100% effective. Dapsone has limited support for preventing necrosis. Nitroglycerin patches counter the vasoconstrictive properties of the venom and lead to hemodilution in the bloodstream and increased bleeding at the site to wash the venom out.

19. **Correct answer: D**
Shellfish poisoning can exhibit symptoms days after ingestion. The toxin contained in shellfish, clams, and oysters is called saxotoxin and is not affected by steaming or cooking. It inhibits sodium channels of membranes, blocking propagation of nerve and muscle action potentials. If the nerves are involved, there may be parasthesias of the lips, tongue, gums, and face. The parasthesias may spread to the trunk and lead to paralysis and respiratory arrest. There is no definite treatment, so care is driven by treating symptoms and providing psychological support.

20. **Correct answer: A**
Cadmium accumulates in the lungs, liver, and kidneys by exposure to cigarette smoke. Cadmium is actually a heavy metal with a half-life of 15–20 years. It is a respiratory irritant and can produce pulmonary edema, interstitial pneumonia, and cardiovascular collapse if inhaled. It is used in the manufacture of storage batteries, alloys, and in electroplating. If cadmium is ingested, the individual will have severe gastrointestinal symptoms within 30 minutes. Most cadmium collects in erythrocytes and kidney tissues. It is not metabolized in the body.

21. **Correct answer: C**
Inhalation anthrax has an incubation period of 7 days to as long as 60 days after exposure. Symptoms are initially vague and flu-like such as malaise, low-grade fever, and nausea. These symptoms quickly progress to profound diaphoresis, chest discomfort, and rhonchi. The mild symptoms occur in the first 5 days of the illness followed by a brief rally. There is then an abrupt onset of high fever and severe respiratory distress. Death occurs as early as 24–36 hours after symptoms begin.

22. **Correct answer: A**
Inhalation anthrax starts with mild, nonspecific symptoms such as malaise, low-grade fever, fatigue, and cough. Untreated, death occurs within 24–36 hours from respiratory failure.

23. **Correct answer: B**
Ciprofloxacin, a fluorquinolone antibiotic, is the drug of choice for inhalation anthrax. Doxycycline, a tetracycline derivative, may also be used, but the dosage is incorrect. Penicillin G is not an option as the bacteria, *Bacillus anthracis*, becomes beta-lactamase

positive, making the penicillin ineffective. Augmentin is not used for this situation, and it is only given orally.

24. **Correct answer: C**
The CDC states that contact precautions are all that is required for inhalation anthrax. Standard precautions may include the use of a face mask if the patient is having a productive cough.

25. **Correct answer: C**
Ricin is made from castor beans and is one of the most toxic substances known. It interferes with protein synthesis and causes cell death. Chewing castor beans may cause some symptoms, but the most lethal form is inhaled. The toxin is not spread by casual contact. The most likely victims would be seen in enclosed areas such as subway trains, buses, or small rooms. It is usually aerosolized with some liquid like water or a weak acid.

26. **Correct answer: B**
Loss of the radial pulse indicates probable compartment syndrome and this is an emergency and pressure must be relieved via an escharotomy, an incision through multiple layers of tissue. Any circumferential burn of the body may lead to impaired function and necessitate an escharotomy.

27. **Correct answer: D**
A carboxyhemoglobin of 18% and a burned chin is indicative of smoke inhalation in this patient. When a sudden flame-up comes near the face, the first instinct is to gasp. This inhalation of superheated air will cause swelling of the tissues in the air passages. This man was probably very near the flame as his chin was burned, and he is at great risk of a compromised airway and may need intubation.

28. **Correct answer: C**
Lactated Ringer's is used for burn patients for a variety of reasons with many of the formulas for burn resuscitation. It is preferred for large volume resuscitation because LR contains 130 mEq/L of sodium compared with normal saline that has 154 mEq/L. LR has a higher pH (6.5) compared to normal saline (5.0). The pH of the LR is close to a normal pH. The patient will be in metabolic acidosis, so the metabolized lactate will buffer the acidosis. LR is also an isotonic crystalloid.

29. **Correct answer: C**
Third-degree full thickness burns destroy nerve endings because they extend into subcutaneous tissue. The tissue may have a whitish color and will be somewhat firm with a leather-like appearance. Sometimes you can see clotted vessels through the eschar.

30. **Correct answer: A**
Dobutamine is an inotrope and will improve the pumping action of the heart. This alpha-, beta1-, and beta2-agonist will increase contractility and cardiac output, with little or no concomitant increase in myocardial oxygen consumption. Dobutamine has a very mild vasodilatory effect, though high doses can cause ischemia.

31. **Correct answer: D**
The probable diagnosis for this patient is mercury poisoning. Fish can contain large amounts of mercury. The concentration in fish can be more than 1,000 times greater than in the surrounding water. People who eat fish as a main component of their diet

may be at risk. Organic mercury compounds are very toxic. They are taken into the body by ingestion, inhalation, skin, and eye contact. These mercury compounds can attack all body systems. They can cause nausea, lack of appetite, abdominal pain, kidney failure, swollen gums and mouth sores, numbness and tingling in the lips, mouth, tongue, hands, and feet, tremors, and seizures. The patient can become very uncoordinated and feel disconnected from his surroundings. He may lose part or all of his vision and hearing. Additional neurologic issues may include memory loss, personality changes, and headache. Organic mercury can pass to a baby via breast milk. Methyl mercury may cause serious birth defects.

32. **Correct answer: D**
Romazicon is a benzodiazepine antagonist and should be given to counteract the effects of Versed. Xanax, Valium, and Ativan are also benzodiazepines.

33. **Correct answer: C**
Cardene cannot be mixed with Ringer's lactate or sodium bicarbonate infusions. According to studies, although the combination does not cause a precipitate, the Ringer's lactate inactivates 15 to 42% of the drug.

34. **Correct answer: C**
Western equine encephalitis is a type of encephalitis caused by an arbovirus (togovirus). An arbovirus means it is carried by arthropods. A horse or small mammal was probably infected and the virus was vectored by a mosquito. This type of encephalopathy is not directly transmitted human to human. This patient is at high risk for aspiration pneumonia and ARDS.

35. **Correct answer: C**
Plague is not transmitted by rats. Plague is transmitted by fleas carrying the *Yersinia pestis* bacterium, and aerosol droplets may spread the disease from person to person. Some countries consider plague as a biologic weapon.

36. **Correct answer: A**
Nonspecific is not a form of anthrax. Cutaneous, pulmonary, and gastrointestinal are all forms of anthrax.

37. **Correct answer: A**
The type of chemical agent that can cause blistering is called a vesicant.

38. **Correct answer: B**
The type of device made by combining radioactive materials and an explosive is known as a radiologic dispersal device.

39. **Correct answer: A**
Watery, rice-like diarrhea, nausea, vomiting, irritability, confusion, and paresthesias around the mouth are symptoms of arsenic poisoning. Additional symptoms include headache, a metallic taste, palpitations, and EKG changes.

40. **Correct answer: D**
A tertiary blast injury is a blast injury that occurs when a body is hurled though the air and struck by another object.

41. **Correct answer: A**
Hemorrhagic contusion is an example of a primary blast injury. A blast injury occurs after an explosion that causes sudden changes in atmospheric pressure.

42. **Correct answer: D**
A fourth-degree full thickness burn involves muscle, fat, fascia, or bone. This type of burn usually occurs as a result of deep thermal or electrical burns.

43. **Correct answer: B**
Hypochloremia and hyponatremia are disadvantages of using 0.5% silver nitrate solution for burn patients.

44. **Correct answer: D**
The area of a burn that has the closest contact with the heat source and sustains the most damage is the zone of coagulation. Coagulation necrosis is usually the result of most burn injuries.

45. **Correct answer: B**
After a patient ingests toxic levels of iron, there is a latent asymptomatic phase that occurs 2–12 hours after ingestion. After about 12 hours the patient may enter the next phase, which is an abrupt cardiovascular collapse.

46. **Correct answer: D**
Ethylene glycol is the toxic ingredient in automobile antifreeze.

47. **Correct answer: B**
Hydrofluoric acid is absorbed even through intact skin, causing local and systemic effects. Hydrofluoric acid is used as a rust remover, metal cleaner, and to etch glass.

48. **Correct answer: A**
In patients receiving high-dose epinephrine, glucose levels should be monitored closely for potential hyperglycemia. There is an even greater risk for hyperglycemia if the patient is diabetic. Potassium, not calcium, chloride, or sodium, should also be monitored for potential hyperkalemia or hypokalemia.

49. **Correct answer: B**
Vascular thrombosis may result from alkaline substances, and liquefaction necrosis will occur. Serious injury results from products with a pH higher than 12.

50. **Correct answer: C**
Oven cleaners contain large amounts of alkali. Additional alkaline substances include dishwasher detergent, laundry detergent, drain openers, and ammonia capsules.

51. **Correct answer: D**
Symptoms of salicylate poisoning include tachycardia and hyperthermia. Additional symptoms include tinnitus, tachypnea, LOC changes, respiratory alkalosis, metabolic acidosis, or mixed acid–base abnormalities. Occult GI tract bleeding may occur.

52. **Correct answer: C**
Deferoxamine is used to treat iron poisoning via chelation. It is also possible the patient may have to be treated with GI tract decontamination, which may include gastric lavage or whole bowel irrigation. Chelation is the bond of elements, not a treatment.

53. **Correct answer: C**
Metabolic acidosis is likely to be seen with an iron overdose. After iron is metabolized, free hydrogen is released and leads to metabolic acidosis.

54. **Correct answer: B**
A trough vancomycin level >20 μg/ml is actually a panic level and if not addressed will cause nephrotoxicity. Ototoxicity usually occurs if levels are prolonged at >30 μg/ml. Vancomycin may cause hypertension, thrombocytopenia, tubular necrosis, colitis, and deafness. The patient may require hemodialysis, hemofiltration, or peritoneal dialysis. Note: Charcoal hemofiltration does not remove vancomycin.

55. **Correct answer: D**
Arsenic poisoning may cause convulsions. Arsenic is found in all human tissues as a trace element. The levels may become elevated with exposure. About 60% of ingested arsenic is excreted in the urine. Arsenic may be found in well water, pesticides, paints, cosmetics, treated wood, and coal. Chronic exposure can lead to various types of cancers.

56. **Correct answer: C**
A pacer should be kept at the bedside for a patient with metoprolol overdose because bradycardia, AV block, and hypotension will probably occur.

57. **Correct answer: B**
This type of burn may be a superficial or a deep second-degree partial thickness burn. The nerve endings are still intact, and this burn is very painful. Sometimes burns can be deceptive. A reddened area that should be diagnosed as a first-degree burn may be overlooked when staff is calculating requirements for fluid and nutrient resuscitation. After a few hours these areas can develop blisters, and are only then recognized as dermal burns. There is a new way of assessing burn levels by using a laser Doppler during the first week of treatment.

58. **Correct answer: D**
The Parkland formula was developed by Dr. Charles Baxter at Parkland Hospital in Dallas, Texas in the 1960s and is still utilized today. It is used nationwide as a standard for fluid resuscitation. There are many other formulas in use, but this one is widely known and will probably be on the PCCN examination. The formula is 4 ml fluid × patient's weight (in kg) × % of burn, so 4 × 70 = 280 × 30 = 8,400 ml fluid requirement for the first 24 hours. Half the calculated volume is given in the first 8 hours, and then the remaining volume is given over the next 16 hours. **Remember to calculate from the time the burn occurred.**

59. **Correct answer: B**
The formula is 4 × 65 = 260 × 45 = 11,700.

60. **Correct answer: C**
As mentioned previously, Ringer's lactate is preferred for large volume resuscitation because LR contains 130 mEq/L of sodium compared with normal saline, which has 154 mEq/L. LR has a higher pH (6.5) compared to normal saline (5.0). The pH of the LR is close to a normal pH. The patient will be in metabolic acidosis, so the metabolized lactate will buffer the acidosis. LR is also an isotonic crystalloid.

61. **Correct answer: A**
Vitamin C is an antioxidant and it is used to counter oxidant-mediated effects on the inflammatory cascade. Animal studies have shown that if the vitamin C is given within 6 hours of the burn, up to 50% of the fluid needed for resuscitation can be eliminated. Always remember that if you have a burn patient you should start at least two large-bore IVs. Another new treatment involves the use of subatmospheric pressure

dressings. These dressings may aid in removing excess fluid and help save areas that would otherwise have to be grafted or removed.

62. **Correct answer: B**
Oxygen deprivation is not considered a direct source of energy that would lead to a patient's injury. It would be considered a cause of injury or death because of sequelae from the resultant lack of oxygen.

63. **Correct answer: C**
Rocky Mountain spotted fever is spread by ticks that carry a rotavirus. Symptoms include a sudden onset fever for 2 to 3 weeks and a rash that may cover the entire body. Treatment must include both chloramphenicol and tetracycline.

64. **Correct answer: C**
Myoglobinuria is rarely seen with lightning burns. AC current usually causes ventricular fibrillation and DC current usually causes asystole. In some cases arrhythmias are delayed for up to 12 hours. The mechanism of lightning strikes is quite complex. There are several ways lightning can injure a person:

A side splash from another object is probably the cause of this patient's injuries. The lightning hits something like a tree and then bounces off.
A direct strike may also have occurred.
Another type of strike can occur when the person is touching an object that is struck.
Ground current effect occurs when energy spreads out across the surface of the earth.
Lightning has two strokes, upward and downward. If they do not meet, energy can be directed outward.

Internal burns are rare. Myoglobinuria rarely occurs. Generally, lightning causes cardiac and respiratory arrest, burns from metals touching the victim (watches, necklaces, earrings), and neurologic damage.

65. **Correct answer: B**
Notify the physician immediately, as the patient may have botulism. Sometimes, families do not have enough education to make proper decisions or understand the nature of a disease. Attempting to elicit an appropriate history can be challenging. It is likely that, because of the presenting symptoms, this patient has botulism.

66. **Correct answer: B**
Possible adverse effects of fentanyl include respiratory depression, chest wall rigidity, apnea, laryngospasm, abdominal distension, loss of bowel sounds, and generalized muscle rigidity.

67. **Correct answer: A**
Possible adverse effects of morphine include respiratory depression, ileus, abdominal distension, delayed gastric emptying, hypotension, bradycardia, and urine retention.

68. **Correct answer: B**
Fentanyl administered intravenously is incompatible with phenytoin, azithromycin, and pentobarbital.

69. **Correct answer: A**
Contraindications for the use of fentanyl include increased intracranial pressure, severe respiratory disease or depression including acute asthma (unless the patient is

mechanically ventilated), and seizures. Additional contraindications include CNS depression, paralytic ileus, severe liver or renal insufficiency, and hyperglycemia (fentanyl may elevate blood glucose). Fentanyl is used in open heart surgery.

70. **Correct answer: A**
Although you may ask all these questions, the first question should be used to determine if this patient was using actual witch hazel for acne or facial cleaning or if she is using the slang term "witch hazel" for heroin. Many street drugs may present with innocuous names. Heroin may also be referred to as smack, nose drops (liquid heroin), dragon rock (mixed with cocaine), A-bomb (mixed with marijuana), big H, brown sugar, brown tape, diesel, and old navy. Monitor for additional signs and symptoms of heroin abuse such as venous tracks, bruising, and burnt fingertips from holding a roll lighter to smoke the heroin.

71. **Correct answer: A**
The sudden collapse of a young woman at a party without explanation is suspicious for gamma hydroxybutyrate (GHB) or ketamine ingestion. These are known date or party rape drugs. Due to the anesthetic and amnesic effects of the drug, an affected female may be unable to describe events leading up to the collapse. To determine exposure the drug screen should be repeated, looking specifically for gamma hydroxybutyrate and/or ketamine.

72. **Correct answer: B**
Activated charcoal does not adsorb metals. Activated charcoal adsorbs most poisons. Activated charcoal cannot be mixed with ice cream or syrups because the charcoal adsorbs many of these agents, rendering it less effective. Single doses of activated charcoal are indicated for serious poison exposures.

73. **Correct answer: A**
Multiple doses of activated charcoal should be used for ingestions of theophylline. Additional drugs for which multiple doses are indicated include digoxin, phenobarbital, and amitriptyline.

74. **Correct answer: D**
A heart rate of more than 80 beats per minute was not identified as a variable for the definition of SIRS.

75. **Correct answer: B**
Ketamine is contraindicated in a patient with altered intracranial pressure because it increases ICP and cerebral blood flow.

76. **Correct answer: C**
Propofol is made from egg phosphates and soybeans. It is incumbent on the nurse to determine if the patient has allergies or sensitivities to these ingredients.

77. **Correct answer: C**
Rewarm the affected part using warm water at 40 to 43.3° C (104–110° F). Keep the affected part elevated and do not place heavy blankets over the area. The skin will be a waxy, whitish color. The patient may also have numbness, tingling, or a burning sensation of the affected area.

78. **Correct answer: D**
In patients with deep frost bite, amputations are not an emergency. An amputation may be performed days or weeks after the injury. Priorities are to remove wet clothing, rewarm the patient, administer warm, noncaffeinated fluids (if the patient has an intact gag reflex), administer analgesics, and consider tetanus prophylaxis.

79. **Correct answer: B**
The primary lesion of syphilis is a painless chancre or lesion generally found on the genitalia. Because of the painless nature of the lesion and the surrounding pubic hair, the lesion may be missed.

80. **Correct answer: D**
Herpes simplex, either type I or II, can cause this patient's symptoms. The cluster of blisters is seen anywhere boxer shorts fit—from the waist to the mid-thigh—although the genitalia is the most common location for both men and women. Syphilis presents with a single, painless lesion in the initial phase. *Molluscum contagiosum* is highly contagious and has flesh-colored, dome-shaped papules with an umbilicated center. Herpes zoster is shingles. Blisters, along with dermatomes, are seen with herpes zoster.

81. **Correct answer: B**
Renal infarction can occur with cocaine intoxication. The proteinuria and RBCs in the urine are indicative of the renal infarction. Cocaine abuse can lead to any infarction, including MI.

82. **Correct answer: D**
This is a fourth-degree burn. Not many people are familiar with this classification. This is a burn that not only involves muscle but it extends through muscle and bone.

83. **Correct answer: C**
The highest risk at this time is compartment syndrome. A circumferential burn may lead to compartment syndrome. Escharotomy is a procedure, not a direct risk. As a nurse you must constantly assess for quality of pulses. Edema may be so great as to completely cut off circulation in a limb and cause a myoglobin-related renal failure. Elevating the limb may help drain fluid and mitigate further edema. If the pulse is lost, it still may not mean compartment syndrome is the cause. It could be due to not replacing lost volume secondary to the burn. Although infection is a risk, it is not the immediate risk.

84. **Correct answer: D**
Wool and silk give off cyanide gas. Nitriles, like the gloves we wear, will burn and give off cyanide. Household plastics like melamine dishes, plastic cups, polyurethane foam in furniture cushions, and many other synthetic compounds may produce lethal concentrations of cyanide when burned under appropriate circumstances. Cyanide inhibits cellular respiration, even with enough oxygen stores. Cellular metabolism changes from aerobic to anaerobic and produces lactic acid. The organs with the highest oxygen requirements are the most affected by cyanide inhalation.

85. **Correct answer: C**
SIRS is a systemic infection that can present in the elderly with hypothermia and even a WBC of 4,000 or 12,000. MODS is usually the result of a direct injury to an organ. A kidney stone or appendicitis should present with pain and tenderness.

86. **Correct answer: B**
Gentamycin is an aminoglycoside, as are tobramycin and amikacin. These drugs are used to combat gram-negative bacterial infections such as *E. coli*, but they must be used with caution because they can cause nephrotoxicity.

87. **Correct answer: B**
Ludwig's angina is a submaxillary infection. It is a cellulitis of the neck and floor of the mouth that usually occurs with, or after, dental disease.

88. **Correct answer: A**
In sepsis, endotoxins stimulate production of tumor necrosis factor (TNF). TNF, in turn, stimulates neutrophil activation and platelet aggregation. In addition, TNF stimulates increased capillary permeability and promotes the release of IL-1, IL-6, and IL-8.

89. **Correct answer: A**
Ammonium chloride can convert to ammonia and HCl in the liver. This conversion will indirectly correct metabolic alkalosis, but the ammonia that is generated can produce encephalopathy.

90. **Correct answer: C**
Recommendations should not include changing all storage boxes to cardboard. In fact, it is recommended that all cardboard be removed from houses and populated areas as soon as possible. Because cardboard is made of wood fibers, when it decays it is similar to a rotting tree stump, a popular haven for the brown recluse. The spider may hide or nest in folds and between layers of cardboard. Sealed plastic containers and bags provide some barriers to habitation. Gloves protect hands from exposure when handling wood and rocks or when working in storage areas such as basements and attics. Yellow or sodium light bulbs do not prevent the spider from nesting, but will limit food availability (lights repel other insects) and make the area less inviting.

91. **Correct answer: A**
Ginseng has been known to increase the QT interval, which would put this patient at greater risk for cardiac rhythm complications. Advise patients to carefully read the label before consuming any sports or high-energy drink, as many of these drinks now contain various herbs and high levels of caffeine. Ginseng may also cause breast tissue enlargement in men, erectile dysfunction, increased menstrual bleeding, and hormone imbalances in those with breast cancer, uterine cancer, and endometriosis. These effects may occur because ginseng has effects similar to those associated with estrogen. Ginseng may also cause complications or interactions with anticoagulation therapy, calcium-channel blockers, and diabetes management, and ginseng increases the potency of some sedatives.

92. **Correct answer: B**
Ergotamine (Ergot) is used as a treatment for migraine headaches. In females, it may be used to promote uterine contraction in childbirth. Because ergotamine promotes contraction of smooth muscles, it can be used to control bleeding.

93. **Correct answer: A**
Bee stings deliver proteins in the venom that act as enzymes. The enzymes lyse the cells and the cellular debris accumulates very quickly and actually clogs the kidneys. The patient then dies from kidney failure. Any patient who has been stung multiple times needs to be monitored for at least 2 weeks following the incident.

94. **Correct answer: A**
A possible side effect of cocaine is malignant hyperthermia.

95. **Correct answer: B**
Pantoprazole sodium (Protonix) IV push injection should be given over 2 minutes or as an infusion over 15 minutes.

96. **Correct answer: B**
Integrilin and heparin IV administration post-PTCA should be discontinued after 20 to 24 hours. Maximum therapy is extended to 96 hours. The dosage should not be weaned or increased as bleeding times and therapeutic effects would be negatively impacted. PO Integrilin is not available.

97. **Correct answer: D**
Rifampin should not be administered to patients receiving diltiazem hydrochloride as the rifampin decreases serum diltiazem levels to undetectable amounts by increasing metabolism of the drug. Nitroglycerin and digoxin therapy may be used concurrently. Insulin use may be required to manage adverse reaction of hyperglycemia, especially in diabetic patients.

98. **Correct answer: C**
The patient should receive prophylactic antibiotics to mitigate possible endocarditis, which may be the cause of his symptoms.

99. **Correct answer: D**
Pulmonary angiograms require iodine-based radiographic contrast dye to be injected into the antecubital or femoral vein via catheter to the pulmonary artery. The pulmonary vasculature can then be visualized. The radioactive iodine crosses the blood–placental barrier, which is why this procedure is contraindicated in pregnancy. Other contraindications include allergy to shellfish, iodine, radiographic dye, and renal insufficiency.

100. **Correct answer: D**
Renal function is possibly decreased, and the patient may have increased ALT and AST The symptoms will abate in 4 days to 2 weeks.

101. **Correct answer: D**
Cocaine is classified as a Schedule II central nervous system stimulant. It is also used as a local anesthetic, a bronchodilator, and a vasoconstrictor. Cocaine compromises the heart's antioxidant defense system, and an overdose can cause an MI. Cocaine can also cause aortic dissection, stroke, intestinal ischemia, hallucinations, and adverse effects on fetuses.

102. **Correct answer: B**
Digital subtraction angiography can be done to diagnose aneurysms, aortic valve stenosis, carotid stenosis, pulmonary emboli, ulcerative plaques, hepatocellular carcinomas, and many other conditions. The procedure carries some risks, including allergic reactions to the contrast dye, anaphylaxis, aphasia, hemiplegia, paresthesia, hemorrhage, infection, renal toxicity, and thromboemboli.

103. **Correct answer: B**
Lithium is an alkali, a metal salt used mostly in the treatment of bipolar disorder and cluster migraine headaches. In bipolar disorder and alcohol withdrawal, lithium works

by altering sodium transport in nerves and muscles, which helps to stabilize mood. Untreated lithium toxicity may lead to seizures, coma and cardiac dysrhythmias when levels reach greater than 2.5 mEq/L. Toxicity usually occurs with levels of 2 mEq/L, but symptoms may be noted at even lower blood levels with certain body chemistries. Initial toxicity is noted when the patient experiences diarrhea, vomiting, drowsiness, muscular weakness, and disorientation. As toxicity and symptoms worsen, nystagmus, ataxia, giddiness, tinnitus, confusion, and blurred vision may be present. Patients must be managed by close monitoring and immediate intervention of dysrhythmias and electrolyte imbalances.

104. Correct answer: A
An aPTT of 52 seconds indicates effective therapeutic eptifibatide (Integrilin) management post-PTCA. Once aPTT is <45 seconds and ACT <150 seconds, the sheath may be removed in anticipation of discharge. ACT of 221 is normal during PTCA procedure, not postprocedure. A platelet level <100,000/mm^3 indicates an adverse reaction and Integrilin therapy should be held.

105. Correct answer: A
Because of air trapping, a person with asthma has a low peak flow rate during expiration.

106. Correct answer: D
The causative organism for Lyme disease is *Borrelia burgdorferi*, a spirochete carried by the deer tick.

107. Correct answer: B
This patient appears to be decompensating and developing hypovolemic shock. He is in sinus tachycardia and his systolic blood pressure is only 84 and his CVP is 4, RR is 26, skin is cool and clammy, and his mentation is diminished.

108. Correct answer: C
Increased peripheral vascular resistance is not an action of diltiazem (Cardizem). By blocking calcium transport into cells, coronary and vascular smooth muscles relax, leading to decreased peripheral vascular resistance and vasodilation. Prolonging AV conduction causes a decrease in heart rate and interrupts reentrant tachycardiacs.

109. Correct answer: A
Octreotide acetate (Sandostatin) decreases gastrointestinal motility, it does not increase motility. The suppression of serotonin, as well as GI and pituitary hormones results in increased gastrointestinal water reabsorption, decreasing dehydration.

110. Correct answer: D
Tachycardia and hypertension are side effects of the concurrent administration of carvedilol and clonidine and are more profound when clonidine is stopped. Hypoglycemia occurs as a side effect with concurrent administration of oral antidiabetic medications. Hypotension and bradycardia are seen with concurrent administration with MAO inhibitors and beta-blockers. Amiodarone administration may lead to heart blocks as well as bradycardia.

111. Correct answer: A
Potassium should be monitored closely while the patient is receiving valsartan (Diovan). Due to the inhibitory action on aldosterone, potassium levels may rise to dangerous levels, leading to arrhythmias.

112. Correct answer: C
Adverse reactions to Duramorph (morphine sulfate) administration include respiratory depression, palpitations, and anemia, as well as hypotension, bradycardia, delayed capillary refill, decreased libido, and increased intracranial pressure.

113. Correct answer: B
Although exercise is an important element in treating hypertension, it is important NOT to exercise during the heat of the day to avoid dehydration. Patients need to maintain hydration with at least 2–3 L of fluid daily to maximize the efficacy of olmesartan medoxomil (Benicar). Patients should avoid alcohol consumption that would contribute to dehydration. Dark urine and decreased urinary output are strong indicators of dehydration or a more ominous sign of acute renal failure.

114. Correct answer: C
Patients should be taught to administer enoxaparin sodium (Lovenox) when lying down. The only injection site area to be used is the abdomen. When injecting the dose, advise the patient not to remove the air bubble in the syringe as the air bubble is used to ensure administration of the full dose. Rubbing the injection site post-administration will increase the likelihood of bruising and should be avoided.

115. Correct answer: B
Pepcid (famotidine) has been found to increase blood alcohol levels by delaying metabolism and may contribute to alcohol related injuries. Patients have been known to underestimate the amount, frequency, and size of consumed alcoholic beverages, but some medications, such as Pepcid, can sustain blood alcohol levels, contributing to risky behaviors. Risk of bleeding is amplified in patients who combine energy drinks containing ginseng or ginkgo balboa with alcohol.

116. Correct answer: A
Vasodilation and positive inotropy are the primary actions of milrinone. Milrinone is a cAMP inhibitor used primarily for congestive heart failure.

117. Correct answer: C
If a patient with hyperthyroidism on metoprolol suddenly stops taking the drug, the patient may experience a thyroid storm. If metoprolol is to be discontinued, the patient should slowly be weaned off while monitoring T3 and T4 levels. Leukopenia and bradycardia are adverse reactions of metoprolol administration.

118. Correct answer: A
If metoprolol dosing exceeds 400 mg daily, the patient should be monitored closely for bronchospasms. If the patient has a history of reactive airway disease, metoprolol dosing may need to be reduced. Patients may also experience fatigue, hallucinations, drowsiness, decreased HDP, and dry eyes and mouth.

119. Correct answer: D
Patients who miss a dose of Pradaxa should not take a dose within 6 hours of a scheduled dose. The nurse should tell the patient to send her medications home and the next dose will be administered by hospital staff when available from pharmacy. The nurse should alert the physician and plan to continue administration as ordered. Please note: As mentioned previously, Pradaxa has been reported to cause fatal bleeding and is under investigation by the FDA. We have included questions on this drug to help you with other key points for the PCCN exam if the drug is still in use.

120. Correct answer: A

As a nurse you would question an order for aspirin for any patient with recent history of varicella outbreak, either as chicken pox or shingles. Administration of aspirin places the patient at risk for Reye's Syndrome. Other patients at risk include any patient recovering from viral infection or a patient who exhibits presence of flu-like symptoms. The specific mechanism for the reaction and precipitation of Reye's Syndrome and aspirin administration is unknown, but failure to receive early treatment may lead to death. Initial symptoms of Reye's syndrome include persistent vomiting, listlessness, drowsiness, personality changes (irritability), and aggressive behavior.

121. Correct answer: B

Creatinine clearance is critical when dosing dabigatran etexilate (Pradaxa). Patients with a creatinine clearance >30 ml/min may be prescribed the full dose of Pradaxa at 150 mg bid. For patients with renal impairment and a creatinine clearance <30 ml/ml, the maximum dose of Pradaxa is 75 mg bid. An activated partial thromboplastin time and INR are used to determine the effectiveness of dabigatran therapy. An ECT (ecarin clotting time) is used to assess bleeding risk if the patient should require emergency surgery.

122. Correct answer: C

The aPPT should be monitored during administration of bivalirudin for early identification of life-threatening bleeding complications. As there is no antidote for bivalirudin overdose, administration via IV injection and infusion should be carefully monitored. Bivalirudin binds to free thrombin and thrombin in existing clots, placing patients at high risk for exsanguination from existing wounds and invasive procedures. In addition, a woman during menses may experience profound bleeding while receiving Angiomax.

123. Correct answer: C

The appropriate dose of prasugrel (Effient) for a patient weighing <60 kg (132 lbs) is 5 mg PO daily. For patients weighing >60 kg (132 lbs), the normal dose is 10 mg PO daily. Effient is metabolized in the liver and for patients weighing <60 kg, there is a potential for increased bleeding.

124. Correct answer: D

An order for fentanyl 0.5 mg IM q 1–2 hours for pain should be questioned immediately as the dose is 10 times the normal dose. Transcription errors lead to potentially life-threatening reactions. Despite the use of electronic medication records, some facilities still must transcribe physician orders to the electronic record, leading to medication errors. Decimal placement can often be missed in scanning and faxing orders to pharmacy. Order clarification by the nurse and pharmacy helps prevent such errors.

125. Correct answer: A

Avoidance of grapefruit or grapefruit juice does not impact digoxin administration or efficacy. High-fiber foods such as beans and brans taken with digoxin will impair digoxin absorption. Digoxin should be taken at the same time every day to avoid missing doses. Most patients understand that the heart rate should be checked prior to taking digoxin, but it is important that the patient also understand that the dose should be skipped if the heart rate is <60 bpm and to notify the prescribing physician as soon as possible.

126. **Correct answer: D**
Effient irreversibly binds with platelets (not thrombin) for the life of the platelet, which is 7–10 days. This is the primary reason why ceasing administration of Effient (prasugrel) will not immediately lead to improvement of life-threatening bleeding disorders.

127. **Correct answer: B**
If a patient receiving transdermal fentanyl (Duragesic) administration is experiencing skin irritation under the patch, the nurse should request concurrent administration of Kenalog (triamcinolone topical spray). The spray can be applied to the skin and the Duragesic patch applied over it to alleviate skin irritation. Kenalog does not inhibit or interfere with transdermal uptake of Duragesic. Although the patient did not complain about the skin irritation, proactive treatment may lead to better patient compliance. It is never appropriate to advise a patient to take any medication in a manner not prescribed. Cutting the patch or constantly moving the patch may interfere with normal uptake of the medication leading to adverse reactions.

128. **Correct answer: A**
This question requires the nurse to know both generic and brand names for commonly used medications. It is easy to confuse the names for many commonly used drugs. Midazolam is also known as Versed and an appropriate dose is 2.5 mg IVP over 2 min just prior to procedure.

129. **Correct answer: A**
The appropriate potency conversion from morphine to fentanyl is 100 mcg of fentanyl equals 10 mg of morphine.

130. **Correct answer: C**
Aspirin inhibits platelet aggregation by inhibiting thromboxane A2 production. Thromboxane A2 stimulates platelet aggregation.

131. **Correct answer: B**
Duragesic patches contain 2 g of sugar and diabetic patients will likely need a slight increase adjustment to insulin therapy to account for the additional sugar intake.

132. **Correct answer: C**
You would anticipate your patient admitted for a lateral MI to be started on aspirin therapy at 325 mg daily to reduce the risk of another MI. Dosage of 81 mg daily has been found insufficient to prevent and treat patients at risk for or after myocardial event. Instead, 160 mg daily has been recommended to prevent or reduce severity of an MI. Dosages exceeding 325 mg per day could quickly lead to salicylate poisoning.

133. **Correct answer: A**
A disadvantage of using negative pressure wound care devices is NPWC cannot be used on wounds associated with malignancies. Advantages of NPWC include promotion of a moist healing environment, removal of barriers to cell migration and proliferation, and removal of interstitial fluid.

MULTISYSTEM REFERENCES

Ahn, C., & Maitz, P. (2010). Volkmann's contracture in high-voltage electrical injury. *European Journal of Plastic Surgery, 33*(6), 323–329.

Ahn, C., Oneill, S., & Maitz, P. (2011). Improving accuracy of burn referrals through the use of an internet-based burns chart. *European Journal of Plastic Surgery, 34*(5), 331–335.

Ahrens, T., Prentice, D., & Kleinpell, R. M. (2011). *Progressive care nursing certification: Preparation, review and practice exams.* St. Louis, MO: McGraw-Hill.

American Association of Critical-Care Nurses. (2006). *AACN core curriculum for critical care nursing.* St. Louis, MO: Saunders.

Ascough, S., Ingram, R. J., & Altmann, D. M. (2012). Anthrax lethal toxin and the induction of CD4 T cell immunity. *Toxins, 4*(10), 878–899.

Atescelik, M., Bozdemir, M. N., Yildiz, M., Gurbuz, S., Ayranci, M., Goktekin, M. C., . . . Eken, C. (2012). QT dispersion in carbon monoxide poisoning. *European Review for Medical and Pharmacological Sciences, 16*(S1), 25–29.

Barbier, J., Bouclier, C., Johannes, L., & Gillet, D. (2012). Inhibitors of the cellular trafficking of ricin. *Toxins, 4*(1), 15–27.

Basalus, M., Said, S. A. M., Danse, P., Woltjer, H. H., & Fast, J. H. (2010). Dobutamine-mediated dynamic left ventricular outflow tract obstruction associated with hypovolemic shock: Value of echocardiography and importance of early recognition and appropriate volume substitution. *Open Cardiovascular Imaging Journal, 2*, 14–17.

Behroozian, R., Bayazidchi, M., & Rasooli, J. (2012). Systemic inflammatory response syndrome and MELD score in hospital outcome of patients with liver cirrhosis. *Middle East Journal of Digestive Diseases, 4*(3), 168–172.

Bitto, A., Polito, F., Altavilla, D., Irrera, N., Giuliani, D., Ottani, A., . . . Squadrito, F. (2011). Melanocortins protect against multiple organ dysfunction syndrome in mice. *British Journal of Pharmacology, 162*(4), 917–928.

Brooks, J. T., Buchacz, K., Gebo, K. A., & Mermin, J. (2012). HIV infection and older Americans: The public health perspective. *American Journal of Public Health, 102*(8), 1516–1526.

Brorsen, A. (2012). *CEN examination review.* Burlington, MA: Jones & Bartlett Learning.

Brorsen, A., & Rogelet, K. (2009). *PCCN certification review.* Sudbury, MA: Jones and Bartlett.

Butcher, M., & Swales, B. (2012). Assessment and management of patients with burns. *Nursing Standard, 27*(2), 50–56.

Cai, X., Long, Z., Lin, L., Feng, Y., Zhou, N., & Mai, Q. (2012). Serum cystatin C is an early biomarker for assessment of renal function in burn patients. *Clinical Chemistry & Laboratory Medicine, 50*(4), 667–671.

Carter, M. R., & Gaskins, S. W. (2010). Incorporating bioterrorism content in the nursing curriculum: A creative approach. *Journal of Nursing Education, 49*(7), 406–409.

Centers for Disease Control and Prevention [CDC]. (2012). West nile virus disease and other arboviral diseases: United States, 2011. *Morbidity & Mortality Weekly Report, 13*, 61.

Chulay, M., & Burns, S. (2010). *Essentials of progressive care nursing* (2nd ed.). St. Louis, MO: McGraw-Hill.

Craig, D. G., Reid, T. W., Martin, K. G., Davidson, J. S., Hayes P. C., & Simpson, K. J. (2011). The systemic inflammatory response syndrome and sequential organ failure assessment scores are effective triage markers following paracetamol (acetaminophen) overdose. *Alimentary Pharmacology & Therapeutics, 34*(2), 219–228.

Papathanassoglou, E., Bozas, E., & Giannakopoulou, M. D. (2008). Multiple organ dysfunction syndrome pathogenesis and care: A complex systems' theory perspective. *Critical Care, 13*(5), 249–259.

Curley, M. A. Q. (2007). *Synergy: The unique relationship between nurses and patients.* St. Louis, MO: Saunders.

Dasgupta, A. (2003). Urinary adulterants and drugs-of-abuse testing. *MLO: Medical Laboratory Observer, 35*(2), 26–29.

De Cori, S., Biancofiore, G., Bindi, L., Cosottini, M., Pesaresi, I., Murri, L., & Mascalchi, M. (2010). Clinical recovery despite cortical cerebral and cerebellar damage in heat stroke. *Neuroradiology Journal, 23*(1), 35–37.

Dewar, D. C., Butcher, N. E., King, K. L., & Balogh, Z. J. (2011). Post injury multiple organ failure. *Trauma, 13*(1), 81–91.

Dodge, M. R. (2010). SIRS: A systematic approach for medical-surgical nurses to stop the progression to sepsis. *MEDSURG Nursing, 19*(1), 11–15.

Donohoe-Dennison, R. (2007). *Pass CCRN* (3rd ed.). St. Louis, MO: Mosby.

Eisen, R. J., Kugeler, K. J., Ettestad, P., Reynolds, P. J., Brown, T., Enscore, R. E., . . . Schotthoefer, A. M. (2012). Changing socioeconomic indicators of human plague, New Mexico, USA. *Emerging Infectious Diseases, 18*(7), 1151–1154.

Feldman, M., Wu, E., Mendoza, M., Lowry, B., Ford, L., & Holloway, I. (2012). The prevalence and correlates of receiving confirmatory HIV test results among newly diagnosed HIV-positive individuals at a community-based testing center. *AIDS Education & Prevention, 24*(5), 445–455.

Fischer, T. Z., & Waxman, S. G. (2012). Extraterritorial temperature pain threshold abnormalities in subjects with healed thermal injury. *Journal of Rehabilitation Research & Development, 49*(4), 515–522.

Fraley, M. (2010). A silent death. *EMS World, 39*(11), 35–42.

Froude, J. W., Thullier, P., & Pelat, T. (2011). Antibodies against anthrax: Mechanisms of action and clinical applications. *Toxins, 3*(11), 1433–1452.

Fry, D. E. (2012). Sepsis, systemic inflammatory response, and multiple organ dysfunction: The mystery continues. *American Surgeon, 78*(1), 1–8.

Gabbe, B. J., Cleland, H. J., & Cameron, P. A. (2011). Profile, transport and outcomes of severe burns patients within an inclusive, regionalized trauma system. *ANZ Journal of Surgery, 81*(10), 725–730.

Gage, E., Hernandez, M. O., O'Hara, J. M., McCarthy, E. A., & Mantis, N. J. (2011). Role of the mannose receptor (CD206) in innate immunity to ricin toxin. *Toxins, 3*(9), 1131–1145.

Gallagher, J. C., Sai, A., Templin, T., & Smith, L. (2012). Dose response to vitamin D supplementation in postmenopausal women: A randomized trial. *Annals of Internal Medicine, 156*(6), 425–437.

Garretson, S., & Malberti, S. (2007). Understanding hypovolaemic, cardiogenic and septic shock. *Nursing Standard, 21*(50), 46–55, 58, 60.

Gibney, K. B., Colborn, J., Baty, S., Bunko Patterson, A. M., Sylvester, T., Briggs, G., . . . Staples, J. E. (2012). Modifiable risk factors for West Nile virus infection during an outbreak--Arizona, 2010. *The American Journal of Tropical Medicine and Hygiene, 86*(5), 895–901.

Greathouse, J. S., Stuart, J. L., & White Jr., W. A. (2012). Difficult airway management following severe gasoline burn injury: A case report. *AANA Journal, 80*(4), 268–272.

Griffiths, G. D. (2011). Understanding ricin from a defensive viewpoint. *Toxins, 3*(11), 1373–1392.

Guy, H., Alyanak, A., & Yılmaz, E. (2011). Cutaneous anthrax: Evaluation of 14 cases. *Klimik Journal, 24*(3), 176–178.

Hane, M., Rubin, E., & Foltin, R. W. (2011). Aripiprazole maintenance increases smoked cocaine self-administration in humans. *Psychopharmacology, 216*(3), 379–387.

Hardin, S., & Kaplow, R. (2005). *Synergy for clinical excellence: The AACN synergy model for patient care.* St. Louis, MO: Saunders.

Hayakawa, M., Katabami, K., Wada, T., Minami, Y., Sugano, M., Shimojima, H., . . . Gando, S. (2011). Imbalance between macrophage migration inhibitory factor and cortisol induces multiple organ dysfunction in patients with blunt trauma. *Inflammation, 34*(3), 193–197.

Herbst, R. T., Harris, E. D., Everhart, D. S., Mendelson, E. T., Jacob, J., & Jones, P. (2011). Cocaethylene formation following ethanol and cocaine administration by different routes. *Experimental and Clinical Psychopharmacology, 19*(2), 95–104.

Hicks, C. W., Xizhong, C., Sweeney, D. A., Yan, L., Barochia, A., & Eichacker, P. Q. (2011). The potential contributions of lethal and edema toxins to the pathogenesis of anthrax associated shock. *Toxins, 3*(9), 1185–1202.

Hranjec, T., Turrentine, F. E., Stukenborg, G., Young, J. S., Sawyer, R. G., & Calland, J. F. (2012). Burn-center quality improvement: Are burn outcomes dependent on admitting facilities and is there a volume-outcome "sweet-spot"? *American Surgeon, 78*(5), 559–566.

Iqbal, S., Clower, J. H., Hernandez, S. A., Damon, S. A., & Yip, F. Y. (2012). A review of disaster-related carbon monoxide poisoning: Surveillance, epidemiology, and opportunities for prevention. *American Journal of Public Health, 102*(10), 1957–1963.

Jacobsen, R. C., & Gratton, M. C. (2011). A case of unrecognized prehospital anaphylactic shock. *Prehospital Emergency Care, 15*(1), 61–66.

Jones & Bartlett Learning. (2011.) *2012 nurse's drug handbook. (*11th ed.). Sudbury, MA: Jones & Bartlett Learning.

Jones, G. (2002). Continuing professional development: Anaphylactic shock. *Emergency Nurse, 9*(10), 29–36.

Jovičić, S., Ignjatović, S., & Majkić-Singh, N. (2012). Biochemistry and metabolism of vitamin D. *Journal of Medical Biochemistry, 31*(4), 309–315.

Judit, K., Jung, J., Simona, G., Azamfirei, L., Sanda-Maria, C., Ruxandra, C., & Szederjesi, J. (2011). Pancreas injury in shock. *Acta Medica Marisiensis, 57*(6), 656–658.

Kannangai, R., David, S., & Sridharan, G. (2012). Human immunodeficiency virus type-2: A milder, kinder virus: An update. *Indian Journal of Medical Microbiology, 30*(1), 6–15.

Kong, V. Y. (2012). A tragic miscommunication: Ethical decision making in burns care. *Online Journal of Health Ethics, 8*(1), 1–10.

Krul, J., & Girbes, A. J. (2011). Gamma-hydroxybutyrate: Experience of 9 years of gamma-hydroxybutyrate (GHB)-related incidents during rave parties in The Netherlands. *Clinical Toxicology, 49*(4), 311–315.

Kumar, O., Pradhan, S., Sehgal, P., Singh, Y., & Vijayaraghavan, R. (2010). Denatured ricin can be detected as native ricin by immunological methods, but nontoxic in vivo. *Journal of Forensic Sciences, 55*(3), 801–807.

Liu, S., Lane, S. D., Schmitz, J. M., Waters, A. J., Cunningham, K. A., & Moeller, F. G. (2011). Relationship between attentional bias to cocaine-related stimuli and impulsivity in cocaine-dependent subjects. *The American Journal of Drug and Alcohol Abuse, 37*(2), 117–122.

Lloyd, E. C., Rodgers, B. C., Michener, M., & Williams, M. S. (2012, January 1). Outpatient burns: Prevention and care. *American Family Physician, 85*(1), 25–32.

Lynn-McHale Wiegand, D. J. (Ed.). (2011). *AACN procedure manual for critical care* (6th ed.). St. Louis, MO: Saunders.

Mailhot, G. (2012). Vitamin D bioavailability in cystic fibrosis: A cause for concern? *Nutrition Reviews, 70*(5), 280–293.

Makranz, C., Heled, Y., & Moran, D. S. (2011). Hypothermia following exertional heat stroke treatment. *European Journal of Applied Physiology, 111*(9), 2359–2362.

Mao, H., Yu, S., Yu, X., Zhang, B., Zhang, L., Hu, J., . . . Xing, C. (2011). Effect of coupled plasma filtration adsorption on endothelial cell function in patients with multiple organ dysfunction syndrome. *International Journal of Artificial Organs, 34*(3), 288–294.

Mazerolle, S., Ruiz, R. C., Casa, D. J., Pagnotta, K. D., Pinkus, D. E., Armstrong, L. E., & Maresh, C. M. (2011). Evidence-based practice and the recognition and treatment of exertional heat stroke, part I: A perspective from the athletic training educator. *Journal of Athletic Training, 46*(5), 523–532.

Mazerolle, S. M., Pinkus, D. E., Casa, D. J., McDermott, B. P., Pagnotta, K. D., Ruiz, R. C., . . . Maresh, C. M. (2011). Evidence-based medicine and the recognition and treatment of exertional heat stroke, part II: A perspective from the clinical athletic trainer. *Journal of Athletic Training, 46*(5), 533–542.

Miners, A. L. (2010). The diagnosis and emergency care of heat related illness and sunburn in athletes: A retrospective case series. *Journal of the Canadian Chiropractic Association, 54*(2), 107–117.

Montiel-Jarquín, Á., Láscarez-Lagunas, I., Sánchez-Gasca, C., Láscarez-Lagunas, L., García-Cano, E., Gómez-Conde, E., . . . Guerrero-Fernández, M. E. (2012). Lactate clearance is a prognostic factor in patients on shock state. *European Journal of General Medicine, 9*(2), 98–103.

Moon, J. M., Shin, M. H., & Chun, B. J. (2011). The value of initial lactate in patients with carbon monoxide intoxication: In the emergency department. *Human & Experimental Toxicology, 30*(8), 836–843.

Morel, N., Chabarttier, C., Merson, L., Lelias, A., Bernard, J. C., Delaunay, F., . . . Janvier, G. (2012). Advantage of using a recombinant activated factor VII in traumatic haemorrhagic shock: The Bordeaux experience. *Journal of Emergencies, Trauma & Shock, 5*(2), 143–148.

Murphy, P., Colwell, C., Pineda, G., & Bryan, T. (2009). Burning issues: By understanding the pathophysiology of burns, providers can give patients their best chance at good outcomes. *EMS Magazine, 38*(10), 83–90.

Murphy, S. (2010). Carbon monoxide poisoning. *Nursing Standard, 24*(40), 50–56.

Nesmith, E. G., Weinrich, S. P., Andrews, J. O., Medeiros, R. S., Hawkins, M. L., Weinrich, M. C., & Jones, R. (2011). Substance use and the systemic inflammatory response syndrome (SIRS) following trauma. *Journal of Trauma Nursing, 18*(2), 79–86.

O'Donovan, K. (2011). Cardiogenic shock complicating myocardial infarction: An overview. *British Journal of Cardiac Nursing, 6*(6), 280–285.

Payne, S., & Cole, E. (2012). Treatment of acute burn blisters in unscheduled care settings. *Emergency Nurse, 20*(5), 32–37.

Peterson, J. L., Miner, M. H., Brennan, D. J., & Rosser, B. R. S. (2012). HIV treatment optimism and sexual risk behaviors among HIV positive African American men who have sex with men. *AIDS Education & Prevention, 24*(2), 91–101.

Picariello, C., Lazzeri, C., Valente, S., Chiostri, M., Attanà, P., & Gensini, G. F. (2010). Kinetics of procalcitonin in cardiogenic shock and in septic shock. Preliminary data. *Acute Cardiac Care, 12*(3), 96–101.

Pierson, D. J. (2012). Does aspirin reduce mortality in the systemic inflammatory response syndrome? *Critical Care Alert, 20*(4), 30–31.

Pincus, S. H., Smallshaw, J. E., Kejing, S., Berry, J., & Vitetta, E. S. (2011). Passive and active vaccination strategies to prevent ricin poisoning. *Toxins, 3*(9), 1163–1184.

Rabjohn, L. V., & Roberts, K. (2012). Burn injuries of the foot and ankle. *Podiatry Management, 31*(3), 199–208.

Rowley-Conwy, G. (2012). Management of minor burns in the emergency department. *Nursing Standard, 26*(24), 60, 62, 64–67.

Sarwar, U., Nicolaou, M., Khan, M. S., & Tiernan, E. (2011). Air-freshener burns: A new paradigm in burns etiology & quest. *International Journal of Preventive Medicine, 2*(4), 291–293.

Schodin, B. A. (2012). Vitamin D: How much is enough, too much, or too little? *Medical Laboratory Observer, 44*(2), 26–30.

Sekhar, K. S., Pradhan, H. K., & Pattnaik, B. (2012). Bioterrorism: How prepared are we? *Indian Journal of Medical Specialties, 3*(1), 43–48.

Shan, M., Hafeez, S., & Mehmood, K. T. (2010). Management of burns. *Journal of Pharmaceutical Sciences & Research,* 2(8), 492–498.

Simpson, C., & Abelsohn, A. (2012). Heat-induced illness. *Canadian Medical Association Journal, 184*(10), 1170.

Smith, C. R., Tucker, J. R., Wilson, B. A., & Clover, J. R. (2010). Plague studies in California: A review of long-term disease activity, flea-host relationships and plague ecology in the coniferous forests of the Southern Cascades and northern Sierra Nevada mountains. *Journal of Vector Ecology: Journal of the Society for Vector Ecology, 35*(1), 1–12.

Song, R., Bian, H., Wang, X., Huang, X., & Zhao, K. S. (2011). Mitochondrial injury underlies hyporeactivity of arterial smooth muscle in severe shock. *American Journal of Hypertension, 24*(1), 45–51.

Spagnolo, F., Costa, M., Impellizzeri, M., Cardamone, R., Falautano, M., Martinelli, V., . . . Volonte, M. A. (2011). Delayed hyperbaric oxygen treatment after acute carbon monoxide poisoning. *Journal of Neurology, 258*(8), 1553–1554.

Srinivasan, A., Song, X., Ross, T., Merz, W., Brower, R., & Perl, T. M. (2002). A prospective study to determine whether cover gowns in addition to gloves decrease nosocomial transmission of vancomycin-resistant enterococci in an intensive care unit. *Infection Control and Hospital Epidemiology, 23*(8), 424–428.

Stephenson, J. A., Gravante, G., Butler, N. A., Sorge, R., Sayers, R. D., & Bown, M. J. (2010). The systemic inflammatory response syndrome (SIRS): Number and type of positive criteria predict interventions and outcomes in acute surgical admissions. *World Journal of Surgery, 34*(11), 2757–2764.

Straight, J. R., Knight, A. R., Zebley, J. L., Anderson, D., & Pierce, J. D. (2007). Fluid resuscitation therapy for hemorrhagic shock. *Journal of Trauma Nursing, 14*(3), 152–162.

Vaughn, M. G., Fu, Q., Perron, B. E., Bohnert, A. S., & Howard, M. O. (2010). Is crack cocaine use associated with greater violence than powdered cocaine use? Results from a national sample. *The American Journal of Drug and Alcohol Abuse, 36*(4), 181–186.

Watcher, R. (2012). *Understanding patient safety* (2nd ed.). Los Altos, CA: Lange.

Werdan, K., Ruß, M., Buerke, M., Delle-Karth, G., Geppert, A., & Schöndube, F. A. (2012). Cardiogenic shock due to myocardial infarction: Diagnosis, monitoring, and treatment. *Deutsches Aerzteblatt International, 109*(19), 343–351.

Wright, J. G., Quinn, C. P., Shadomy, S., & Messonnier, N. (2010). Use of anthrax vaccine in the United States: Recommendations of the Advisory Committee on Immunization Practices (ACIP), 2009. *MMWR Recommendations & Reports, 59*(RR-6), 1–30.

Zhaochun, C., Moayeri, M., & Purcell, R. (2011). Monoclonal antibody therapies against anthrax. *Toxins, 3*(8), 1004–1019.

Zhenyu, L., Yanbing, L., Hao, T., Bin, L., Zhibin, C., Jingguo, W., . . . Zhongfu, M. (2010). Effect of anaphylactic shock on suppressors of cytokine signaling. *Immunological Investigations, 39*(7), 740–753.

Zimbudzi, E., Stuart, R. L., Korman, T. M., & Kotsanas, D. (2011). Contamination of renal patients' hospital chart covers with vancomycin-resistant enterococci: Handle with care. *Australasian Medical Journal, 4*(10), 538–541.

Zimmerman, E., Frieberg, E. M., DeBord, J., Akingbola, O., Yang, S. G., & Yosypiv, I. V. (2012). Acute onset of multi-organ system dysfunction. *Clinical Pediatrics, 51*(1), 96–98.

Section 12

Behavioral/Psychosocial

SECTION 12: BEHAVIORAL/PSYCHOSOCIAL QUESTIONS

1. **Supporting and respecting the culture, beliefs, and values of the progressive care patient is known as**
   A. Standard of care
   B. Moral agency
   C. Duty
   D. Advocacy

2. **Many times nurses experience conflicts when asked to assist patients with decision making. The obligation to assist the patient in making a decision when the patient does not have sufficient data or expertise is called**
   A. Paternalism
   B. Moral agency
   C. Interdependence
   D. Assumptive thinking

3. **In health care, actions are right or wrong based on a set of rules and morals. This ethical approach is known as**
   A. Social contact theory
   B. Deontology
   C. Moral agency
   D. Natural law

4. **If your patient is seeking freedom from a sense of worthlessness and loneliness, the patient is at the ________________ level of Maslow's Hierarchy of Needs.**
   A. Self-actualization
   B. Esteem and recognition
   C. Love and belonging
   D. Safety and security

5. **Individuals who are driven toward unacceptable behaviors and who redirect their energy into more socially acceptable behaviors are using a psychological defense mechanism called**
   A. Resolution
   B. Compensation
   C. Repression
   D. Sublimation

6. **Alcohol abuse may lead to a deficiency in micronutrients that in turn may cause depression and suicidal behavior. One of these micronutrients is**
   A. Potassium
   B. Copper
   C. Sodium
   D. Selenium

7. **The false belief that something is wrong with one's body or body part is called**
   A. Malingering
   B. Hypochondriasis
   C. Transference
   D. Somatic delusion

8. **A 20 year old was admitted for observation after fighting at a friend's house. She has a right fractured humerus, a right Colles' fracture, mild concussion, and right orbital fracture. When paramedics arrived, she was found talking to herself, resisted medical care, and stated she could heal herself. During your assessment you find the patient withdrawn, irritable, fatigued, and indecisive about what to do with her clothing. Your next action should be to**
   A. Request a drug screen
   B. Request a psychologist evaluation for schizophrenia
   C. Request a social worker to assess the patient's home life
   D. Evaluate the patient for feelings of suicide

9. **A false perception that is not grounded in reality and not accounted for by external stimuli is called**
   A. A fugue
   B. A hallucination
   C. An idea of reference
   D. Disorientation

10. **Your patient is a college student and was admitted to your unit after ingesting about 50 extra-strength acetaminophen tablets. Until now he has refused to say why he ingested the drug. About an hour after arrival, you find him crying. When you ask him why he is crying, he tells you he was sexually assaulted by an unknown male 3 weeks ago and he is afraid this will brand him a homosexual. Which of the following responses is the most therapeutic?**
    A. "Don't worry, you'll get over this and be okay"
    B. "Let me get the psychologist to come talk with you tomorrow"
    C. "Why do you believe this will make you a homosexual?"
    D. "What is wrong with being a homosexual?"

11. **Binge eating, mutilation, obesity, drug abuse, and alcoholism are all examples of**
    A. Self-destructive behavior
    B. Psychotic behavior
    C. Neurosis
    D. A fugue

12. **As the educator for your progressive care unit, you note an increased frequency of patients with underlying mental disorders being admitted. You overhear some negative comments regarding nursing assignments for these patients. You ask the nurses to complete a self-awareness survey regarding their beliefs and understanding of mental health issues. You should use this information to**
    A. Determine which nurses should never care for patients with mental health issues
    B. Change nursing assignments immediately
    C. Determine which nurses should be written up and counseled
    D. Create an education program for the nurses to increase understanding of mental health issues and learn how to access resources

13. **Your staff in the progressive care unit has just completed an unsuccessful code on a 20 year old woman. Due to an unexpected cardiac event, the patient did not survive. Chaplain services are called in to assist with a nursing staff debriefing. Staff members experiencing which of the following emotions are at highest risk for psychological stress?**
    A. Anger
    B. Fear
    C. Anxiety
    D. Denial

14. **Your patient is a gang member and heavy alcohol abuser. During a fight almost 24 hours ago, the patient was shot in the leg and hand. His gang members left him at the entrance to the ED with a note explaining the injuries sustained the previous night. You observe the patient thrashing around in the bed, and he is suddenly awake when you enter the room. He is shaking, has vomited, and is tachycardic, hypertensive, and talking to people not in the room. You suspect he is**
    A. Exhibiting signs of paranoid schizophrenia
    B. Experiencing delirium tremens
    C. Experiencing sepsis
    D. Experiencing drug withdrawal

15. **Within a Chinese family, cultural values and practices may include which of the following beliefs?**
    A. Chi is an external energy
    B. Disease is caused by disharmony with society
    C. Medicinal herbs are important
    D. Family involvement in limited

16. **Signs and symptoms of anorexia nervosa may include**
    A. Tachycardia
    B. Absent menses
    C. Hyperthermia
    D. Hyperactivity

17. Your patient is being evaluated for adult ADHD. Which of the following conditions or abnormalities is expected to be present if he has ADHD?

A. A cousin with hyperthyroidism

B. Eye problems

C. A heart murmur

D. None

18. Mr. K. is waiting for surgery for a fractured tibia. Despite being heavily medicated for pain, he continually demands to have his cell phone and a computer pad in his room. His wife says Mr. K. spends too much time on the computer at home. The patient insists he only spends about an hour after work on the computer and texting his friends. Mr. K. probably suffers from

A. Internet addiction

B. Bipolar disorder

C. Depression anxiety

D. Separation anxiety

19. Which of the following statements is untrue regarding responses to posttraumatic stress disorder?

A. Patients are less likely to socialize

B. Patients may have decreased ability to complete home or work tasks

C. Patients may become irritable and hostile

D. Patients may exhibit regressive behaviors

20. Which of the following statements is true about posttraumatic stress disorder?

A. Only war veterans experience PTSD

B. PTSD is easy to diagnose

C. Multiple traumatic events heighten the risk of PTSD

D. Patients become less aggressive

21. M. and H. are the parents of a 20 year old with leukemia. Their daughter just died. Initially, the parents stay a little while in the PCU waiting room and have a glazed expression while at their daughter's bedside. As a nurse, you recognize their response as

A. Adaptation to the environment

B. The initial steps to coping

C. The initial response to a crisis

D. Normal and does not need to be addressed

22. During discharge teaching, you notice multiple bruises on the arms and reddened areas on the neck of your patient's sister. You suspect she is being physically abused. What other indicator would support your assessment?

A. Extroverted behavior

B. Denial of abuse when asked directly

C. She volunteers information

D. Hesitance to discuss home situation

23. You are caring for a patient who was the driver in a motor vehicle accident in which a child was killed. She is combative and restless, hyperventilating, tachycardic, and has an elevated blood pressure. She states, "I've got to leave

here... they'll arrest me...they'll lock me up...I can't believe this... there is no way out." You should tell her

A. "They should arrest you, you killed a child."
B. "Calm down. It wasn't your fault."
C. "Stop it. You are working yourself up. Look at me and focus on what I am telling you to do."
D. "Just relax. They can't arrest you because you are a patient here."

24. **Your patient, a drug abuser with cirrhosis, has returned again to your unit after failing rehabilitation. Although you previously had a friendly and open relationship, he will not look at you and only answers minimally to questions. You tell him**
    A. "I can't believe you wasted the opportunity at the rehabilitation center."
    B. "I know you want to stay drug-free but now you will have a permanent criminal record."
    C. "Why don't we work together to find new resources for you to use when you are tempted to take one of these drugs?"
    D. "I am proud of how long you stayed sober. Let's try again."

25. **Your patient was admitted to the PCU after fainting at work secondary to bradycardia and malnutrition. She is 67 inches tall but weighs only 93 pounds. You find her crying, sitting on the edge of her bed. She tells you that she is worried the intravenous fluid will make her gain weight. What is the most effective way to manage this problem?**
    A. Have her boyfriend talk to her
    B. Ask if she wants to speak to her minister
    C. Ask the physician for a dietary consult
    D. Ask for a patient conference with the healthcare team and family

26. **You are obtaining a patient's history when you notice multiple rotted teeth. You suspect bulimia nervosa. The patient tells you she regularly purges after meals so she can meet the weight standards for her job. What family dynamics would you expect to find associated with bulimia nervosa?**
    A. No significant family dynamics are noted with bulimia nervosa
    B. A family history of drug abuse or psychiatric disorders
    C. A strong sense of ego
    D. Poor scholastic performance

27. **Depression often devastates families and often goes undiagnosed and misunderstood by families, the public, and the medical community. Which of the following statements is also true regarding depression?**
    A. Depression is only seen in maltreated individuals
    B. Depression is easy to diagnose
    C. The elderly do not respond to antidepressant therapy
    D. Depression is recurrent and may increase in severity

28. **In the United States, Asperger's syndrome is considered to be which of the following types of disorders?**
    A. Developmental delay disorder
    B. Autistic spectrum disorder

C. Pervasive developmental disorder
D. Attention deficit disorder

29. **W. has sickle-cell anemia and is a frequent patient in your progressive care unit. You were told in report that W.'s siblings were escorted out of the unit for arguing in the hallway about financial difficulties and responsibilities. During your assessment, W. appears to have difficulty concentrating on your questions and is withdrawn and restless. When attempting to engage her in activities, she refuses and states that she "wants to be alone." You should**
A. Respect her wishes and go care for your other patient
B. Leave the room to contact her husband
C. Straighten her room while looking for sharp objects or potential dangers
D. Leave the room to contact the patient's physician

30. **Your patient was admitted from the ED for appendicitis. She is grimacing and will not allow you to assess her abdomen. The hospitalist ordered Demerol for pain. Approximately 10 minutes after administration of the Demerol, the patient is combative, has pulled her IV out, has torn off her IV dressing, and is screaming at the staff. Your next action should be to**
A. Apply restraints by yourself as additional staff may scare the patient
B. Wear personal protective equipment to enter her room to apply restraints
C. Call security to help subdue the patient
D. Use a Posey restraint system to subdue the patient

31. **The fear of crowds is known as**
A. Acrophobia
B. Agoraphobia
C. Arachnophobia
D. Aschizophobia

32. **Your patient is explaining his history to you when he simply stops speaking and looks around the room. His behavior is known as**
A. Rude
B. Affect
C. Blocking
D. Amnesia

33. **Simultaneous existence of contradictory or contrasting emotions toward a person or object is known as**
A. Apathy
B. Double bind
C. Depersonalization
D. Ambivalence

34. **Which of the following medications is not considered an antimanic drug?**
A. Klonopin
B. Tegretol
C. Lithium
D. Tofranil

35. Which of the following is classified as an antianxiety drug?

A. Restoril
B. Elavil
C. Sinequan
D. Tofranil

36. Your patient cut his forearm and requires several stitches. He begins to hallucinate midway through the procedure. He is demanding, loud, and very insistent. His behavior worsens and disrupts the staff. You could categorize his behavior as

A. Paranoid
B. Self-absorbed
C. Deteriorating
D. Overanxious

37. Your patient's family is frustrated that their family member has not improved during the week since being placed on Elavil. The patient has remained depressed, so the family brought the patient to the hospital to determine the cause of the continuing depression. As a progressive care nurse, you know

A. The Elavil dose is not high enough to be therapeutic
B. Elavil is causing an idiosyncratic reaction in this patient
C. The patient must not be taking the medication
D. Elavil may take up to 3 weeks to become effective

38. A patient undergoing an assessment for an ear injury becomes agitated because his friend was not allowed to accompany him to the treatment area. Despite reassurances that the exam will not take long, the patient throws a chair into the wall and begins disconnecting the suction and oxygen apparatus from the wall. Your first priority is to

A. Call a code
B. Be firm and establish clear limits on behavior
C. Leave the room
D. Sedate the patient

39. Which of the following drugs is classified as an MAO inhibitor?

A. Nardil
B. Cogentin
C. Artane
D. Akineton

40. A side effect after administration of an antipsychotic drug that causes muscle spasms is known as

A. Dystonia
B. Expression
C. Latency
D. Delusion

41. Your patient has been taking an antipsychotic medication. She is now suffering from drooling, muscle tremors, and has difficulty walking. This patient is exhibiting

A. Boundary effects
B. Extrapyramidal effects

C. Dystonic effects
D. Latent effects

42. **Your 22 year old patient inhaled a large amount of cocaine. He is now complaining of paresthesias and "something small like little pieces of rock crawling under my skin." This condition is a type of psychosis and is known as**
A. Magnan's sign
B. Drummond's sign
C. Cullen's sign
D. Wilder's sign

43. **Acetaminophen overdose may cause hypoglycemia and should be treated with a**
A. Continuous IV infusion of D_5W at 100 cc/hour
B. Bolus of D10, continuous infusion of 0.45% normal saline
C. Bolus of D50, continuous infusion of D_5W
D. Continuous IV infusion of Lactated Ringer's

44. **Your patient is undergoing alcohol withdrawal and exhibits diplopia, peripheral neuropathy, confusion, recent memory loss, and hyperexcitability. You suspect that this patient is suffering from**
A. Jorn's syndrome
B. Leucine deficiency
C. Increased caritine levels
D. Wernicke–Korsakoff syndrome

45. **Bath salts contribute to multiple overdoses. Bath salts are very addictive psychoactive chemicals that are presumed to include synthetic cocaine and an ecstasy variety in their components. Symptoms of bath salts overdose would not include**
A. Hallucinations and delusions
B. Self-injury behavior and suicide attempts
C. Profound lethargy
D. Extreme agitation

46. **The effects of the high dosage of bath salts are similar to the trip of amphetamines, cocaine, and methamphetamine. Treatment of bath salts overdose would include**
A. Phenylalanines
B. Phentermines
C. Benzodiazepines
D. Ephedrines

47. **An antidote for ethylene glycol toxicity is**
A. Digoxin
B. Anisindione
C. Fomepizole
D. Narcan

48. **GHB (Ecstasy) overdoses can lead to amnesia in approximately what percentage of cases?**
A. 13%
B. 21%

C. 24%
D. 32%

49. Factors that may affect results of urine morphine levels would not include

A. Poppy seed ingestion may produce false-positive results
B. 10 mg MS IV may be detectable in urine up to 84 hours
C. Use of stealth adulterant to cause negative results in a positive sample
D. High levels of lymphocytes will mask morphine in urine

50. Your patient is experiencing delirium tremens. Nursing interventions include keeping the room well lit and minimizing stimulation. Staff members continuously reorient the patient to time, place, and person. Haldol has been given as ordered, and the patient is in four-point restraints. Which of these nursing interventions should be discontinued?

A. Reorientation
B. Medication administration
C. Restraints
D. Controlling stimulation

51. Your patient is a young woman with diffuse abdominal pain and confusion. Just after admission, she had generalized seizures and bradycardia. Opioid overdose was suspected and she was given naloxone with only minimal effect. The patient is now lethargic, but does tell you she is a "body packer" to help pay for beauty school. She becomes hypotensive and bradycardic. Appropriate therapy includes

A. Bowel irrigations, intubation, mechanical ventilation, anticonvulsants
B. Sodium bicarbonate activated charcoal, hemodialysis
C. Antiemetics, gastric lavage, bronchodilators
D. Activated charcoal, sodium bicarbonate, vasopressors

52. When treating salicylate overdose, which of the following goals is appropriate for this condition?

A. A hypocalcemic state
B. Urine pH of 7 to 8
C. Resolution of jaundice
D. Entry of salicylate into the CNS

53. Bath salts withdrawal symptoms are similar to methamphetamine withdrawal. These symptoms would include

A. Agitation
B. Euphoria
C. Increased appetite
D. Melancholy

54. The word is used to describe observable behavior that represents the expression of a subjectively experienced feeling state (emotion) is known as

A. Lability
B. Affect
C. Constricted
D. Blunt

55. Excessive motor activity that accompanies and is associated with a feeling of inner tension, and is usually nonproductive and repetitious, is called

A. Displacement
B. Assertion
C. Paranoia
D. Agitation

56. Your patient has dementia. The physician places a pen in the patient's hand while the patient has their eyes closed. The patient is unable to recognize the object as a pen. This failure to recognize objects despite intact sensory function is known as

A. Cognition
B. Conversion
C. Displacement
D. Agnosia

57. Patients with dementia often lose their ability to taste. An inability to taste is known as

A. Dysgeusia
B. Dysgnathia
C. Micrognathia
D. Macrognathia

58. An organ that is part of the limbic system and involved in some aspects of memory, control of the autonomic functions, and in emotional expression is the

A. Pituitary gland
B. Hippocampus
C. Locus coeruleus
D. Pineal gland

59. Which of the following drugs has a half-life of approximately 24 hours and requires continuous doses of naloxone?

A. Demerol
B. Heroin
C. Cocaine
D. Methadone

60. The triad of symptoms usually associated with opioid overdose is

A. Respiratory depression, meiosis, and coma
B. Obtundation, hypotension, and ventricular arrhythmias
C. Confusion, slurred speech, and seizures
D. Stupor, respiratory alkalosis, and hypotension

61. The specific antidote for a benzodiazepine overdose is

A. Calcium chloride
B. Flumazenil
C. Atropine
D. Calcium gluconate

62. The specific antidote for methamphetamine is

A. Desipramine
B. Alkalinizing agents

C. There is no antidote
D. Naloxone

63. **Patients who are undergoing alcohol withdrawal are frequently hypoglycemic. Treatment should include**
A. Bolus of D10W, q 2 hour blood glucose monitoring
B. TPN with high concentrations of sugars, q 2 hour blood glucose monitoring
C. Maintenance fluids of $D_{25}W$ at 125 ml/h peripherally
D. Thiamine, then bolus with D50, then infusion of D_5W

64. **Which of the following illegal drugs is the most commonly abused?**
A. Marijuana
B. Toluene
C. Cocaine
D. Heroin

65. **The useful organization and incorporation of both new and old data, experience, and emotional capacities into the personality is called**
A. Introspection
B. Solidarity
C. Introversion
D. Integration

66. **Patients who have schizophrenia sometimes exhibit opposition or resistance, either covertly or overly, to outside suggestions or advice. This behavior is known as**
A. Projection
B. Negativism
C. Manipulation
D. Antagonism

67. **You are assessing a 25 year old patient who appears euphoric and confused. While looking around the room, you note a chewed up pacifier on the bed. Why would the pacifier be significant?**
A. It was left from a previous patient
B. The patient may have been using the pacifier prior to your entering the room
C. The pacifier was caught in the railing and torn
D. The patient's children were in the room just before you arrived

68. **The drug of choice for the treatment of tricyclic antidepressant overdose is**
A. Atropine
B. Imipramine
C. Doxepin
D. Sodium bicarbonate

69. **A cyclic antidepressant that may cause cardiovascular effects and will probable cause status epilepticus is**
A. Amoxapine
B. Amitriptyline
C. Desipramine
D. Doxepin

70. A patient intoxicated with methamphetamine would exhibit which of the following conditions?

A. Elevated liver enzymes
B. Bradycardia
C. Hypothermia
D. Hypotension

71. Lithium is used as an antipsychotic medication to treat bipolar disorder. Lithium toxicity is deadly. Which of the following statements is true regarding lithium toxicity?

A. Toxicity may occur if blood levels reach 1 mEq/L
B. Signs of lithium toxicity include constipation, hypertonicity, and giddiness
C. Untreated lithium toxicity may lead to seizures, coma, and cardiac dysrhythmias
D. Lithium toxicity may be treated safely on a medical–surgical floor

72. Your patient gave birth 2 months ago to a healthy baby boy. She has been suffering from postpartum depression. She was admitted with hallucinations, agitation, ventricular arrhythmias, and a possible seizure (witnessed by her husband). She has been taking a tricyclic antidepressant. Which of the following drugs is classified as a tricyclic antidepressant?

A. Amitriptyline
B. Gentamicin
C. Clonidine
D. Fluvastatin

73. Continuing with the scenario above, the patient's husband said the last time the patient took one of prescribed doses of her amitriptyline was last evening. A blood level was drawn in the ED and considered a trough level. This patient's treatment should include

A. Hemodialysis
B. Sodium bicarbonate
C. Syrup of Ipecac
D. Trazodone

74. Methamphetamine is officially classified as a(n)

A. Stimulant
B. Euphoric
C. Hallucinogen
D. Antidepressant

75. The use of alkalinizing agents for the treatment of methamphetamine overdose is

A. Not necessary
B. Only to be used if seizures are present
C. Contraindicated
D. The only method to treat the resultant muscle spasms

76. The primary symptoms of cocaine toxicity include hyperthermia, hyperactivity, tachycardia, and hypertension. These symptoms may be managed by administration of

A. Morphine
B. Fentanyl

C. Codeine
D. Ativan

77. Which of the following conditions is least likely to affect an elderly patient's ability to counter psychiatric emergencies?
A. Altered or reduced problem-solving and coping mechanisms
B. Stable health
C. Increased loss of or limited support systems
D. Greater financial pressures or limited resources

78. A woman who is 8 months pregnant was severely injured in an automobile accident. Her condition has been declining over the past week. The husband has been informed of the probable demise of his wife. The patient was made a "Do not resuscitate" and moved to the PCU because she requires more care than the staff on the orthopedic unit can provide. In addition, the physician suspects fetal demise and has notified the husband of this possibility. The husband wants to bring their only other child, an 8 year old boy, into the PCU to visit his mother. The PCU has a policy that children must be 12 years old to visit. What is an appropriate nursing action at this time?
A. Sneak the child in during night shift
B. Take a picture of the mother for the child
C. Arrange a patient care conference as soon as possible to discuss options
D. Inform the husband that the visiting policy is strictly enforced

79. Your patient is a 52 year old father of six, who has suffered a heart attack and requires immediate coronary artery bypass graft. His children and wife are present as well as multiple other family members and church members. You overhear his wife and children speaking about complete insurance coverage; they state that the patient's employer has approved significant sick time for his recovery and has offered him the chance to work from home if additional home recuperation time is required. You are determining the level of psychiatric distress in this family. Your first priority is to
A. Administer psychotic medications
B. Examine the range and effectiveness of coping mechanisms
C. Work with any available family members, friends, or religious support systems
D. Determine if there is a crisis

80. Your patient is the lone survivor of a car crash that killed her parents and two siblings. She is recovering from a pneumothorax, hemothorax, and a left fractured tibia. She has been extremely depressed and withdrawn. You are discussing medications, psychiatric therapy, and the increased risk of suicide and suicidal behavior with the patient's distant relatives. The family members make each of the following statements. Which of the statements is false?
A. "If she is considering suicide, she will make statements or give warnings of suicide."
B. "We should trust our instincts if we feel she is in danger."
C. "As she recovers from her depression, she is at greater risk of suicide."
D. "If she talks about suicide or asks about pills, then she is just voicing the thought and will not attempt suicide."

81. Continuing with the scenario from the previous question, as the patient recovers from her injuries, her behavior and moods change rapidly. Which of the following behaviors is most concerning to you as the nurse and indicates possible suicidal behavior?

A. Drug seeking with multiple requests for pain medications and sedatives
B. Withdrawal from conversation and interaction
C. Crying and statements of helplessness
D. Screaming at her distant relatives

82. Your patient is a 46 year old admitted to the PCU after a barroom brawl in which he suffered multiple minor stab wounds. He is angry and verbally assaults the staff. The goal of anger management for this patient would not include

A. Confronting the patient directly with whatever made him angry
B. Discussing what in particular made the patient angry
C. Discussing with the patient alternative and positive ways to express his feelings
D. Developing positive ways for the patient to express his feelings when confronted with frustrating situations in the future

83. Your patient had a three-vessel CABG procedure and sustained a small stroke during the procedure. The stroke left some residual numbness in the left arm. The family is quite agitated and does not agree with the patient's advance directives. The family informs you that they want everything done for the patient and to ignore the patient's request for no resuscitative measures. Which of the following nursing interventions would be appropriate at this time?

A. Inform the family that the physician will meet with them to discuss treatment options
B. Tell the patient about the family's concerns
C. Notify the physician that all orders are to come from the family
D. Inform the family that the patient is fully capable of making decisions

84. Your patient is scheduled for implantation of a VAD. About 20 minutes prior to the scheduled start of the procedure, she informs you that she has concerns about side effects and the procedure itself. Your best nursing intervention would be to

A. See if the patient signed the consent form for the procedure
B. Notify the physician that the patient does not have a full understanding of the procedure
C. Cancel the procedure
D. Answer the patient's questions yourself

85. A car carrying four teenagers went off a bridge and killed all but one of the teens. Today, a second EEG was done and brain death was confirmed for the fourth teen. The family was approached about organ donation. They requested that the patient remain in the PCU for at least 7–8 days until the older sister can return from a war zone. The appropriate nursing response would be to

A. Tell the family other patients are waiting for the bed
B. Notify the physician to tell the family organ donation must be made within 24 hours
C. Notify social services and arrange for emergency compassionate leave for the sister
D. Wait until the family leaves to procure the organs

86. Your patient suffered a concussion. She is currently unable to recognize familiar faces. This symptom is not explained by defective visual acuity or reduced consciousness or alertness. Her condition is called

A. Symbolization
B. Thought insertion
C. Transference
D. Prosopagnosia

87. Which of the following patients are most likely to exhibit signs of posttraumatic stress disorder (PTSD)?

A. A 15 year old runaway boy
B. A 25 year old female who witnessed a murder
C. A 37 year old man arrested for his first DUI
D. A 68 year old lady who experienced a 3.5 earthquake

88. As a part of your assessment of a patient experiencing posttraumatic stress disorder, which of the following symptoms are most likely to occur?

A. Denial that anything is wrong
B. Total recall of the event
C. Duration of symptoms longer than one week
D. Willingness to discuss the incident

89. While examining a veteran who was a prisoner of war, what behavior would you expect to observe?

A. A well-kept patient who has had the same job for 15 years
B. An anxious man who keeps asking where his car keys are
C. A patient who is unkempt and becomes agitated when asked the date
D. A street person who lost their job 6 months ago

90. The stage between normal forgetfulness due to aging and the development of dementia is called

A. Loss of problem solving
B. Mild cognitive impairment
C. Pre-Alzheimers
D. Delirium

91. Getting lost on familiar routes, having difficulty balancing a checkbook, and misplacing items may be signs of

A. Delirium
B. Dementia
C. Depression
D. Confusion

92. A mood state characterized by pessimistic thinking, lowered self-esteem, sadness, and guilt is called

A. Fugue
B. Delirium
C. Withdrawal
D. Depression

93. **Patients with posttraumatic stress disorder may experience recurrence of a memory, feeling, or perceptual experience from the past. This condition is known as a**
   A. Disintegration
   B. Euthymia
   C. Flashback
   D. Fantasy

94. **A model of health and illness that suggests that links among the nervous system, the immune system, behavioral styles, cognitive processing, and environmental factors can put people at risk for illness is called a (an)**
   A. Integration model
   B. Centration model
   C. Synergy model
   D. Biopsychosocial model

95. **A key to prevention of excess mortality and morbidity in patients at risk for alcohol withdrawal is the appropriate use of an instrument designed to assess the level of risk for alcohol withdrawal. An example of an instrument to assess risk of alcohol withdrawal is the**
   A. Bevington scale
   B. P.O.L.A.R.I. scale
   C. AWSS scale
   D. CIWA-AR scale

SECTION 12: BEHAVIORAL/PSYCHOSOCIAL ANSWERS

1. **Correct answer: D**
   Supporting and respecting the culture, beliefs, and values of the progressive care patient is known as advocacy.

2. **Correct answer: A**
   The obligation to assist the patient in making a decision when the patient does not have sufficient data or expertise is called paternalism. The nurse has the duty to do no harm (non- maleficence) and should not take away the patient's autonomy.

3. **Correct answer: B**
   In health care, actions are right or wrong based on a set of rules and morals. This ethical approach is known as deontology. Deontology emphasizes duty (obligation) to another human being.

4. **Correct answer: B**
   If your patient is seeking freedom from a sense of worthlessness and loneliness, the patient is at the esteem and recognition level of Maslow's Hierarchy of Needs.

5. **Correct answer: D**
   Individuals who are driven toward unacceptable behaviors and who redirect their energy into more socially acceptable behaviors are using a psychological defense mechanism called sublimation.

6. **Correct answer: D**
   Alcohol abuse may lead to a deficiency in micronutrients that in turn may cause depression and suicidal behavior. One of these micronutrients is selenium.

7. **Correct answer: D**
   The false belief that something is wrong with one's body or body part is called somatic delusion. Malingering is the deliberate manufacturing of an illness to prolong treatment. Hypochondriasis is morbid concern with one's body or health in the absence of a physical cause.

8. **Correct answer: D**
   You should first evaluate the patient's feelings, paying close attention to any statements indicating a risk for suicide or injury to staff. Morgan is now exhibiting signs of depression after a manic episode. Patients with psychotic elements exhibited with mania, depression, or both may be misdiagnosed with schizophrenia, anxiety disorder, and/or drug abuse. Patients with bipolar disorder may swing between moods over minutes, hours, or days. Symptoms include hallucinations, delusions, and aggressive or violent behavior. Careful history may reveal a trend of manic and depressive episodes that would clarify Morgan's true condition and lead to faster and correct treatment. A social worker should be involved, but ensuring immediate patient and staff safety is the primary concern.

9. **Correct answer: B**
   A false perception that is not grounded in reality and not accounted for by external stimuli is called a hallucination.

10. **Correct answer: C**

This patient has opened up to you, and it is important to maintain the communication. Finding out why he feels homosexuality is bad gives insight to the suicide attempt. There are many other legal and ethical issues that have to be handled with this case. It is obvious he will need psychological counseling. After your conversation you must follow your hospital's policy/procedure manual about reporting such incidents. "Don't worry, you'll get over this and be okay" and "Let me get the psychologist to come talk with you tomorrow" are not therapeutic, and they negate his feelings. Asking, "What is wrong with being a homosexual?" could be perceived as threatening.

11. **Correct answer: A**

Binge eating, mutilation, obesity, drug abuse, and alcoholism are all examples of self-destructive behavior. Self-destructive behaviors are those that over time will shorten or threaten length and quality of life.

12. **Correct answer: D**

You ask the nurses to complete a self-awareness survey regarding their beliefs and understanding of mental health issues. You should use this information to create an education program for the nurses to increase understanding of mental health issues and learn how to access resources. Surveys can be used to anonymously identify staff perceptions and determine educational opportunities. Mental health issues impact every person at some point in their lives. Whether due to a catastrophic event or ongoing psychological issues, it is important that nurses understand their own biases regarding mental health and be able to identify resources when caring for this population. If the nurses believe the survey will be used punitively, then data may be skewed to what the staff believe the surveyor is looking for, not the truth. Instead of changing assignments immediately, it is best to use the opportunity for education and professional growth.

13. **Correct answer: C**

Anger, fear, and denial are normal emotions in this situation, but staff members that feel anxiety are at the greatest risk. Anxiety is a common emotion found in psychological emergencies. Anxiety involves uncertainty of the unknown and may limit the person's ability to identify resources or initiate appropriate coping mechanisms. Debriefings after codes, both successful and unsuccessful, are therapeutic and allow staff to verbalize emotions in a safe and stable environment. As a team, the staff may identify ways to support families and each other during crisis and emergency situations.

14. **Correct answer: B**

The timing of this patient's symptoms is consistent with alcohol withdrawal or delirium tremens (DTs). DTs usually are seen 12 to 24 hours after last ingestion of alcohol as blood alcohol levels drop. Effects may peak up to 15 days after DTs begin. Fluids, vitamins, nutrition, and short-term pharmacologic treatments are appropriate. The severity of symptoms is affected by the amount and duration of alcohol ingestion as well as underlying physical health, other drugs, and existing psychological status. There are no indications at this time that the patient is septic or has schizophrenia. There may be underlying drug withdrawal symptoms.

15. **Correct answer: C**

Many cultures may have beliefs and practices that may influence medical management of the patient in the hospital setting. The Chinese often use medicinal herbs and religious beliefs regarding internal energy known as a person's chi to manage health. Cultural beliefs must be acknowledged as influential in patient care regardless of staff beliefs.

16. **Correct answer: B**
Patients with anorexia nervosa may have a diminished or absent menses. Other signs and symptoms may include bradycardia, hypothermia, fatigue, GERD, electrolyte abnormalities, hair loss, and loss of tooth enamel.

17. **Correct answer: D**
In most cases, no additional abnormalities are found. However, if there is a family history of ADHD, there is a higher probability of an individual having ADHD.

18. **Correct answer: A**
There is actually a diagnosis of Internet addiction. The American Psychiatric Association is developing criteria for this diagnosis. Criteria currently recognized are: lying about time spent on the Internet, avoiding friends or family to be on the Internet, anxiety when the Internet is not available, and increasing hours spent on the Internet. Academic and work performance often suffers. Internet addiction rehabilitation centers are becoming more prevalent. Mr. K. needs a referral to a mental health practitioner. At present, it is believed that approximately 9 million Americans fulfill the criteria for IA and 30% of those with IA have one or more comorbid psychiatric disorders.

19. **Correct answer: B**
Patients with PTSD may have diminished concentration and are unable to concentrate on home or work tasks. Patients often regress, have increased anxiety, become aggressive, suffer panic attacks, avoid family, and reenact the event frequently. Patients with PTSD are more likely to attempt suicide than their peers without PTSD.

20. **Correct answer: C**
Posttraumatic stress disorder may result in many different symptoms. If the patient experiences multiple traumatic events, the risk for developing PTSD increases. Additional causes of PTSD can include physical or sexual abuse, neglect, harassment, death of a significant other, accidents, war, terrorist attacks, disasters, or life-threatening illnesses/injuries. PTSD may also be caused by witnessed domestic violence, suicide, or murder.

21. **Correct answer: C**
The death of their daughter is causing the parents to experience the initial response to a crisis. The death may have been expected eventually, but now involves an environment and circumstances beyond the parent's experience or ability to cope. The crisis may last for weeks depending on available support systems, the healthcare team, parent education, culture, and spiritual intervention.

22. **Correct answer: B**
Abuse may be suspected if the sister denies abuse in the presence of bruising, injury to bones, and ecchymosis around the throat. Many abused women and children have stories of a positive home life and excuses to explain injuries due to clumsiness. Due to the likely introverted personalities of abused individuals, it is important to establish a safe zone and trust to encourage honest communication and to begin assistance to escape the abuse.

23. **Correct answer: C**
The goal at this point is to regulate the patient's breathing and stabilize vital signs. Using a firm and quiet voice with simple sentences can help the severely anxious patient focus and diffuse the anxiety. Severely anxious individuals are less able to see options and cope at this stage. Goals should include decreasing any unnecessary stress and remaining available to the patient for communication. The statement, "Calm down. It wasn't your fault" speaks to facts not known. Statements like, "They should arrest you, you killed a child" are judgmental.

24. **Correct answer: C**
"Why don't we work together to find new resources for you to use when you are tempted to take one of these drugs?" is the appropriate statement. Sometimes patients are "frequent flyers" and relationships are developed with certain progressive care staff. The patient may feel as if he has failed the nurse by not remaining sober and that assistance may be withdrawn. This statement does not judge the patient and shows the patient the help is still available by initiating communication and encouraging the patient to talk about his struggles with staying away from drugs.

25. **Correct answer: D**
This patient has anorexia. It is very difficult to treat anorexia nervosa and often requires a team approach. This patient and her significant others may need psychological counseling as well as medical and nutritional assistance. The important concern for the progressive care nurse is the impact the anorexia has on the body and the patient's recovery. The typical anorexic may have multiple complications of one or more body systems. She may have symptoms such as cardiac arrhythmias, EKG abnormalities, amenorrhea, esophagitis, anemia, dehydration, electrolyte imbalances, peripheral neuropathy, hematuria, and osteopenia.

26. **Correct answer: B**
Family dynamics you would expect to find associated with bulimia nervosa include a strong family history of similar disorders, drug abuse, and psychiatric disorders. Bulimia nervosa is often seen in patients who are overachievers, trying to please those around them. These patients often do very well in school and have above-average intelligence. They also have poor self-esteem or self-image problems.

27. **Correct answer: D**
Depression is recurrent and may increase in severity. Many cases report that after the first depressive episode, as many as 40% of individuals will experience another episode within 2 years. Often, these patients are diagnosed with multiple psychiatric disorders such as anxiety disorder, dysthymic disorders, disruptive behavior, or substance abuse. Depression may be seen in any patient, although environmental factors such as maltreatment can contribute to risk of depression. A patient with chronic illness, infection, or certain biochemical factors is also at risk for depression. Depression is difficult to diagnose unless there is an understanding of depression and risk factors. Unfortunately, depression can be just as severe in children and teens as in adults and is associated with approximately 80% of childhood and teen suicides. Undiagnosed and untreated depression can continue into adulthood impacting personal and professional relationships and the ability to function successfully in society.

28. **Correct answer: C**
Asperger's syndrome is a pervasive developmental disorder. Patients affected by this disorder are eccentric in their behavior and social interactions. Men are affected by this disorder at a 4:1 ratio over women. There is no known cause of Asperger's syndrome, but it often occurs with fragile X syndrome, hypothyroidism, and neurofibromatosis. The condition is generally diagnosed between 3 and 11 years of age. About one-fourth of those affected grow out of their condition by adulthood.

29. **Correct answer: C**
This patient is exhibiting signs of depression and should not be left alone until you have determined she is not a danger to herself or others. While straightening her room you should note any potential items that could be used to harm herself or others. If the items can be removed, do so; if not, attempt to lessen the danger. The patient's depression may have been brought on by many factors such as her prolonged and recurrent illness, family financial and emotional stress, and feelings of guilt or anger regarding her frequent hospital visits. Only after ensuring the patient's safety should the nurse leave the room to contact the physician, social worker, case manager, charge nurse, and manager. If the patient's mental health continues to deteriorate, she may need constant observation for suicide or restraints applied. The patient's husband will need to be contacted and updated, but it is important that the staff have a clear plan of action with him. This includes family support, financial guidance, specialist support, and, most importantly, a plan for W.'s mental and physical health.

30. **Correct answer: B**
When entering this patient's room or any patient's room to apply restraints, wear appropriate personal protective equipment to protect yourself against exposure to bodily fluids. The patient most likely has had a psychotic reaction to the Demerol and has exposed her IV site and removed her IV, resulting in a potential for exposure to bodily fluids. When attempting to place restraints on a combative patient, regardless of the age, at least four staff members should be present—one for each limb. The family should not be asked to participate in placement of the restraints as they are untrained and it may be seen as a betrayal by the patient. Instead, family members should remain at a safe distance to avoid injury or interference with healthcare providers. A Posey is not the best choice because it leaves the patient's hands free to continue pulling on IV lines. Whenever restraints are in use, be vigilant to document continued need of restraints, type used, time placed, vital signs including airway, breathing, and circulation before and after restraints are placed, time of removal, and reassessments. Be sure to follow your facility's restraint protocols and policies. Patient and staff safety is paramount.

31. **Correct answer: B**
The fear of crowds is known as agoraphobia. A phobia is a fear or dread of an act, an object, or a situation that is usually not realistically dangerous. However, the patient perceives that danger exists.

32. **Correct answer: C**
When a patient simply stops talking and there is a gap or interruption in speech that is related to absent thoughts or distractions, it is known as blocking.

33. **Correct answer: D**
Simultaneous existence of contradictory or contrasting emotions toward a person or object is known as ambivalence.

34. **Correct answer: D**
Tofranil is an antidepressant. Tegretol, klonopin, and lithium are all antimanic drugs.

35. **Correct answer: A**
Restoril is classified as an antianxiety drug. Elavil, sinequan, and tofranil are all classified as tricyclic medications.

36. **Correct answer: C**
Because this patient's behavior is escalating, the correct categorization of the behavior is "deteriorating." The patient may be exhibiting some paranoid tendencies, but the cause of the hallucinations is unknown at this time.

37. **Correct answer: D**
Elavil and tricyclics in general may take up to 3 weeks to become effective. It is appropriate to reassure the patient and the family and make certain all parties verbalize understanding.

38. **Correct answer: B**
This patient is acting out his frustration. It is important to act immediately to set firm clear goals and limits to behavior. It is crucial you remain with the patient until he calms down, then attempt to discuss his feelings. Obviously, if you believe you or the patient is in imminent danger, call for help.

39. **Correct answer: A**
Nardil is classified as an MAO inhibitor. Parnate and marplan are also MAO inhibitors. Cogentin, artane, and akineton are antiparkinson drugs.

40. **Correct answer: A**
A side effect after administration of an antipsychotic drug that causes muscle spasms is known as dystonia.

41. **Correct answer: B**
The patient's drooling, muscle tremors, and difficulty walking are similar to those of patients who suffer from Parkinson's disease and are known as extrapyramidal effects.

42. **Correct answer: B**
This condition is a type of psychosis and is known as Drummond's sign. Cocaine users have paresthesias, psychoses, and imagine they have a foreign body, in the shape of a powder or fine sand, under the skin that it is constantly changing its position.

43. **Correct answer: C**
Acetaminophen overdose may cause hypoglycemia and should be treated with a bolus of D_{50}, and a continuous infusion of D_5W. Hypoglycemia occurs because of the hepatotoxic effects of acetaminophen. Infusions must also be based on blood glucose results.

44. **Correct answer: D**
The patient undergoing alcohol withdrawal and who exhibits diplopia, peripheral neuropathy, confusion, recent memory loss, and hyperexcitability has Wernicke–Korsakoff syndrome. Wernicke–Korsakoff syndrome is a thiamine deficiency and a metabolic encephalopathy.

45. **Correct answer: C**
Symptoms of bath salts overdose would not include profound lethargy. Symptoms of bath salts overdose include arrhythmias, paranoia, extreme agitation, superhuman strength and combativeness, and hypertension.

46. **Correct answer: C**
The effects of the high dosage of bath salts are similar to the trip of amphetamines, cocaine, and methamphetamine. Treatment of bath salts overdose would include benzodiazepines.

47. **Correct answer: C**
An antidote for ethylene glycol toxicity is fomepizole. Ethylene glycol is a compound found in antifreeze. After ingestion, it is converted to oxalic acid, which is excreted by the kidneys. This causes crystals in the urine, acidosis, tetany, and renal failure. Hemodialysis and peritoneal dialysis will remove ethylene glycol.

48. **Correct answer: A**
GHB (Ecstasy) overdoses can lead to amnesia in approximately 13% of cases. Ecstasy can also cause ataxia, central nervous system depression, coma, bradycardias, hypothermia, hypotension, hypothermia, respiratory depression, and respiratory acidosis.

49. **Correct answer: D**
Factors that may affect results of urine morphine levels would not include high levels of lymphocytes. The stealth adulterant masks morphine in the urine. Poppy seed ingestion may produce false-positive results. When heroin is taken, it breaks down into morphine. Ten milligrams of morphine is detectable in urine for 84 hours and can be measured in corpses for about a week.

50. **Correct answer: C**
Restraints should only be used if alternative methods for behavioral correction are ineffective. There is no indication that the patient is violent or has caused any threat to staff or self. Restraints should only be used as a last resort to prevent injury to self and staff. Reorientation, medication, and controlling external stimulation are all effective methods for controlling behavior.

51. **Correct answer: A**
"Body packer" is a term used for people who transport narcotics in body cavities. In this case, it is probable that a packet may have ruptured. Bowel irrigations, intubation, mechanical ventilation, and anticonvulsants may be required as treatments for this patient. More doses of naloxone may be necessary, along with supportive treatment for opioid overdose. Be alert for bradycardia, hypotension, respiratory depression, and hypothermia.

52. **Correct answer: B**
A urine pH of 7 to 8 is an appropriate goal for a patient treated for salicylate overdose.

53. **Correct answer: D**
Bath salts withdrawal symptoms are similar to methamphetamine withdrawal. These symptoms would include melancholy, fatigue, decreased appetite, difficulty sleeping, psychotic behaviors, anxiety, and depression.

54. **Correct answer: B**
The word is used to describe observable behavior that represents the expression of a subjectively experienced feeling state (emotion) is known as affect. Types of affect include flat, labile, euthymic, irritable, constricted, blunted and inappropriate.

55. **Correct answer: D**
Excessive motor activity that accompanies and is associated with a feeling of inner tension and is usually nonproductive and repetitious is called agitation. As nurses, we observe agitation frequently in patients who fidget, wring their hands, pull on clothes or bedding, and who are unable to lie or sit still.

56. **Correct answer: D**
The failure to recognize objects despite intact sensory function is known as agnosia and is often seen in patients with dementia.

57. **Correct answer: A**
Patients with dementia often lose their ability to taste. An inability to taste is known as dysgeusia.

58. **Correct answer: B**
An organ that is part of the limbic system and involved in some aspects of memory, control of the autonomic functions, and in emotional expression is the hippocampus.

59. **Correct answer: D**
Methadone has a half-life of approximately 24 hours and requires continuous doses of naloxone. The continuous doses prevent respiratory depression until the methadone is eliminated from the patient's system.

60. **Correct answer: A**
Respiratory depression, meiosis, and coma are the triad of symptoms associated with opioid overdose.

61. **Correct answer: B**
Flumazenil is a specific antidote for benzodiazepine overdose. This drug should not be used on patients who overdose on tricyclic antidepressants because of an increased risk of seizures.

62. **Correct answer: C**
There is no specific antidote for methamphetamine. It is only possible to treat symptoms as they appear. Desipramine may cause sustained activity of amphetamines in the brain. Alkalinizing agents may potentiate the actions of amphetamines.

63. **Correct answer: D**
Patients who are undergoing alcohol withdrawal are frequently hypoglycemic. Treatment should include thiamine, then bolus with D50, and then start an infusion of D_5W.

64. **Correct answer: A**
Marijuana is the most commonly abused illegal drug in the world. In many countries and some states, medicinal marijuana has been legalized and closely regulated. For more information regarding statistics for a specific area and current ranking, the U.S. government websites at http://www.dea.gov and http://www.nida.nih.gov are updated frequently. Toluene is the addictive chemical in glue.

65. **Correct answer: D**
The useful organization and incorporation of both new and old data, experience, and emotional capacities into the personality is called integration.

66. **Correct answer: B**
Patients who have schizophrenia sometimes exhibit opposition or resistance, either covertly or overly, to outside suggestions or advice. This behavior is known as negativism.

67. **Correct answer: B**
A chewed-up pacifier and presentation of euphoria and confusion should lead the staff to consider Ecstasy addiction and abuse. Ecstasy, or methylenedioxymethamphetamine (MDMA), causes trismus, or teeth grinding. Users may chew on pacifiers to preserve teeth and hide the grinding from others.

68. **Correct answer: D**
Sodium bicarbonate is used to treat tricyclic overdose. Imipramine and doxepin are both tricyclics.

69. **Correct answer: A**
Amoxapine is a cyclic antidepressant that may cause cardiovascular effects and will probably cause status epilepticus. The patient often requires intubation and muscular paralysis because of seizures.

70. **Correct answer: A**
A patient intoxicated with methamphetamine exhibits elevated liver enzymes, tachycardia, hyperthermia, and hypertension.

71. **Correct answer: C**
Untreated lithium toxicity may lead to seizures, coma, and cardiac dysrhythmias when levels reach greater than 2.5 mEq/L. Toxicity usually occurs with levels of 2 mEq/L, but symptoms may be noted at even lower blood levels with certain body chemistries. Initial toxicity is noted when the patient experiences diarrhea, vomiting, drowsiness, muscular weakness, and disorientation. As toxicity and symptoms worsen, nystagmus, ataxia, giddiness, tinnitus, confusion, and blurred vision may be present. Patients must be managed by close monitoring and immediate intervention of dysrhythmias and electrolyte imbalances.

72. **Correct answer: A**
Amitriptyline is classified as a tricyclic antidepressant. A tricyclic antidepressant acts by blocking norepinephrine and serotonin uptake in the central nervous system. They also have anticholinergic properties. The really interesting thing about this group of drugs is that they metabolize in the liver to one of the other tricyclics. You must test for levels of all the tricyclics because the one you are testing for may have metabolized and exacerbated the effect on the patient.

73. **Correct answer: B**
This patient's treatment should include sodium bicarbonate. ABG results should guide the amount to be given. Hemodialysis will not remove amitriptyline from the system. Syrup of Ipecac is not indicated, especially because the patient ingested the medication last evening. You may give hypertonic saline for hypotension.

74. **Correct answer: C**
Methamphetamine is officially classified as a hallucinogen by *The Diagnostic and Statistical Manual of Mental Disorders*. The World Health Organization (WHO) published a list that shows methamphetamine as the second-most-abused chemical substance. The drug may be ingested, smoked, injected, inserted into the anus or urethra, or

snorted. Street names include crystal meth, big blue, base, and ice. The base of the drug is pseudoephedrine or ephedrine mixed with common ingredients. The mixture is often highly explosive and the first warning a meth lab is nearby is when it blows up.

75. **Correct answer: C**
Alkalinizing agents may potentiate the actions of amphetamines, so their use is contraindicated. As mentioned previously, there is no specific antidote for methamphetamine. It is only possible to treat symptoms as they appear.

76. **Correct answer: D**
Ativan may be used to control the symptoms of cocaine toxicity.

77. **Correct answer: B**
Stable health is least likely to affect an elderly patient's ability to counter a psychiatric emergency. Often elderly persons have unstable health that contributes to psychiatric crisis and emergency. Many elderly individuals have limited support systems. Time and circumstances may result in loss of loved ones by death or distance. They often have altered or reduced problem-solving and coping mechanisms. Limited ability to work, disabilities, greater financial pressures, or limited resources and funds may also lead to greater emotional and psychiatric distress because of financial issues.

78. **Correct answer: C**
The most appropriate nursing action would be to arrange a patient care conference as soon as possible to discuss options. This is the best nursing response because it ensures that all members of the healthcare team can join in the decision. Visiting policies vary, but are primarily designed to protect children from disease and from being overwhelmed by equipment and the PCU milieu. Under the circumstances, you would probably want to sneak the kid in on night shift, but many factors should be weighed here. This visit could have a profound effect on the child's last memory of his mother. The conference will weigh the child's maturity and coping ability. He and the father will probably lose the mother and the sibling. There is no simple answer.

79. **Correct answer: D**
In any potential psychiatric emergency or crisis, it is important to determine if one actually exists. In this scenario, the patient has an extensive and involved support system, financial stability, and effective coping mechanisms, so a psychiatric crisis is not likely to develop. It is still important to carefully monitor for any change in status.

80. **Correct answer: D**
"If she talks about suicide or asks about pills, then she is just voicing the thought and will not attempt suicide." is not an accurate statement. Careful consideration and observation should be given to any person voicing any thought or plan regarding suicide. Many individuals will provide warnings about their suicidal thoughts, thereby providing those in the family or in proximity the opportunity to intervene. Such warnings are often cries for help and intervention. Family members should pay close attention to any impression or instinct that the person is considering suicide. As individuals enter and exit depression, they are at greatest risk for suicide as they have sufficient mental focus to form a plan and energy or motivation to carry it out.

81. **Correct answer: C**
Feelings of helplessness or hopelessness indicate psychotic emergencies. Extreme anxiety or ability to recognize options should alert staff and family that the person is at

greater risk of suicide, because suicide may be seen by the patient or individual as the only option. The other answers indicate depression and/or levels of grief and emotional expression.

82. **Correct answer: A**
The goal of anger management for this patient would not include confronting the patient directly with whatever made him angry. Direct confrontation with the object of anger may further exacerbate the situation and limit the person's ability to deal positively with the situation. Instead, engage the person in a conversation regarding the stressor and assist him in identifying feelings and options.

83. **Correct answer: D**
Sometimes family members do not have enough education to make proper decisions. In this case, the family needs to know that the patient is still capable of making decisions and that his wishes will be honored.

84. **Correct answer: B**
Even if the patient signed a consent form, she does not appear to be certain about the procedure or is not fully informed. The nurse must act as advocate and notify the physician.

85. **Correct answer: C**
The appropriate nursing response would be to notify social services. In the best possible world, the military could arrange for compassionate leave for the military service member. Hospital personnel certainly should not simply go ahead and try to procure organs as soon as the family leaves.

86. **Correct answer: D**
Your patient suffered a concussion. She is currently unable to recognize familiar faces. This symptom is not explained by defective visual acuity or reduced consciousness or alertness. Her condition is called prosopagnosia and often resolves when the brain injury heals.

87. **Correct answer: B**
A person who witnesses an intense event is at risk for PTSD. The symptoms may last months or even years. Other factors that influence how the person responds include their mental state at the time of the event, the intensity of the event, and any medical complications.

88. **Correct answer: A**
Denial is often seen in people with PTSD. Most people with PTSD will have trouble recalling the event and even omit significant details. Other symptoms include avoidance of people and places that remind them of the traumatic event; flattened affect, flashbacks, nightmares, and hallucinations may also occur. Symptoms must last more than a month to establish PTSD.

89. **Correct answer: C**
Patients with PTSD may exhibit anxiety, agitation, or even delusions. A stable person is able to maintain a job for many years. Other behaviors may include forgetfulness, suicidal ideation, depression, and fear.

90. **Correct answer: B**
The stage between normal forgetfulness due to aging and the development of dementia is called mild cognitive impairment. People with MCI have mild problems with

thinking and memory that do not interfere with everyday activities. They are often aware of the forgetfulness. Not everyone with MCI develops dementia.

91. **Correct answer: B**
Getting lost on familiar routes, having difficulty balancing a checkbook, and misplacing items may be signs of dementia. Additional early signs of dementia are inability to learn new information or routines, losing interest in things previously enjoyed, personality changes and loss of social skills.

92. **Correct answer: D**
A mood state characterized by pessimistic thinking, lowered self-esteem, sadness, and guilt is called depression.

93. **Correct answer: C**
Patients with posttraumatic stress disorder may experience recurrence of a memory, feeling, or perceptual experience from the past. This condition is known as a flashback.

94. **Correct answer: D**
A model of health and illness that suggests that links among the nervous system, the immune system, behavioral styles, cognitive processing, and environmental factors can put people at risk for illness is called a biopsychosocial model.

95. **Correct answer: D**
An example of an instrument to assess risk of alcohol withdrawal is the Clinical Institute Withdrawal Assessment of Alcohol Scale, Revised (CIWA-Ar). The CIWA-Ar measures 10 symptoms. Mild withdrawal is indicated by a score of less than 8. Autonomic arousal (moderate) withdrawal is indicated by a score between 8 and 15. Scores of 15 or more indicate impending delirium tremens. Appropriate use of this scale helps staff individualize and modify treatment regimens as needed. The CIWA-Ar categories and ranges are as follows:

Agitation	(0–7)
Anxiety	(0–7)
Auditory disturbances	(0–7)
Clouding of Sensorium	(0–4)
Headache	(0–7)
Nausea/Vomiting	(0–7)
Paroxysmal Sweats	(0–7)
Tactile disturbances	(0–7)
Tremor	(0–7)
Visual disturbances	(0–7)

BEHAVIORAL/PSYCHOSOCIAL REFERENCES

Agar, M., Draper, B., Phillips, P., Phillips, J., Collier, A., Harlum, J., & Currow, D. (2012). Making decisions about delirium: A qualitative comparison of decision making between nurses working in palliative care, aged care, aged care psychiatry, and oncology. *Palliative Medicine, 26*(7), 887–896.

Ahrens, T., Prentice, D., & Kleinpell, R. M. (2011). *Progressive care nursing certification: Preparation, review and practice exams*. St. Louis, MO: McGraw-Hill.

Ali, S., Patel, M., Jabeen, S., Bailey, R. K., Patel, T., Shahid, M., . . . Arain, A. (2011). Insight into delirium. *Innovations in Clinical Neuroscience, 8*(10), 25–34.

American Association of Critical-Care Nurses. (2006). *AACN core curriculum for critical care nursing*. St. Louis, MO: Saunders.

Andrejaitiene, J., & Sirvinskas, E. (2012). Early post-cardiac surgery delirium risk factors. *Perfusion, 27*(2), 105–112.

Angela, C. (2011). Identification and management of in-hospital drug-induced delirium in older patients. *Drugs & Aging, 28*(9), 737–748.

Arend, E., & Christensen, M. (2009). Delirium in the intensive care unit: A review. *Nursing in Critical Care, 14*(3), 145–154.

Baker, A. L., Kavanagh, D. J., Kay-Lambkin, F. J., Hunt, S. A., Lewin, T. J., Carr, V. J., & Connolly, J. (2010). Randomized controlled trial of cognitive-behavioural therapy for coexisting depression and alcohol problems: Short-term outcome. *Addiction, 105*(1), 87–99.

Balas, M. C., Rice, M., Chaperon, C., Smith, H., Disbot, M., & Fuchs, B. (2012). Management of delirium in critically ill older adults. *Critical Care Nurse, 32*(4), 15–26.

Balas, M. C., Vasilevskis, E. E., Burke, W. J., Boehm, L., Pun, B. T., Olsen, K. M., . . . Ely, E. W. (2012). Critical care nurses' role in implementing the "ABCDE bundle" into practice. *Critical Care Nurse, 32*(2), 35–48.

Ballard, C., Kahn, Z., & Corbett, A. (2011). Treatment of dementia with Lewy bodies and Parkinson's disease dementia. *Drugs & Aging, 28*(10), 769–777.

Bisschop, P. H., de Rooij, S. E., Zwinderman, A. H., van Oosten, H. E., & van Munster, B. C. (2011). Cortisol, insulin, and glucose and the risk of delirium in older adults with hip fracture. *Journal of the American Geriatrics Society, 59*(9), 1692–1696.

Boettger, S., Friedlander, M., Breitbart, W., & Passik, S. (2011). Aripiprazole and haloperidol in the treatment of delirium. *Australian & New Zealand Journal of Psychiatry, 45*(6), 477–482.

Britton, M. E. (2011). Drugs, delirium and older people. *Journal of Pharmacy Practice & Research, 41*(3), 233–238.

Brorsen, A. (2012). *CEN examination review*. Burlington, MA: Jones & Bartlett Learning.

Brorsen, A., & Rogelet, K. (2009). *PCCN certification review*. Sudbury, MA: Jones and Bartlett.

Burge, D., Kent, W., Verdon, J., Voogt, S., & Haines, H. M. (2010). Nurse practitioners are well placed to lead in the effective management of delirium. *Australian Journal of Advanced Nursing, 28*(1), 67–73.

Buschert, V. C., Friese, U., Teipel, S. J., Schneider, P., Merensky, W., Rujescu, D., . . . Buerger, K. (2011). Effects of a newly developed cognitive intervention in amnestic mild cognitive impairment and mild Alzheimer's disease: A pilot study. *Journal of Alzheimer's Disease, 25*(4), 679–694.

Buxton, J. A., & Dove, N. A. (2008). The burden and management of crystal meth use. *Canadian Medical Association Journal, 178*(12), 1537–1539.

Carlson, E., Dalenberg, E. B., & McDade-Montez, C. (2012). Dissociation in posttraumatic stress disorder part I: Definitions and review of research. *Psychological Trauma: Theory, Research, Practice, and Policy, 4*(5), 479–489.

Chulay, M., & Burns, S. (2010). *Essentials of progressive care nursing* (2nd ed.). St. Louis, MO: McGraw-Hill.

Clegg, A., Young, J., & Siddiqi, N. (2012). Delirium in cardiac patients: A clinical review. *British Journal of Cardiac Nursing, 7*(3), 111–115.

Conley, D. M. (2011). The gerontological clinical nurse specialist's role in prevention, early recognition, and management of delirium in hospitalized older adults. *Urologic Nursing, 31*(6), 337–342.

Critical Care Nurse. (2012). Delirium assessment and management. *Critical Care Nurse, 32*(1), 79–82.

Critical Care Nurse. (2012). EB55: Detecting delirium in patients in the surgical intensive care unit: Implementing the Confusion Assessment Method-Intensive Care Unit tool. *Critical Care Nurse, 32*(2), 5–6.

Critical Care Nurse. (2012). EB117: Using the evidence to decrease delirium. *Critical Care Nurse, 32*(2), e66–e67.

Critical Care Nurse. (2012). EB120: Who's delirious: Leading the way in identifying delirium in critically ill patients across a 13-hospital network. *Critical Care Nurse, 32*(2), 3–4.

Cruickshank, C. C., & Dyer, K. R. (2009). A review of the clinical pharmacology of methamphetamine. *Addiction, 104*(7), 1085–1099.

Curley, M. A. Q. (2007). *Synergy: The unique relationship between nurses and patients*. St. Louis, MO: Saunders.

Czincz, J., & Hechanova, R. (2009). Internet addiction: Debating the diagnosis. *Journal of Technology in Human Services, 27*(4), 257–272.

Donohoe-Dennison, R. (2007). *Pass CCRN* (3rd ed.). St. Louis, MO: Mosby.

Ervin, K., & Koschel, A. (2012). Dementia care mapping as a tool for person-centred care. *Australian Nursing Journal, 19*(10), 32–55.

Etgen, T., Sander, D., Bickel, H., & Forstl, H. (2011). Mild cognitive impairment and dementia: The importance of modifiable risk factors. *Deutsches Aerzteblatt International, 108*(44) 743–750

Fisher, G. G., Franks, M. M., Plassman, B. L., Brown, S. L., Potter, G. G., Llewellyn, D., . . . Langa, K. M. (2011). Caring for individuals with dementia and cognitive impairment, not dementia: Findings from the aging, demographics, and memory study. *Journal of the American Geriatrics Society, 59*(3), 488–494.

Förster, S., Buschert, V. C., Teipel, S. J., Friese, U., Buchholz, H. G., Drzezga, A., . . . Buerger, K. (2011). Effects of a 6–month cognitive intervention on brain metabolism in patients with amnestic MCI and mild Alzheimer's disease. *Journal of Alzheimer's Disease, 26*(S3), 337–348.

Geda, Y. E., Silber, T. C., Roberts, R. O., Knopman, D. S., Christianson, T. J., Pankratz, V. S., . . . Petersen, R. C. (2012). Computer activities, physical exercise, aging, and mild cognitive impairment: A population-based study. *Mayo Clinic Proceedings, 87*(5), 437–442.

Gesin, G., Russell, B. B., Lin, A. P., Norton, H. J., Evans, S. L., & Devlin, J. W. (2012). Impact of a delirium screening tool and multifaceted education of nurses' knowledge of delirium and ability to evaluate it correctly. *American Journal of Critical Care, 21*(1), e1–e11.

Gofton, T. E. (2011). Delirium: A review. *Le Journal Canadien Des Sciences Neurologiques, 38*(5), 673–680.

Gravely, A. A., Cutting, A., Nugent, S., Grill, J., Carlson, K., & Spoont, M. (2011). Validity of PTSD diagnoses in VA administrative data: Comparison of VA administrative PTSD diagnoses to self-reported PTSD Checklist scores. *Journal of Rehabilitation Research & Development, 48*(1), 21–30.

Guenther, U., Weykam, J., Andorfer, U., Theuerkauf, N., Popp, J., Ely, E. W., & Putensen, C. (2012). Implications of objective vs. subjective delirium assessments in surgical intensive care patients. *American Journal of Critical Care, 21*(1), e12–e20.

Handsaker, S., Dempsey, L., & Fabby, C. (2012). Identifying and treating depression at the end of life and among the bereaved. *International Journal of Palliative Nursing, 18*(2), 91–97.

Haney, M., Rubin, E., & Foltin, R. W. (2011). Aripiprazole maintenance increases smoked cocaine self-administration in humans. *Psychopharmacology, 216*(3), 379–387.

Hardin, S., & Kaplow, R. (2005). *Synergy for clinical excellence: The AACN synergy model for patient care.* St. Louis, MO: Saunders.

Harvard Women's Health Watch. (2011). When patients suddenly become confused: Hospital delirium is common and often goes unrecognized. *Harvard Women's Health Watch, 18*(9), 1–3.

Herbst, R. T., Harris, E. D., Everhart, D. S., Mendelson, E. T., Jacob, J., & Jones, P. (2011). Cocaethylene formation following ethanol and cocaine administration by different routes. *Experimental and Clinical Psychopharmacology, 19*(2), 95–104.

Hernandez, L., Eaton, C. A., Fairlie, A. M., Chun, T. H., & Spirito, A. (2010). Ethnic group differences in substance use, depression, peer relationships, and parenting among adolescents receiving brief alcohol counseling. *Journal of Ethnicity in Substance Abuse, 9*(1), 14–27.

Hoe, J., & Thompson, R. (2010). Promoting positive approaches to dementia care in nursing. *Nursing Standard, 25*(4), 47–56.

Holowka, T. M., Marx, D. M., Kaloupek, B. P., & Keane, D. G. (2012). PTSD symptoms among male Vietnam veterans: Prevalence and associations with diagnostic status. *Psychological Trauma: Theory, Research, Practice, and Policy, 4*(3), 285–292.

Jones & Bartlett Learning. (2011). *2012 nurse's drug handbook. (*11th ed.). Sudbury, MA: Jones & Bartlett Learning.

Kelly, M. A., Morse, J. Q., Stover, A., Hofkens, T., Huisman, E., Shulman, S., & Pilkonis, P. A. (2011). Describing depression: Congruence between patient experiences and clinical assessments. *British Journal of Clinical Psychology, 50*(1), 46–66.

Kleim, E., Ehlers, B., & Glucksman, A. (2012). Investigating cognitive pathways to psychopathology: Predicting depression and posttraumatic stress disorder from early responses after assault. *Psychological Trauma: Theory, Research, Practice, and Policy, 4*(5), 527–537.

Krul, J., & Girbes, A. R. J. (2011). Gamma-hydroxybutyrate: Experience of 9 years of gamma-hydroxybutyrate (GHB)-related incidents during rave parties in The Netherlands. *Clinical Toxicology, 49*(4), 311–315.

Lilly, M. M., & Valdez, C. E. (2012). Interpersonal trauma and PTSD: The roles of gender and a lifespan perspective in predicting risk. *Psychological Trauma: Theory, Research, Practice, and Policy, 4*(1), 140–144.

Lin, P. P., Lin, L. C., Shyu, Y. I. L., & Hua, M. S. (2011). Predictors of pain in nursing home residents with dementia: A cross-sectional study. *Journal of Clinical Nursing, 20*(13/14), 849–857.

Liu, S., Lane, S. D., Schmitz, J. M., Waters, A. J., Cunningham, K. A., & Moeller, F. G. (2011). Relationship between attentional bias to cocaine-related stimuli and impulsivity in cocaine-dependent subjects. *The American Journal of Drug and Alcohol Abuse, 37*(2), 117–122.

Lynn-McHale Wiegand, D. J. (Ed.). (2011). *AACN procedure manual for critical care* (6th ed.). St. Louis, MO: Saunders.

MacDonald, D. S., Braslavsky, S. W. S., Camicioli, A., Dixon, R., & Roger, A. (2012). Mild cognitive impairment is associated with selected functional markers: Integrating concurrent, longitudinal, and stability effects. *Neuropsychology, 26*(2), 209–223.

Martinez-Horta, S., & Kulisevsky, J. (2011). Is all cognitive impairment in Parkinson's disease "mild cognitive impairment"? *Journal of Neural Transmission, 118*(8), 1185–1190.

National Institute of Mental Health. (2009). How is bipolar disorder treated? *National Institute of Mental Health Online*. Retrieved from http://www.nimh.nih.gov/health/publications/bipolar-disorder/how-is-bipolar-disorder-treated.shtml

Nazarko, L. (2011 May). Understanding dementia: Diagnosis and development. *British Journal of Healthcare Assistants, 5*(5), 216–220.

Ouldred, E., & Bryant, C. (2011). Delirium: prevention, clinical features and management. *Nursing Standard, 25*(28), 47–56.

Peacock, R., Hopton, A., Featherstone, I., & Edwards, J. (2012). Care home staff can detect the difference between delirium, dementia and depression. *Nursing Older People, 24*(1), 26–30.

Perry, M. (2012). A guide to vascular dementia. *Practice Nurse, 42*(14), 25–29.

Phillips, S., & Phillips, A. (2011). Dementia: A growing problem for older people with diabetes? *Practice Nursing, 22*(10), 526–531.

Pinkston, J. B., Alekseeva, N., & González, T. E. (2009). Stroke and dementia. *Neurological Research, 31*(8), 824–831.

Read, A., Colder, J. P., Merrill, C. R., Ouimette, J. E., White, P., & Swartout, J. (2012). Trauma and posttraumatic stress symptoms predict alcohol and other drug consequence trajectories in the first year of college. *Journal of Consulting and Clinical Psychology, 80*(3), 426–439.

Saczynski, J. S., Marcantonio, E. R., Quach, L., Fong, T. G., Gross, A., Inouye, S. K., & Jones, R. N. (2012). Cognitive trajectories after postoperative delirium. *The New England Journal of Medicine, 367*(1), 30–39.

Schmitter–Edgecombe, A., McAlister, M., & Weakley, C. (2012). Naturalistic assessment of everyday functioning in individuals with mild cognitive impairment: The day-out task. *Neuropsychology, 26*(5), 631–641.

Scott, S., Sampson, E. L., & Jones, L. (2012). The Compassion programme: Looking at improving end-of-life care for people with advanced dementia. *International Journal of Palliative Nursing, 18*(5), 212–217.

Smid, R. J., van der Velden, G. E., Gersons, P. G., & Kleber, B. P. R. (2012). Late-onset posttraumatic stress disorder following a disaster: A longitudinal study. *Psychological Trauma: Theory, Research, Practice, and Policy, 4*(3), 312–322.

Tao, R., Huang, X., Wang, J., Zhang, H., Zhang, Y., & Li, M. (2010). Proposed diagnostic criteria for Internet addiction. *Addiction, 105*(3), 556–564.

Traynor, V., Inoue, K., & Crookes, P. (2011). Literature review: Understanding nursing competence in dementia care. *Journal of Clinical Nursing, 20*(13/14), 1948–1960.

U.S. Drug Enforcement Administration. (2010). Drug abuse prevention and control. *United States Drug Enforcement Administration Online.* Retrieved from http://www.usdoj.gov/dea/pubs/csa.html

Van Rompaey, B., Schuurmans, M. J., Shortridge-Baggett, L. M., Truijen, S., Elseviers, M., & Bossaert, L. (2009). Long term outcome after delirium in the intensive care unit. *Journal of Clinical Nursing, 18*(23), 3349–3357.

Vaughn, M. G., Fu, Q., Perron, B. E., Bohnert, A. S., & Howard, M. O. (2010). Is crack cocaine use associated with greater violence than powdered cocaine use? Results from a national sample. *The American Journal of Drug and Alcohol Abuse, 36*(4), 181–186.

Watcher, R. (2012). *Understanding patient safety* (2nd ed.). Los Altos, CA: Lange.

Watkinson, S. (2011). Managing depression in older people with visual impairment. *Nursing Older People, 23*(8), 23–28.

Westerby, R., & Howard, S. (2011). Early recognition and diagnosis. *Practice Nurse, 41*(16), 42–47.

Wortmann, D., Park, J. H., & Edmondson, C. L. (2011). Trauma and PTSD symptoms: Does spiritual struggle mediate the link? *Psychological Trauma: Theory, Research, Practice, and Policy, 3*(4), 442–452.

Wylie, L., Hollins, M., Marland, G., Martin, C. R., & Rankin, J. (2011). The enigma of post-natal depression: An update. *Journal of Psychiatric & Mental Health Nursing, 18*(1), 48–58.